Barts and The London
Queen Mary's School of Medicine and Dentistry
WHITECHAPEL LIBRARY, TURNER STREET, LONDON E1 2AD
020 7882 7110

4 WEEK LOAN
Books are to be returned on or before the last date below,
otherwise fines may be charged.

2 3 OCT 2007

RANG'S CHILDREN'S FRACTURES

Third Edition

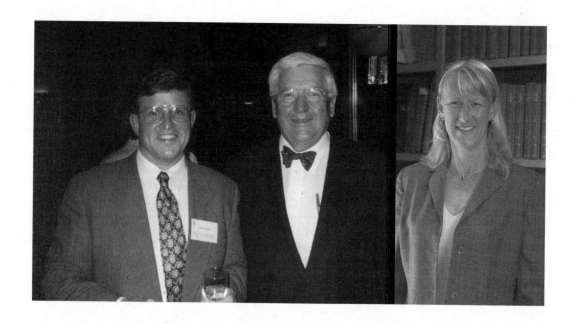

Dennis R. Wenger, M.D., Mercer Rang, M.D., and Maya E. Pring, M.D.

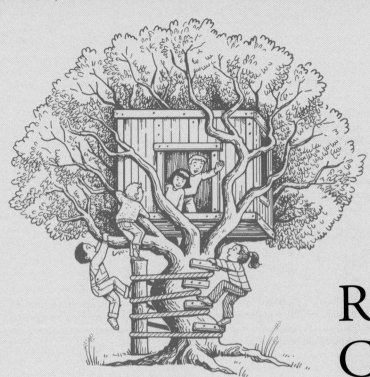

RANG'S CHILDREN'S FRACTURES

Third Edition

Mercer Rang, M.D.
Professor of Orthopedic Surgery
University of Toronto

Maya E. Pring, M.D.
Associate Staff—Orthopedics
Children's Hospital—San Diego

Dennis R. Wenger, M.D.
Director, Pediatric Orthopedic Training Program
Children's Hospital—San Diego
Clinical Professor of Orthopedic Surgery
University of California—San Diego

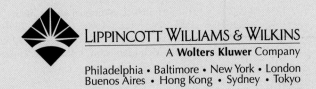

LIPPINCOTT WILLIAMS & WILKINS
A **Wolters Kluwer** Company

Philadelphia • Baltimore • New York • London
Buenos Aires • Hong Kong • Sydney • Tokyo

Acquisitions Editor: Robert Hurley
Managing Editor: Stacey Sebring
Project Manager: Fran Gunning
Senior Manufacturing Manager: Benjamin Rivera
Marketing Director: Sharon Zinner
Design Coordinator: Doug Smock
Production Services: Nesbitt Graphics, Inc.
Printer: Edwards Brothers

© 2005 by LIPPINCOTT WILLIAMS & WILKINS
530 Walnut Street
Philadelphia, PA 19106 USA
www.LWW.com

Printed in the USA

Library of Congress Cataloging-in-Publication Data
Rang, Mercer.
　　Rang's children's fractures / Mercer Rang, Maya Pring, Dennis Wenger; foreword by Robert Salter. — 3rd ed.
　　　　p. cm.
　　Rev. ed. of: Children's fractures. 2nd ed. ©1983.
　　ISBN 0-7817-5286-8
　　1. Fractures in children.　I. Pring, Maya.　II. Wenger, Dennis R.
(Dennis Ray)　III. Title.　IV. Title: Children's fractures.
　　[DNLM: 1. Fractures—Child.　WE 180 R196r 2006]
RD101.R33　2006
617.1'5'083—dc22

2005007039

Care has been taken to confirm the accuracy of the information presented and to describe generally accepted practices. However, the authors, editors, and publisher are not responsible for errors or omissions or for any consequences from application of the information in this book and make no warranty, expressed or implied, with respect to the currency, completeness, or accuracy of the contents of the publication. Application of the informa-tion in a particular situation re-mains the professional responsibility of the practitioner.

The authors, editors, and publisher have exerted every effort to ensure that drug selection and dosage set forth in this text are in accordance with current recommendations and practice at the time of publication. However, in view of ongoing research, changes in government regulations, and the constant flow of information relating to drug therapy and drug reactions, the reader is urged to check the package insert for each drug for any change in indications and dosage and for added warnings and precautions. This is particularly important when the recommended agent is a new or infrequently employed drug.

Some drugs and medical devices presented in the publication have Food and Drug Administra-tration (FDA) clearance for limited use in restricted research settings. It is the responsibility of the health care provider to ascertain the FDA status of each drug or device planned for use in their clinical practice.

The publishers have made every effort to trace the copyright holders for borrowed material. If they have inadvertently overlooked any, they will be pleased to make the necessary arrangements at the first opportunity.

To purchase additional copies of this book, call our customer service department at (800) 638-3030 or fax orders to (301) 824-7390. Lippincott Williams & Wilkins customer service rep-resentatives are available from 8:30 am to 6:30 pm, EST, Monday through Friday, for telephone access. Visit Lippincott Williams & Wilkins on the Internet: http://www.lww.com.

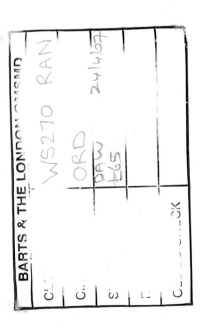

Contents

Contributors

LCDR Jeffrey A. Cassidy
Medical Corps, United States Navy Reserves
Director of Pediatric Orthopaedic Services
Naval Medical Center, San Diego

Henry G. Chambers, M.D.
Chief of Staff
Children's Hospital—San Diego
Associate Clinical Professor of Orthopedics
University of California—San Diego

CAPT Bruce L. Gillingham
Medical Corps, United States Navy
Director for Surgical Services
Pediatric Orthopaedic Surgeon
Naval Medical Center, San Diego

François D. Lalonde, M.D.
Associate Staff—Orthopedics
Children's Hospital—San Diego
Assistant Clinical Professor of Orthopedics
University of California—San Diego

Scott J. Mubarak, M.D.
Director, Pediatric Orthopedic Clinical Program
Children's Hospital—San Diego
Clinical Professor of Orthopedics
University of California—San Diego

Peter O. Newton, M.D.
Director, Scoliosis Program
Program Consultant, Surgical Research
Children's Hospital—San Diego
Associate Clinical Professor of Orthopedics
University of California—San Diego

Philip Stearns, C.P.N.P.
Director, Nurse Practitioner and Physician Assistant Program
Department of Orthopedics
Children's Hospital—San Diego

C. Douglas Wallace, M.D.
Medical Director of Orthopedic Trauma
Children's Hospital—San Diego
Assistant Clinical Professor of Orthopedics
University of California—San Diego

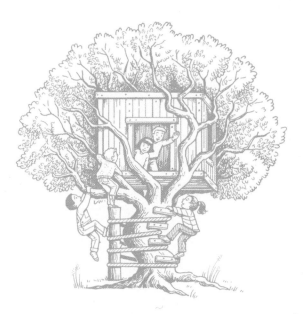

Foreword

It was in 1955 that Dr. Walter Blount wrote his splendid CLASSIC entitled *Fractures in Children* in which he emphasized that fractures in children were definitely different from fractures in adults.

During the ensuing 50 years, numerous books on this important subject have been written by eminent pediatric orthopedic surgeons. Of these books, the most widely read as well as the most enjoyed have been the first and second editions (1974 and 1983) of *Children's Fractures* written solely by the late Dr. Mercer Rang.

Tragically and poignantly, Dr. Rang passed away in October 2003 after a courageous battle against a prolonged illness.

I deem it a special privilege to have recruited Mercer to the Orthopaedic Staff of the Hospital for Sick Children in Toronto in 1967 where he became a warm friend and an admirable colleague for the rest of his life. His most enduring and endearing as well as appreciated quality was his remarkable skill as a teacher through both the spoken and written word.

Prior to Dr. Rang's illness, he and his good friend Dr. Dennis Wenger had already co-authored a superb book entitled *The Art and Practice of Children's Orthopedics*. Also before Mercer's illness, this pair of gifted teachers had already begun the onerous task of co-authoring the third edition of *Children's Fractures*. Surely there can be no finer tribute to Mercer Rang than Dennis Wenger's perpetuation of this book with an additional author, Maya Pring.

Although neither the first nor the second editions contained a Foreword, the Preface that Mercer wrote for the second edition was so delightfully typical of his whimsical humor that I felt the first paragraphs should be included in his memory in this Foreword:

A parable: The child in the back of the car has a broken arm. The driver stops to ask directions, "Excuse me, can you tell me the way to the Children's Hospital, please?"

A well-meaning pedestrian steps forward to offer advice: "It's really very easy." He begins to describe the usual way, rattling through the roads and landmarks to be noted. Before this information has had time to sink in he begins again with another route, "This is the best way; I read it in last week's paper." He moves his hands to indicate turns and so on, before realizing that his instructions have not been comprehended. "Well, perhaps you should take the easiest route. It's about 4 miles straight down the road."

Directions about fracture care are a little like this.

Together, the late Dr. Mercer Rang and the current authors, Dr. Dennis Wenger and Dr. Maya Pring, have created an outstanding book that is an entirely appropriate successor to Mercer's first two editions.

Woven throughout the tissue of this exemplary book is the thread of that uncommon sense, namely, common sense. As in the previous two editions, the illustrations are impressive. Indeed, most of the line drawings were rendered by Mercer Rang's artistic hand.

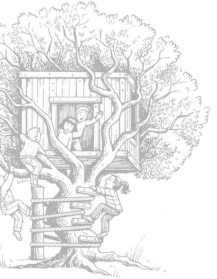

Recent advances in the management of children's fractures since the second edition of Mercer's book (1984) have been described in detail. Examples of such advances include the initial cast treatment of femoral shaft fractures in infants and very young children as well as the open reduction and internal fraction of femoral shaft fractures in older children, the closed reduction and percutaneous pinning of supracondylar fractures of the humerus, and the flexible intramedullary flexible nails for diaphyseal fractures.

Every person who treats children's fractures will be enormously grateful to the late Mercer Rang as well as to Dennis Wenger and Maya Pring for writing this most admirable book. It should become an essential reference book in the emergency department of every hospital in which children's fractures are treated.

This exemplary book is certainly a fitting memorial to the late Dr. Mercer Rang.

ROBERT B. SALTER
Toronto

Preface

The world of children's fracture care has changed remarkably since the 1973 first edition of this textbook. When Mercer Rang was recruited from Kingston, Jamaica, to the Hospital for Sick Children in Toronto in 1967, one of his assignments was to study fracture care in children. At that time, the only significant textbook on children's fractures was that of Walter Blount, which had last been published in 1955.

Mercer Rang recognized this void and also understood that contemporary orthopedic residents needed to know more than the principles that Walter Blount had espoused, if they were to provide state of the art care for children. (It should be noted that Blount's text said nothing about growth plate injuries.) The A-O ideas from Switzerland made their first North American appearance in Canada (especially Toronto and Montreal) in the late 1960s and early 1970s and Rang was quick to recognize that some of their principles applied to children's injuries. This is particularly true of forearm fractures in children over age 10 who up until that time had been primarily treated with closed reduction with almost any degree of angulation accepted. It became apparent that older children had little potential for remodeling and required adult treatment methods.

The first edition of this text briefly presented the tradition of children's fracture treatment and also presented new thinking and new ideas. Rang was able to illustrate and explain children's fractures in a way that was clearer and more entertaining than anything that had been presented before. The success of the text was immediate, becoming a standard reference throughout the orthopedic world. This was further aided by Rang's brilliant speaking style, which made all who heard him speak want to buy the book.

A second equally successful edition was published in 1983. Several years had elapsed before thought was given to a third edition. A significant impetus for the third edition came from Mr. Robert Hurley, Executive Editor at Lippincott, Williams & Wilkins, who felt that a practical textbook of this type should be updated and continued. Although occupied with other pursuits, Mercer and I had further discussions in response to Mr. Hurley's request and made the decision to proceed. Work began in early 2002. By that time Children's Hospital—San Diego had a large clinical and research unit devoted to treatment of children's fractures, and it was decided that the revision of the text should be based in our center with appropriate input from Toronto.

We decided on three authors to represent the eras of orthopedic experience: a senior sage, an experienced intermediary, and the dynamic intellect and energy of youth. Dr. Maya Pring, a native of Colorado and a graduate of the Mayo Clinic orthopedic training program, completed her fellowship at Children's Hospital—San Diego and has been on staff here for several years. She brings a level of experience, intellect, and energy to the subject of children's fractures that energizes this edition.

As in the first and second edition, this text is designed as a basic introduction to the diagnosis and treatment of children's fractures. It is not intended to be a comprehensive reference and should not be used as such. To emphasize this, a coda at the end of the text lists the many outstanding comprehensive children's fracture texts that are currently available and that provided valuable information for this revision.

The book is designed for medical students, physician's assistants, residents, emergency room doctors, general orthopedists, and children's orthopedists.

Many new features have been added. In the introductory chapters, we comment briefly on the differences between children's and adult's injuries and also discuss evolving trends toward efficient fracture treatment systems, many of which are being developed in children's hospitals in North America. Chapters 3 and 4 deal with practical matters of fracture description, fracture communication, conscious sedation methods and specific techniques for managing a safe, high-volume fracture reduction system.

We have added a chapter on casts in children since we see so many problems in this area and find that many physicians are not fully versed on the matter. The diagnostic chapters try to present in a simple and practical way the most common injuries in each of the anatomic areas in a child. We do not focus on advanced techniques and rare problems. We close with a chapter on cultural trends and the epidemiology of fractures that reviews fracture prevention efforts and then presents reasons for the increasing incidence of children's fractures in North America.

The result is a third edition which we believe provides a concise, practical, and contemporary view of children's orthopedics. We have focused on a style somewhere between that of a traditional orthopedic text and a typical college textbook. I have always been struck by the friendliness and ease of use of contemporary textbooks used in high schools and universities and tried to emulate them. Mercer Rang and I first worked on this approach in our textbook *The Art and Practice of Children's Orthopedics.*

In closing, I want to pay homage to my great mentor, Mercer Rang, who introduced me to clear thinking and educational style as relates to all of children's orthopedics. Sadly, Mercer developed an illness and passed away in October 2003 and was unable to see the final rendition of this text. He was instrumental in its planning and organization, writing and illustrating many of the chapters. We are saddened by his passing and the world has lost both a kind man and an orthopedic giant. I want to personally thank Helen Rang and her lovely family, who have been both understanding and cooperative in this difficult transition. We dedicate this text to the spirit of Mercer Rang, whose grace and style made orthopedic education a brilliant art form.

DENNIS R. WENGER, M.D.
San Diego

Acknowledgments

We are grateful to our colleagues, both in Toronto and San Diego, for their assistance and interest in revising this text. A special thanks goes to Robert Salter in Toronto whose organizational skills, research efforts, and energy helped to develop the Hospital for Sick Children in Toronto as one of the world's leading pediatric orthopedic centers. Also, our thanks to Drs. William Cole and John Wedge in Toronto, who continue this spirit.

The fracture treatment philosophy, which evolved at the Hospital for Sick Children in Toronto, is now widely used throughout the world. Children's Hospital—San Diego has greatly benefited from transmission of this knowledge, and we fortunately have been able to expand and further develop the field. We want to specifically thank our contributors, each who in some way have a connection to our Toronto base.

Dr. Scott Mubarak had his fellowship training in Toronto and has continued to have a strong clinical and research interest in all areas of children's orthopedic trauma. Dr. Bruce Gillingham was also a Toronto fellow with Mercer Rang, and both he and Dr. Cassidy have strengthened this text with their chapter on spine fractures. Our San Diego colleagues, Dr. Henry Chambers, Dr. Peter Newton, Dr. Douglas Wallace, and Dr. François Lalonde (all trained by Hospital for Sick Children—Toronto influenced staff) have greatly strengthened this book, both by co-writing chapters and by allowing us to use their cases to illustrate points.

A special thanks goes to Mr. Philip Stearns, a nurse practitioner at Children's Hospital—San Diego, who was the founding member and leader of a pioneering cadre of nurse practitioners and physician assistants who help provide efficient fracture care in a new and innovative way. Philip has helped to write several chapters and is a leader in defining a new field in orthopedic surgery. These concepts are outlined in Chapter 4.

We also want to thank Mr. J.D. Bomar, the audio-visual coordinator in the orthopedic department, who was responsible for all images and, more importantly, for much of the layout of this text. Also, we want to thank Karen Noble, Administrative Assistant to Dr. Wenger in San Diego, whose intellect, work ethic, and innate organizational skills were central to completing this project.

We also wish to thank Ms. Stacey L. Sebring, Developmental Editor at Lippincott, as well as Mr. Robert Hurley, Executive Editor at Lippincott, who have guided this process. We want to thank them not only for the traditional editorial skills, but in addition for their allowing us the freedom to produce a text with a layout that differs from traditional medical books.

We also thank our families for the time lost to them. Their understanding that the creative process has great rewards, and sometimes "trumps" other activities, confirms their sophistication.

Finally, we wish to thank Helen Rang and her wonderful family for their kindness, patience, and consideration as this project has evolved in a transitional period.

DENNIS R. WENGER, M.D.
San Diego

MAYA E. PRING, M.D.
San Diego

MERCER RANG, M.D.
Toronto (1926-2003)

1

Children Are Not Just Small Adults

Mercer Rang ❧ *Dennis Wenger*

INTRODUCTION

Fractures in children differ from those in adults. Because the anatomy, biomechanics, and physiology of a child's skeleton are very different from those of an adult, in children you will see differences in fracture pattern, problems of diagnosis, and treatment methods. This chapter introduces the many differences encountered when comparing children's fractures to adult injuries.

ANATOMIC DIFFERENCES

Much of a young child's skeleton is composed of radiolucent growth cartilage; thus often injury can only be inferred from widening of the growth plate or from displacement of adjacent bones on plain or stress films. The periosteum is thicker and stronger and produces callus more quickly and in greater amount than in adults.

> "The most savage controversies are those about matters as to which there is no good evidence either way"
> — BERTRAND RUSSELL

1

"Fractures in children differ from those in adults"

BIOMECHANICAL DIFFERENCES

Biomechanics of Bone

Many years ago, it was thought that fractures were less common in children as compared to adults because "the proportionate excess of the animal over the earthy constituents" protected the bone and allowed it to bend instead of breaking. Subsequently, it has been determined that haversian canals occupy a greater portion of the cortex, making young bone more porous (Fig. 1-1) and more flexible than adult bone. In effect, a child's bone is more like Gruyère cheese than cheddar and can tolerate a greater degree of deformation than an adult's bone can.

The pores in the cortex of a child's bone may limit the extension of a fracture line in the same way that a hole drilled through the end of a crack in a window will prevent the crack from extending. Compact adult bone fails in tension, whereas the more porous nature of a child's bone allows failure in compression as well.

DESCRIPTIVE TERMS— CHILDREN'S FRACTURES

The porous character of a child's bone noted previously accounts for the various fracture types (Fig. 1-2). The following commonly used terminology, although somewhat overlapping (and not always agreed on), has become part of the essential language of children's fractures.

Fracture Severity Descriptions

Buckle or Torus Fracture   Compression failure of bone produces a buckle fracture, which is also called a torus fracture because of its resemblance to the raised band around the base of an architectural column. These fractures occur near the metaphysis, where porosity is greatest, particularly in younger children. Disabled teenaged children, who do not bear weight and hence have porous bones, may also sustain buckle fractures.

Traumatic Bowing of Bone   Bending of bones, most commonly recognized in the ulna and fibula, can occur without any evidence of acute angular deformity (Fig. 1-3). If you try to break a child's forearm, either postmortem or during osteoclasis, you will find that the bones may be bent 45° or more before the telltale sound of a fracture is heard. If you stop before the bone fractures, you will

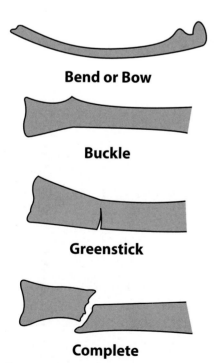

Figure 1-1   Microradiographs of the distal radial diaphysis of an adult and of a child 8 years old. The haversian canals are larger in the child. Children's bones are more porous than adults'.

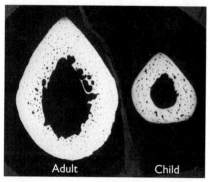

Bend or Bow

Buckle

Greenstick

Complete

Figure 1-2   Fracture types in children.

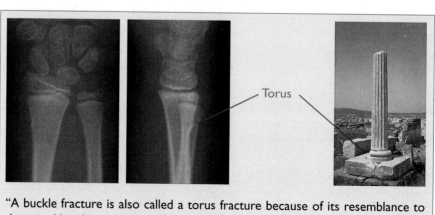

Torus

"A buckle fracture is also called a torus fracture because of its resemblance to the raised band around the base of an architectural column"

find that it will slowly, but incompletely, straighten itself out over several minutes. Such is the mechanism for traumatic bowing.

This phenomenon has also been described as plastic deformation of bone. In dogs, the bone deforms because microscopic shear fractures—at about 30° to the long axis—develop on the concave aspect of the bone. Because there is no true fracture there is no hemorrhage, no periosteal new bone formation, and no remodeling.

Greenstick Fracture   When a bone is angulated beyond the limits of bending, a greenstick fracture occurs (Fig. 1-4). This is a failure of the tension side of the bone; the compression side bends. A greenstick fracture occurs when the energy is sufficient to start a fracture but insufficient to complete it. The remaining bone undergoes plastic deformation. At the moment of fracture there is considerable displacement—as in most fractures—and then elastic recoil of the soft tissues improves the position. The fracture can hinge open again subsequently, owing to muscle pull. Complete closure of the fracture defect, which is prevented by jamming of spicules, can usually only be achieved by completing the fracture and momentarily overcorrecting the angulation.

Complete Fracture   Complete fractures are rarely comminuted in children (Fig. 1-5). This may be because a child's bone is more flexible than that of an adult. Some of the force of impact is dissipated in bending the bone, whereas in adults the kinetic energy of impact is entirely used to disrupt the intermolecular bonds in the bone.

Fracture Patterns

The treatment of fractures is helped by an understanding of the differences between fast and slow fractures, and between spiral and oblique fractures.

The surface of a slow fracture is rough, like a stubbly lawn, whereas a fast fracture is smooth. Young bone and a rough fracture surface make it easier to keep the ends hitched.

Spiral Fractures   The direction of force decides the direction of the fracture line (Fig. 1-6). A spiral fracture, produced by a twist, has an intact periosteum hinge along the straight, axial part of the fracture. If you can find where this is, you can determine whether the fracture can be reduced by clockwise or counterclockwise rotation and the intact periosteal hinge will help maintain reduction. These fractures are not held by the three-point pressure principle applicable to transverse fractures and are better held by a "crank-handle" cast (several right angles), which controls rotation (Fig. 1-7).

"When a bone is angulated beyond the limits of bending, a greenstick fracture occurs"

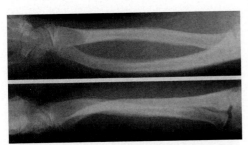

Figure 1-3   Traumatic bowing of the ulna in a child.

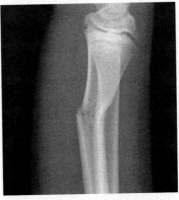

Figure 1-4   Greenstick fracture in a child.

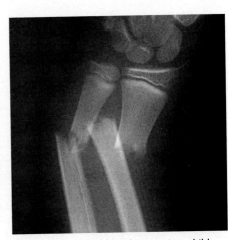

Figure 1-5   Complete fracture in a child.

Oblique Fractures An oblique fracture, due to axial overload, usually propagates at about 30° to the axis of the bone because the periosteum is widely torn; these fractures are unstable and are best reduced by distraction—a straight pull. They are held either in traction or by a cast applying potentially risky circumferential pressure. Longitudinal loading obviously displaces the fracture (Fig. 1-8).

Transverse Fractures A transverse fracture results from angulation with the periosteum torn on one side as a fragment of bone buttonholes through. A se-

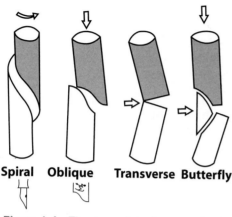

Spiral Oblique Transverse Butterfly

Figure 1-6 The shape of the fracture tells you how it was produced. Spiral fractures are shaped like a pen nib. Oblique fractures are like a ski jump.

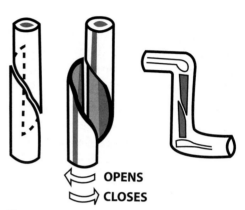

OPENS
CLOSES

Figure 1-7 Spiral fracture. There is an axial periosteal hinge providing longitudinal stability. A crank-handle cast prevents displacement.

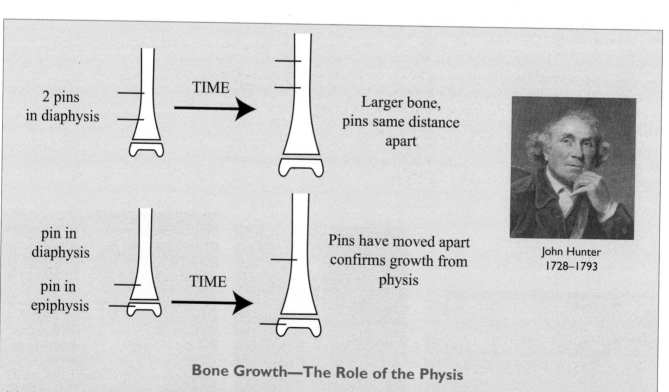

2 pins in diaphysis

TIME

Larger bone, pins same distance apart

pin in diaphysis

pin in epiphysis

TIME

Pins have moved apart confirms growth from physis

John Hunter
1728–1793

Bone Growth—The Role of the Physis

John Hunter of London was the leader of the movement to place the discipline of surgery in a scientific basis. He helped translate "barber surgeons" into trained surgeons with a scientific background, setting the stage for formation of the Royal College of Surgeons. His early animal studies demonstrated that longitudinal growth occurs at the physis.

verely displaced transverse fracture is often best reduced by increasing the deformity to 90°, so that the end can be unbuttoned; by pulling hard in this 90° angulation position; and then (still pulling) by straightening the bone. A three-point pressure cast will best maintain the reduction (Fig. 1-9).

Butterfly Fractures A butterfly fracture is due to a combination of axial overload and angulation (Fig. 1-10). When the fracture is produced by a blow, the butterfly fragment lies on the side of the bone that was struck. The periosteum is most damaged on the opposite side, and the fractures are unstable. When the butterfly fragment is small, three-point pressure may hold the fracture, but usually distraction is required.

THE PHYSIS

The physis (growth plate), once known as conjugal cartilage (joins or "conjugates" adjacent bone) was confirmed to be the center for bone growth by John Hunter, the renowned British surgical scientist. In the early 1700s while enjoying a pork dinner with a friend, he noted slightly "colored" transverse lines at the ends of a young pig's bone (the pig had been fed garbage contaminated by madder—a dye for cloth—which was selectively deposited in the growing pig's physis).

Suspecting this as the area where bones grow longitudinally, he then conducted experiments, by placing transverse pins in growing animal bones. Those placed at a certain distance apart in the diaphysis (mid-bone) remained similarly spaced over time. When one pin was placed in the epiphysis and the other in the diaphysis, the pins separated over time, clarifying that longitudinal growth came from the physis (growth plate).

PHYSEAL TERMINOLOGY

In describing the physis (growth plate) and adjacent bone, we will use traditional terminology (Fig. 1-11). Minimal reference to classic language (Greek) clarifies the terms that center on the physis (growth plate). Growth "plate" describes the shape of the physeal growth cartilage, in that it is shaped like a small dish (not very thick, varying diameters).

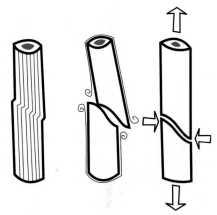

Figure 1-8 An oblique fracture. An overloaded column fails in this fashion.

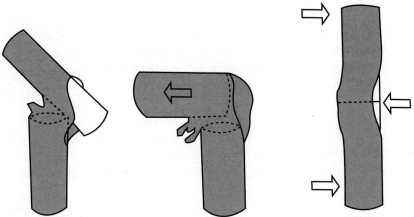

Figure 1-9 A transverse fracture. Reduction requires retracing the path of the injury. It is held by three-point pressure.

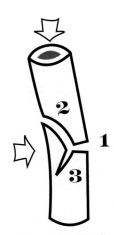

Figure 1-10 Butterfly fracture. The numbers indicate the order in which the fractures occur.

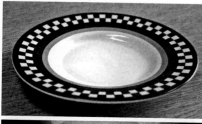

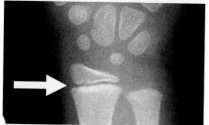

Figure 1-11   The physis (growth plate).

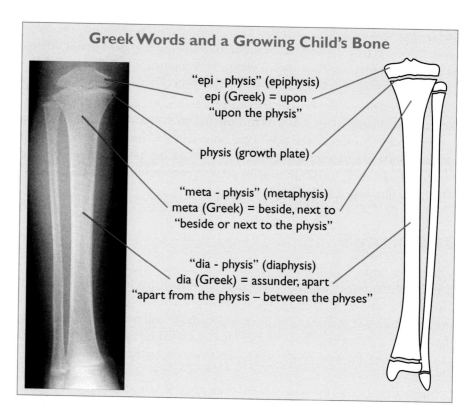

Greek Words and a Growing Child's Bone

"epi - physis" (epiphysis)
epi (Greek) = upon
"upon the physis"

physis (growth plate)

"meta - physis" (metaphysis)
meta (Greek) = beside, next to
"beside or next to the physis"

"dia - physis" (diaphysis)
dia (Greek) = assunder, apart
"apart from the physis – between the physes"

The adjacent bone is named by its association with the physis. The articular end of the bone is positioned "upon" the physis thus is called the epiphysis (epi = upon).

Physeal Language Errors

The most difficult remaining descriptive problem relates to the clinical use of the term epiphysis when one really means physis. One still hears the term "epiphyseal fracture" when the speaker really means "physeal fracture." Fractures can involve the epiphysis, but when they do, there is appropriate language to describe them. Learning accurate, clear, internationally accepted language for the description of injuries within and about the physis remains integral to mastering children's orthopedics.

Physeal Biomechanics

"One still hears the term 'epiphyseal fracture' when the speaker really means 'physeal fracture'"

Ruysch (1713) was one of the earliest experimentalists to find that considerable force is required to separate the epiphysis from the metaphysis because they are firmly connected externally by the periosteum and internally by mamillary processes. In 1820, James Wilson showed that a longitudinal force of 550 pounds was required to detach the epiphysis from the metaphysis, but that if the periosteum was divided first the force required was only 119 pounds. A few years later, in 1845, Salmon again demonstrated the importance of periosteum. Although he could separate the epiphysis of a newborn's distal femur by hyperextending the knee, he could not produce displacement until he cut the periosteum.

In 1898, John Poland wrote *Traumatic Separation of the Epiphysis,* a book of 900 pages that summarized what was known about the epiphysis to that time. Since then, very little new information has been added, and those interested in children's fractures should read his book. Poland was probably the first to show experimentally that it was easy to produce epiphyseal separation but difficult to produce dislocations in children (Fig. 1-12). He wrote, "This is easily understood when the comparatively weak conjugal neighborhood in the young subject is realized. The violence producing the two forms of injury—epiphyseal separation in children and dislocations in adults—is frequently of the same character." (This quotation is better understood if you appreciate that the growth plate was once called conjugal cartilage, because it joins two bones intimately together.) Poland concluded that ligaments are stronger than growth cartilage.

At least one attachment of a ligament is to an epiphysis. Hence, when a valgus force is applied to the knee of a child, for example, the distal femoral growth plate gives way, whereas in an adult the medial ligament will rupture or detach.

Growth cartilage has the consistency of hard rubber. When the plate is thick, the epiphysis can be rocked slightly on the metaphysis because of the elasticity of the plate. This property not only protects the bone from injury but appears to protect the joint surface from the type of crushing injury that is common in adults.

In 1950, Harris revived interest in biomechanical testing of the growth plate. Applying a lateral force to an epiphysis, he found that the hormonal environment greatly influences the strength of the bond between the epiphysis and the metaphysis.

Bright and Elmore studied the force required to separate the upper tibial epiphysis in a rat (Fig 1-13) and found that the age of the animal and direction in which the force is applied are both important factors. The plate is most resistant to traction and least resistant to torsion. Furthermore, the epiphysis can be displaced 0.5 mm before separation begins. In a subsequent paper, they showed that small cracks developed within the physis when 50% of the force required to separate the plate was applied.

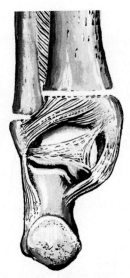

Figure 1-12 Strong ligaments attached to the epiphysis account for epiphyseal separation being more frequent than joint dislocations. Poland was the first to emphasize that strong ligaments attached to the epiphysis account for epiphyseal separation being more frequent than joint dislocations.

PERIOSTEAL BIOMECHANICS

The periosteum is much thicker, stronger, and less readily torn in a child than in an adult and continuity of the periosteum determines whether or not a fracture displaces. When displacement occurs, the intact hinge of periosteum can help or hinder reduction.

PHYSIOLOGICAL DIFFERENCES

Growth Remodeling

Growth provides the basis for a greater degree of remodeling than is possible in an adult. As a bone increases in length and girth, the deformity produced by a fracture is corrected by asymmetric growth of the physis and the periosteum (Fig. 1-14). Karaharju and associates studied fractures in puppies' tibiae that had been plated with angulation. The physis grew asymmetrically to straighten up the articular surface. Most of the correction occurred early.

Remodeling occurs most efficiently in younger children and if the deformity is in the axis of rotation of the adjacent joint. Thus in a 3-year-old child, a distal radius fracture left in bayonet apposition (lateral view) will straighten itself over the next year (Fig. 1-15).

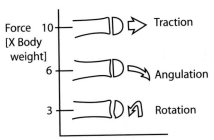

Figure 1-13 Load required to separate the proximal tibial epiphysis of a rat using forces applied at different angles to the growth plate. (Based on Bright RW, Elmore SM. Physical properties of epiphysieal plate cartilage. Surg Forum 19:463, 1968.)

The bump of a malunion is corrected by periosteal resorption; the concavity is filled out by periosteal new bone. This is an example of Wolff's law, which may be mediated by piezoelectric potentials. The compression side of a loaded bone develops a negative potential, which is a stimulus to bone formation.

Remodeling (perhaps better thought of as realignment), which restores the function of a bone to normal, must be distinguished from rounding off, which improves the radiograph but does little for the patient (Fig. 1-16), often leaving the joint to function at an abnormal angle.

Overgrowth

A fracture through the shaft of a long bone stimulates longitudinal growth, probably because of the increased nutrition to growth cartilage produced by the hyperemia associated with fracture healing. In practice, an undisplaced fracture of the shaft of the femur will, in the course of a year or two, cause the femur to be about 1 cm longer than its opposite member. An incomplete, asymmetric metaphyseal fracture (especially proximal tibia) can cause undesirable progressive angulation over the year following fracture, causing deformity so severe that on occasion it requires surgical correction.

Progressive Deformity

Permanent damage to the growth plate will produce shortening (Fig. 1-17) or progressive angular deformity. Such complications have been recognized for many years, and, in 1888, Lentaigne even diagnosed this condition in an Egyptian mummy.

Nonunion

Nonunion is an adversary almost unknown to the children's orthopedic surgeon. In fact, when it does occur, especially in the distal tibia, one thinks of associated disease as the cause (congenital pseudarthrosis due to neurofibromatosis). Displaced intra-articular fractures and the rare shaft fracture with gross interposition may not unite, but otherwise union is easily achieved. As in adults, femoral neck and scaphoid (carpal navicular) fractures may go on to nonunion. The reason for ready union in children is not known for certain, but perhaps the periosteum is actively (not dormantly) osteogenic and clearly children have an excellent vascular supply to most fractures.

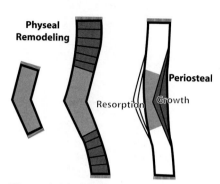

Physeal Remodeling

Periosteal

Resorption   Growth

Figure 1-14   The basis of remodeling.

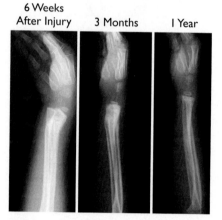

6 Weeks After Injury   3 Months   1 Year

Figure 1-15   Five-year-old child with a distal radius fracture that healed in a mal-reduced position. At 3 months the deformity persists. One year later the radius is straighter.

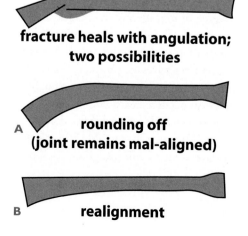

fracture heals with angulation; two possibilities

A   **rounding off (joint remains mal-aligned)**

B   **realignment**

Figure 1-16 Remodeling has two meanings. A) Rounding off does not help the patient; radiologists call this remodeling to lure the physician into inappropriate optimism. B) Realignment or "straightening itself out" is the real meaning of remodeling.

Speed of Healing

Children heal quickly; therefore reduction should be secured early. The orthopedic surgeon does not have as long to deliberate over a fracture in a child as compared to an adult.

Refracture

Refracture occurs under several circumstances:

1. Early, when the cast is removed too soon.
2. Late, when the fracture has healed with deformity so that the fracture is a stress concentrator (Fig. 1-18).
3. Late fracture in cases where the cast was maintained for the advised time period and the fracture is well aligned.

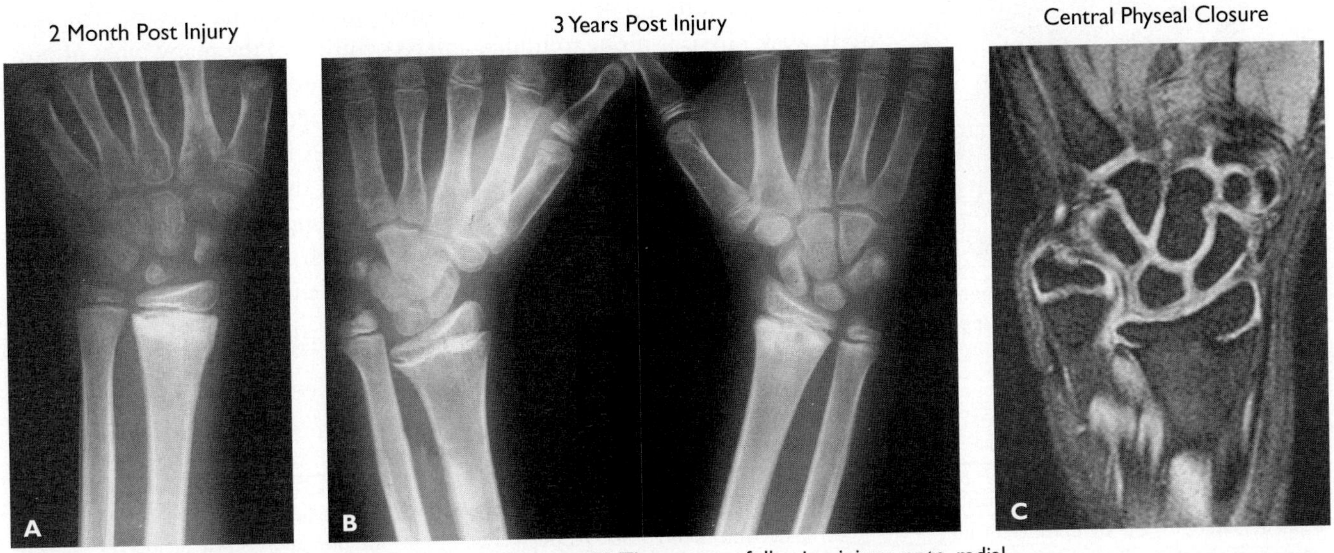

2 Month Post Injury   3 Years Post Injury   Central Physeal Closure

Figure 1-17 A) Salter-Harris I left distal radius fracture. B) Three years following injury, note radial physeal closure and ulnar overgrowth. C) MRI confirms physeal arrest.

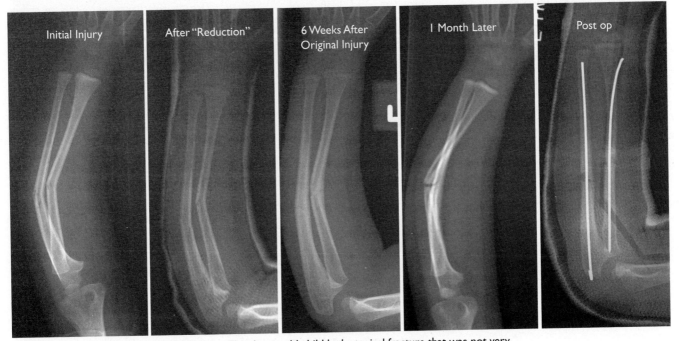

Initial Injury   After "Reduction"   6 Weeks After Original Injury   1 Month Later   Post op

Figure 1.18 Classic example of refracture. This 4-year-old child had a typical fracture that was not very well reduced. One month after cast removal, a mild fall led to refracture. The patient was taken to the OR for reduction and fixation.

We commonly see the latter in children who pursue vigorous activities (skate boarding, motocross, etc., Fig. 1-19).

Studies in rabbit bones show four biomechanical healing stages, each which can allow refracture:

Stage I: The sticky stage—refracture through the original fracture site with low stiffness.

Stage II: Early union—refracture through the original site with high stiffness.

Stage III: Refracture occurs partly through the original fracture site and partly through intact bone.

Stage IV: Refracture entirely through intact bone.

SUMMARY

Children's fractures differ from similar adult injuries in many ways. The relatively weak physis is prone to injury, and recognition of the many types of physeal injury, with application of modern treatment methods, is central to the art and practice of children's fracture treatment. The vigor of growth, with its corresponding excellent blood supply to bone, ensures healing in most children's fractures. Refracture, thought to be uncommon in the past, is a regular occurrence in the modern era that emphasizes "extreme sports." Overall, the biology of the child's musculoskeletal system, blessed with the positive attributes of growth, makes treatment a pleasant, positive experience.

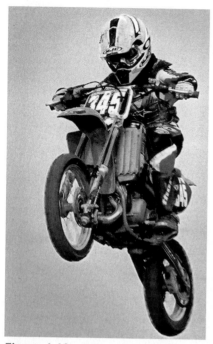

Figure 1-19 Refracture is common in children who pursue aggressive sports. (Photo courtesy of R. Knudson.)

Suggested Readings

Altner PC, Grana L, Gordon M: An experimental study of the significance of muscle tissue interposition on fracture healing. Clin Orthop 111:269, 1975.

Arunachalarun VSP, Griffiths JC: Fracture recurrence in children. Injury 7:37, 1975.

Borden S: Traumatic bowing of the forearm in children. J Bone Joint Surg 56A:611, 1974.

Bright RW, Burstein AH, Elmore SM: Epiphyseal plate cartilage. A biomechanical and histological analysis of failure modes. J Bone Joint Surg 56A:688, 1974.

Currey JD, Butler G: Mechanical properties of bone tissue in children. J Bone Joint Surg 57A:810, 1975.

Diab, M: Lexicon of Orthopedic Etymology. Harwood Academic Publishers. 1999.

Edvardson P, Syversen SM: Overgrowth of the femur after fractures of the shaft in childhood. J Bone Joint Surg Br 1976;58: 339-344.

Gordon JE: New Science of Strong Materials or Why You Don't Fall Through the Floor. London, Penguin Books, 1968.

Harris WR: The endocrine basis for slipping of the upper femoral epiphysis. J Bone Joint Surg 32B:5, 1950.

Hirsch C, Evans FG: Studies on some physical properties of infant compact bone. Acta Orthop Scand 35:300, 1965.

Karaharju EO, Ryoppy SA, Makinen RJ: Remodelling by asymmetrical epiphyseal growth. J Bone Joint Surg 58B:122, 1976.

Mabrey JD, Fitch RD: Plastic deformation in pediatric fractures: mechanism and treatment. J Pediatr Orthop 1989;9:310-314.

Poland J: Traumatic Separation of the Epiphysis. London, Smith, Elder, 1898.

Pritchett JW: Growth plate activity in the upper extremity. Clin Orthop 1991; 268: 235-242.

Shapiro F, Aoltrop ME, Glimcher MJ: Organization and cellular biology of the perichondral ossification of Ranvier. A morphological study in rabbits. J Bone Joint Surg 59A:703, 1977.

Treharne RW: Review of Wolff's law and its proposed means of operation. Orthop Review 10:35, 1981.

Tschantz P, Taillard W, Ditesheim PJ: Epiphyseal tilt produced by experimental overload. Clin Orthop 123:271, 1977.

White AA, Punjabi MM, Southwick WO: The four biomechanical states of fracture repair. J Bone Joint Surg 59A:188, 1977.

Wolff J: The classic: concerning the interrelationship between form and function of the individual parts of the organism. Clin Orthop 1988;228:2-11.

2

The Physis and Skeletal Injury

Mercer Rang   *Dennis Wenger*

INTRODUCTION

Many fractures in children would heal well, whether they were looked after by a professor in a university hospital or by Robinson Crusoe on a deserted island. Fractures through the physis (growth plate) are a different story.

EPIPHYSEAL FRACTURES

Fractures of the true epiphysis usually involve the growth plate but occasionally occur in isolation. They may be classified as follows (Fig. 2-1):

- Avulsion at the site of ligamentous attachment
- Comminuted compression fracture
- Displaced osteochondral fragment

> *"The physis alone accounts for much of why children's orthopedics has become a sub-specialty"*
> — *ANONYMOUS*

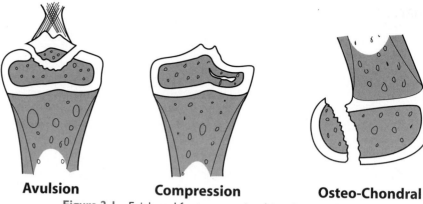

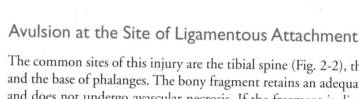

Avulsion   **Compression**   **Osteo-Chondral**

Figure 2-1   Epiphyseal fractures not involving the growth plate.

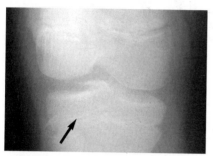

Figure 2-2   Anterior tibial spine fracture in a child who had a bicycle accident.

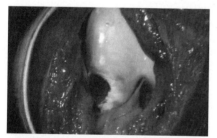

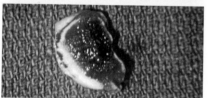

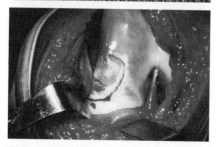

Figure 2-3   Osteochondral fracture of the lateral femoral condyle secondary to acute traumatic patellar dislocation. The fragment was large enough that it could be surgically repositioned.

Avulsion at the Site of Ligamentous Attachment

The common sites of this injury are the tibial spine (Fig. 2-2), the ulnar styloid, and the base of phalanges. The bony fragment retains an adequate blood supply and does not undergo avascular necrosis. If the fragment is displaced, union is rare because synovial fluid inhibits callus formation. The displaced fragment may block joint movement or may leave the joint unstable because of functional ligamentous lengthening. These problems justify accurate reduction: sometimes requiring open reduction.

Osteochondral Fragments

Osteochondral fragments are most commonly scalped off the distal femur, the patella, the capitellum (humerus), and the radial head. A displaced fragment produces the problems of a loose body and articular cartilage injury. If the fragment is large and from an important part of the joint, it should be replaced and fixed anatomically (Fig. 2-3). If small, it should be removed. Often, the fragment has little bone attached and is difficult to see on x-ray (especially radial head and capitellum).

PHYSEAL (GROWTH PLATE) INJURIES

Injuries to the growth plate form perhaps one third of skeletal trauma in children. The possible consequences of such injuries include progressive angular deformity, progressive limb-length discrepancy, and joint incongruity. Although damage to the growth plate has the potential for causing many disastrous problems, in fact, the area repairs well, and problems after injury are uncommon when treated well. When growth is disturbed, the reason is one of the following:

- Avascular necrosis of the physis
- Crushing or infection of the physis
- Formation of a bone bridge between the bony epiphysis and the metaphysis
- Hyperemia producing local overgrowth

The problems and the means of their prevention can only be understood by an appreciation of the anatomy and the healing reactions in the growth plate area.

Anatomy

The growth plate is a cartilaginous disc situated between the epiphysis and the metaphysis. The germinal cells are attached to the epiphysis and have a blood supply from epiphyseal vessels (Fig 2-4). Repeated multiplication of these cells provides the cell population for the rest of the plate. The daughter cells multiply further, secreting a cartilage matrix, and increase in size, thereby producing growth. The matrix calcifies. Metaphyseal vessels enter the cell columns, remove a little matrix, and lay down bone on the cartilage matrix to form metaphyseal bone.

With a fracture, the plane of separation is most frequently the junction between calcified and uncalcified cartilage. A transverse section through the growth plate in this region demonstrates the small amount of structural matrix present, which probably accounts for the relative weakness of the area. The important germinal part of the plate—indeed the greater thickness of the plate—remains mostly with the epiphysis. This plane of separation is relatively bloodless, so that an epiphyseal separation often has little associated swelling.

However, when the plane of fracture separation has been examined carefully, the anatomic fracture line is often less "pure." It has been noticed that it may pass between the epiphysis and the germinal layer. Johnston and Jones performed biopsies of fractures requiring open reduction and found that the fracture line often passes between the epiphysis and the germinal layer.

This is particularly the case in fractures through the physes that have significant natural undulations (a "hilly terrain") such as the distal femur and distal tibia (Fig. 2-5). These undulations may be evolutionary design features that prevent easy disruption of the physis but when it finally is forced to give, the shearing action may predispose to a fracture. If reduction is not anatomic, there will be epiphyseal-to-metaphyseal bone contact, which may form a bar across the physis. Obviously, if much of the germinal layer is disturbed, there is a chance for growth arrest.

Blood Supply to the Epiphysis

The blood supply of the epiphysis is important. Dale and Harris showed that there are two fundamental types of epiphyses (Fig. 2-6) according to how they receive their blood supply. The prognosis after physeal injury is greatly determined by this factor.

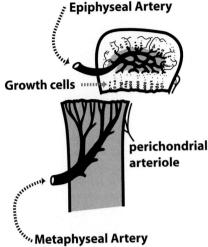

Figure 2-4 Blood supply of the growth plate. Damage to the epiphyseal artery can destroy the plate. Damage to the metaphyseal artery is less important.

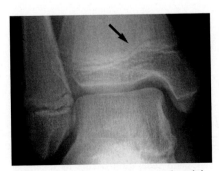

Figure 2-5 The irregularity and undulations in certain physes may increase the risk for physeal closure with fracture (e.g., "Kump's bump"—distal tibial physis).

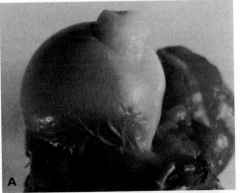

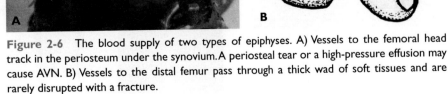

Figure 2-6 The blood supply of two types of epiphyses. A) Vessels to the femoral head track in the periosteum under the synovium. A periosteal tear or a high-pressure effusion may cause AVN. B) Vessels to the distal femur pass through a thick wad of soft tissues and are rarely disrupted with a fracture.

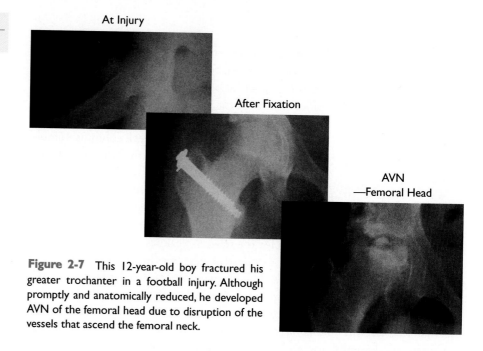

At Injury

After Fixation

AVN
—Femoral Head

Figure 2-7 This 12-year-old boy fractured his greater trochanter in a football injury. Although promptly and anatomically reduced, he developed AVN of the femoral head due to disruption of the vessels that ascend the femoral neck.

Epiphyses Totally Clad with Cartilage (such as head of femur, head of radius). Total interruption of the blood supply to the germinal cells may follow fracture separation. Avascular necrosis of the plate and epiphysis, and arrest of longitudinal growth naturally follow (Fig. 2-7).

Epiphyses with Soft Tissue Attachments (most physeal injuries—distal radius, distal tibia, distal femur, etc.). When these are separated, the soft tissue hinge will remain attached to the epiphysis, so that the circulation to the epiphysis remains intact. The germinal cells are not injured, and longitudinal growth continues unscathed.

HEALING REACTIONS OF THE PHYSIS AND EPIPHYSIS

Dale and Harris have published the most credible description of growth plate separation. The plate separates mostly between the calcified and uncalcified layers of the growth plate. For a week or two, the hiatus is filled by fibrin. Initially,

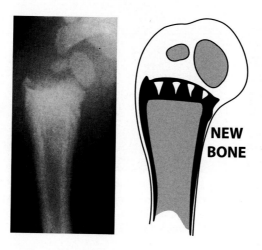

NEW BONE

Figure 2-8 Healing after growth plate separation occurs by means of new bone formed by the growth plate and by the periosteum. This can be seen clearly 3 weeks after the initial injury.

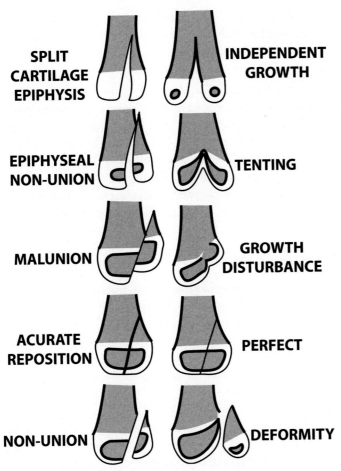

Figure 2-9   Healing patterns of Type IV injuries.

the physis becomes wider, because growth cartilage continues to be produced without invasion by metaphyseal vessels. After about 2 weeks, the vessels begin to invade the cartilage columns again. The physis becomes narrower once more, and the healing occurs without leaving a scar. In this way, the growth plate heals more quickly than a fracture through bone (Fig. 2-8). The repair of an injury at right angles to the plane of the growth plate shows more variation (Fig. 2-9).

Cartilaginous Epiphysis   If they remain displaced, both portions of the epiphysis continue to grow separately, producing a double-ended bone.

Ossified Epiphysis   If the fracture surfaces are not in contact, both fragments continue to grow for some time. Eventually, premature arrest of growth adjacent to the fracture line takes place.

If the fracture surfaces are approximated but without anatomic reduction of the growth plate, a bridge of callus will form between the epiphysis on one side and the metaphysis on the other. This bony bridge produces a brake on growth. When the bridge is at the center of the epiphysis, the two outside edges will continue to grow, resulting in tenting of the end of the bone. When the bridge is toward one margin of the growth plate, a progressive, angular deformity develops.

If the fracture is accurately reduced so that there is coaptation of the growth plate, there will be a small scar at the site of growth plate injury, but this is not sufficient to disturb growth.

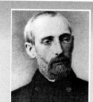
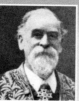

Prolonged Immobilization or Early Motion?

The controversy regarding whether fractures should be casted for a long time or removed early were championed by the above experts. Thomas believed that fracture immobilization should be enforced, prolonged, and uninterrupted to ensure fracture healing. Lucas-Championniere vigorously opposed principles of treatment of fractures by prolonged rest. He advocated early motion and is considered one of the founding fathers of modern fracture brace treatment that allows early mobilization of joints. A-O principles and Salter's CPM ideas follow this concept.

Effect of Internal Fixation Small Kirschner wires passed through the center of the plate do not interfere with growth. If they are passed near the margin of the plate, growth is occasionally disturbed. Threaded pins or screws across the plate act as effectively as Blount's staples in inhibiting growth.

Repair of Articular Surfaces Cartilage defects in a joint invite intra-articular adhesions. Salter and associates have shown that continuous passive motion (CPM) not only discourages adhesions but stimulates more rapid and complete healing of full-thickness defects in rabbits. Motion—not immobilization—for injured joint surfaces would seem wise; however, often early motion will increase the chance for pseudarthrosis. Finding the happy medium is the art. CPM is rarely required following primary treatment of children's joint fractures (as opposed to adults who are much more likely to become stiff).

SALTER-HARRIS CLASSIFICATION

The Salter-Harris classification of growth plate injuries remains the most practical and commonly used. Founded on the pathology of injury, the classification is well suited to an accurate verbal description of a fracture and provides an excellent guide to rational treatment (Table 2-1). Most growth plate injuries can be easily classified, leaving very few fractures to produce arguments at fracture rounds. The classification should be studied in the original, as it is one of the classic papers in orthopedics.

There have been others. In 1898, Poland illustrated the common variations of separation (Fig. 2-10). The Weber classification (from the A-O) provides the extreme of simplicity (Fig. 2-11). In very general terms, a Weber Type A (equivalent to Salter-Harris I or II) can be treated conservatively, and a Type B (equivalent to Salter-Harris III or IV) requires surgery.

The antithesis of the Weber classification is that of Ogden who proposed nine types of physeal injuries (including intra-articular fractures, osteochondral avulsions, etc.). His system may be useful for research studies but has proven to be too complex for easy memorization (and thus everyday clinical use). Most classification systems in medicine that have more than three or four subgroups cannot be readily memorized, and used on a day-to-day basis.

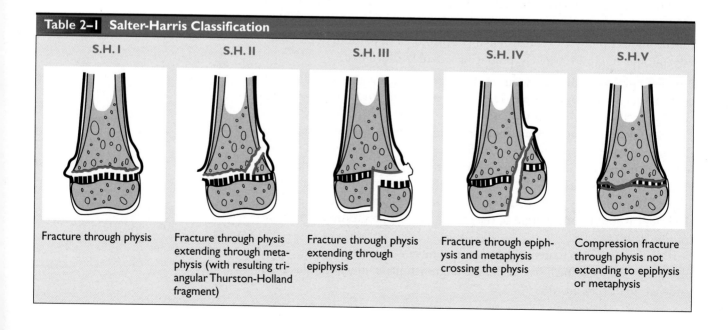

Table 2–1 Salter-Harris Classification

S.H. I	S.H. II	S.H. III	S.H. IV	S.H. V
Fracture through physis	Fracture through physis extending through metaphysis (with resulting triangular Thurston-Holland fragment)	Fracture through physis extending through epiphysis	Fracture through epiphysis and metaphysis crossing the physis	Compression fracture through physis not extending to epiphysis or metaphysis

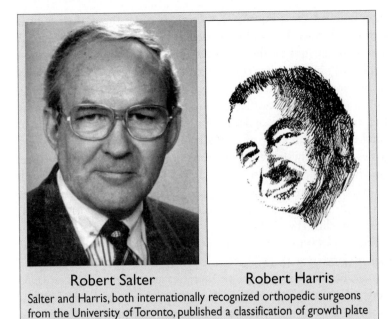

Robert Salter　　Robert Harris

Salter and Harris, both internationally recognized orthopedic surgeons from the University of Toronto, published a classification of growth plate fractures in 1963 that remains the most commonly used worldwide.

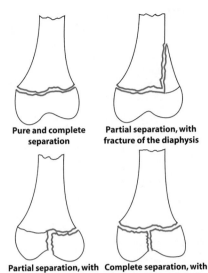

Pure and complete separation　　**Partial separation, with fracture of the diaphysis**

Partial separation, with fracture of the epiphysis　　**Complete separation, with fracture of the epiphysis**

Figure 2-10 Poland's classification of growth plate injuries (1898).

Only simple, practical classifications gain wide acceptance (and get dictated into medical records and correspondence). Thus the classic Salter-Harris classification system remains the most commonly used worldwide.

Fracture Types (Salter-Harris)

Type I In a Type I fracture (Fig. 2-12), the epiphysis separates completely from the metaphysis. The germinal cells (the growth cells) remain with the epiphysis, and the calcified layer remains with the metaphysis. If the periosteum is not completely torn, there may be little or no displacement. The radiograph in these circumstances may be normal and the diagnosis is made on clinical suspicion (Fig. 2-13).

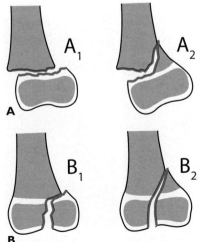

Figure 2-11 This extremely simple classification was described by Weber and Brunner in St. Gallen, Switzerland. **Type A** can be treated with closed reduction. **Type B** requires surgery (in most cases).

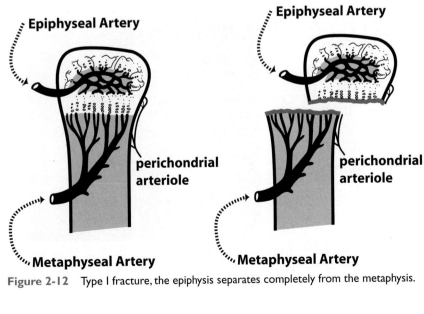

Figure 2-12 Type I fracture, the epiphysis separates completely from the metaphysis.

Most parents look on these injuries as sprains, because there often is little swelling and little deformity. You will be alerted to them by tenderness over the growth plate and should not be disturbed by the absence of radiologic signs. Stress radiographs may be taken if accurate diagnosis is imperative but are rarely performed in the modern era (pain issues, how much stress?, what is learned?). Diagnosis of separation of an unossified epiphysis in a very young child is more difficult and is made on clinical signs, the presence of soft tissue swelling, or possible swelling noted on an x-ray or with ultrasound.

Type I injuries are usually the result of a shearing, torsion, or avulsion force. Apophyses can also be separated with a Type I pattern (base of fifth metatarsal, medial epicondyle) with an avulsion force the likely mechanism. Pathologic Type I injuries occur in scurvy, rickets, disorders associated with hormonal imbalance, and osteomyelitis (Fig. 2-14).

When the periosteum is torn, displacement is easily reduced without any satisfying crepitus and often with little sensation that the fragment is snapping back into position, because the two fracture surfaces are covered with cartilage.

Early healing occurs within 3 weeks, and problems are rare. Exceptions include a displaced fracture of the proximal femoral physis with subsequent avascular necrosis, which has a grim prognosis. Nonunion of a separated medial epicondyle is not uncommon and may cause subsequent instability.

It is often difficult to distinguish between a Type I injury of the growth plate (which has an excellent prognosis) and a Type V injury (in which the plate is crushed) which has a poor prognosis. The history of injury is the best guide with Type V injuries produced by axial compression. These injuries will need to be followed more closely regarding subsequent physeal closure.

Type II The cleavage plane of a Type II injury (Fig. 2-15) passes through much of the plate before the fracture angles through the metaphysis. The fracture is produced by lateral displacement force, which tears the periosteum on one side but leaves it intact in the region of the triangular metaphyseal fragment, known as the Thurston-Holland fragment after the radiologist who first described it.

The fracture is easily reduced, and overreduction is prevented by the intact periosteum. The cartilage-covered surfaces usually prevent the sensation of

S.H. I

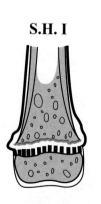
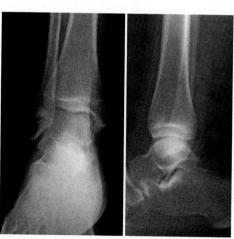

Figure 2-13 Typical Salter-Harris I fracture of the distal fibula. The x-rays appear normal but the patient has focal tenderness over the physis (not over adjacent ligaments) confirming the diagnosis.

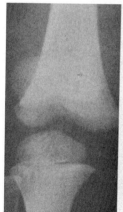
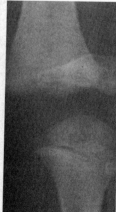

Figure 2-14 Separation of both distal femoral epiphyses. For 6 weeks this boy, aged 3 years, had been treated with antibiotics and steroids for fever and multiple joint pain. By the time a diagnosis of osteomyelitis was reached, the epiphyses had separated.

S.H. II

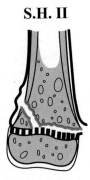

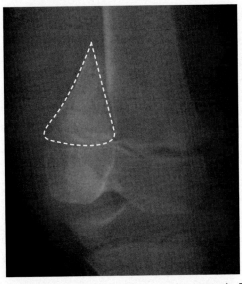

Figure 2-15 Classic Salter-Harris II fracture of the distal femur with a triangular Thurston-Holland sign (outlined). Even with anatomic reduction, nearly 40% of distal femoral physeal fractures will have subsequent physeal closure.

S.H. III

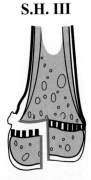

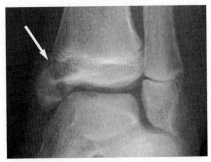

Figure 2-16 Classic Type III fracture of medial malleolus in a child.

crepitus as the fragment is pushed into position. When the radial head is separated, for example, it may be impossible to judge the success of a reduction by clinical means.

Occasionally, the shaft of a bone will become trapped in the buttonhole tear of the periosteum. This is most common at the shoulder if there is a large, metaphyseal fragment poking through a small periosteal tear. If the degree of displacement is unacceptable, open reduction is sometimes required. Also, distal femoral fractures may require open reduction plus K-wire fixation (and have a high risk for physeal closure).

Type III Type III injuries are most commonly seen in partially closed growth plates such as the distal tibia. The plane of separation passes along with the growth plate for a variable period before entering the joint through a fracture of the epiphysis. The fracture is intra-articular and requires accurate reduction to prevent malarticulation.

Open reduction is often required, but the fragment should not be dissected free of its blood supply. The most common site is at the distal end of the tibia, toward the end of growth, when the medial half of the plate is closed (Tillaux fracture). Growth disturbances, therefore, are not a problem. Another common site is the medial malleolus; however, often a tiny Thurston-Holland fragment remains attached, making a Type III versus Type IV call difficult (Fig. 2-16).

Type IV The fracture line in a Type IV injury passes from the joint surface, across the growth plate, and into the metaphysis (Fig. 2-17). The most common example is a fracture of the lateral condyle of the humerus; medial distal tibial fractures (medial malleolus) are also common (but as just noted, this can be a Type III).

This is an injury for which a surgeon can do a great deal. Left alone, this injury will produce joint stiffness and deformity owing to loss of position, nonunion, and growth disturbance. The fracture must be accurately reduced, usually by open reduction and internal fixation, both to secure a smooth joint surface and to close the fracture gap. This allows cell-to-cell apposition of the growth plate and ensures that growth is not disturbed as well as minimizes the risk for nonunion.

S.H. IV

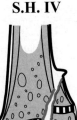

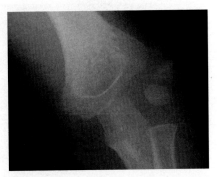

Figure 2-17 Classic Salter-Harris IV fracture of the lateral condyle of the distal humerus requiring open reduction.

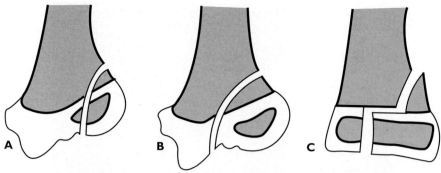

Figure 2-18 Not all Type IV injuries are the same. A) When the fracture line crosses a bony epiphysis, the risk of bony callus bridging the growth plate and causing a growth disturbance is great if accurate reduction is not achieved. B) When the fracture line passes through a cartilaginous epiphysis, bridging is less likely. C) A stepped fracture line sometimes allows a stable closed reduction.

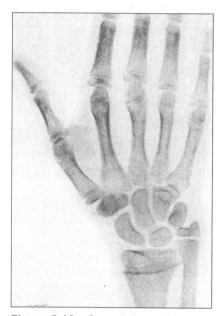

Figure 2-19 One of the earliest radiographs of a Type V injury was published by Poland in 1898. The growth plate of the radius has closed, and the radius has not grown. Note ulnar overgrowth.

At other sites, the growth plate cannot be seen clearly, and when there is doubt about whether it is accurately reduced, some have suggested that the surgeon should improve the view by removing the metaphyseal fragment (medial distal tibia). The gap can be filled with fat to discourage bridging. There are several subvarieties of this injury that are not generally known (Fig. 2-18).

Type V Concepts about Type V injuries are changing (Fig. 2-19). In the original concept, the plate is crushed, thereby extinguishing further growth. All or part of the plate may be affected. A compression injury of the plate may seem like nothing more than a sprain at first, and only later will the true nature of the lesion be recognized.

At other times, a Type I or Type II injury is obvious initially; then pressure from the most prominent corner of the metaphysis produces a crushing injury, to the chagrin of the surgeon and to the detriment of the patient. Also, a Type V injury can occur in an occult manner. In association with a long bone fracture (Fig. 2-20) patients with severe injury mechanisms should often be followed for at least a year to be sure that physeal closure has not occurred. In the case of an occult closure, the clinical exam may be more important (limb-length change, angular deformity) than the x-ray which will be initially directed at the injury site (midshaft femur) rather than the physis.

Since the work of Langenskiold, Bright, and Peterson on growth arrest owing to bony bridging, the classical concept of a Type V injury needs reexam-

At Injury	After Healing	Late Physeal Closure	S.H. V

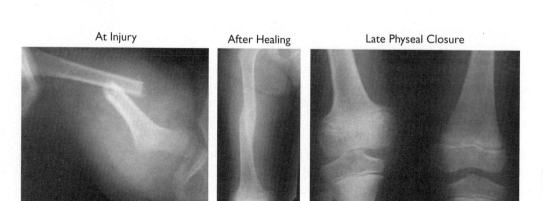
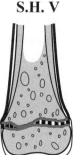

Figure 2-20 This 8-year-old girl fell from a balcony and was thought to have a simple right midshaft femoral fracture and was treated with a spica cast. Three years later, her right femur was found to be short due to occult distal femoral physeal closure. Hresko et al. and Bowler et al. have described this phenomenon (see Suggested Readings).

ining. When a small area of the growth plate is damaged, there is a race to replace the defect. Either regenerated growth cartilage or bone may win. Growth is threatened if bone forms. The surgeon's focus should be on the bridge rather than the crush, if only because the bridge can be treated.

All significant growth plate injuries should be followed for at least 6 months and perhaps a year because growth disturbance is a possibility. The cost for follow-up examination and x-rays as well as the added x-ray exposure make mandatory follow-up less critical in mild injuries (Type I, Type II in younger children with mild fracture mechanisms). Again, the art of practice is required.

In such cases, we state that "Physeal closure is possible but very unlikely. If your limb seems to be getting shorter or appears to angulate over time, see your family doctor for confirmation and referral to orthopedics." PRN returns are often unwise in dictations; instead tell the patient, "If you detect or suspect any problem, please return to see me" and dictate "The patient is encouraged to return if either the patient or the family doctor note any abnormalities."

Type VI A scalping injury to the edge of the physis produces a perichondral ring injury, removing both the edge of the physis and associated perichondral ring of Ranvier (Fig. 2-21). Injuries of the medial malleolus, from lawn mower injuries, are the most common cause in the midwestern part of the United States (where children help their parents with lawn mowing chores—or at least share the ride). Such lawn mowing injuries are much less common in the southwestern United States where hired adults (gardeners) operate most lawn mowers.

Often, there is associated skin loss and the avulsed bone fragment is not recoverable (ground to bits at the scene of the accident). These injuries are difficult to treat and almost routinely lead to physeal closure. Plastic surgery assistance may be needed to get skin coverage and subsequent operations may be needed to deal with physeal closure.

The perichondrial ring may also be lifted from the distal femoral condyle by the lateral collateral ligament, and this too carries the risk of bridging unless it's accurately replaced. A progressive varus deformity follows because bone replaces the perichondrium.

Stress Injuries of the Growth Plate

The concept of stress fracture through the growth plate was introduced by Godshall and others. It is a natural development, from the observation by Bright and associates, that shear cracks in the growth plate are seen when the load applied to the plate is 50% of that necessary to separate the plate. Continued injury could be expected to inhibit healing. Godshall and associates described pain in the knee, inability to run, and circumferential tenderness around the distal femoral growth plate. X-ray films showed widening of the growth plate. After 12 weeks of rest, the lesion healed. These lesions are seen in gymnasts (distal radius) and baseball pitchers (proximal humerus, elbow) (Fig. 2-22). Osgood-Schlatter disease offers a further example.

GUIDE TO THE CARE OF PHYSEAL INJURIES

Defining the Exact Line of the Fracture

This is usually obvious, but some injuries can be very difficult, particularly in the young child with little or no ossification in the epiphysis. Multiple views, with comparative views of the opposite side, may help. (An orthopedist should

"All significant growth plate injuries should be followed for at least 6 months and perhaps a year because growth disturbance is a possibility"

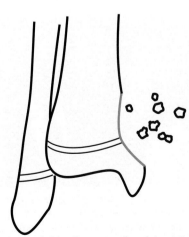

Figure 2-21 Diagram of scalping injury (Type VI) of medial malleolus as might be seen with a lawn mower injury.

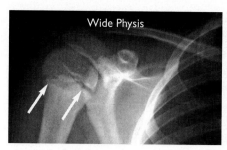
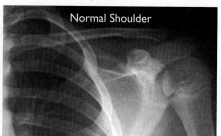

Figure 2-22   X-rays of a 12-year-old male baseball pitcher who tried to pitch every day. He presented with right shoulder pain. The physis shows widening (really thickening) due to chronic repetitive stress.

selfishly think that humans are made symmetrical for the purpose of radiographic comparison.) Stress films are occasionally considered and arthrography may be helpful.

CT scans and particularly MRI studies have greatly improved our diagnostic capacity. The demanding parent, who insists on an MRI study (sometimes annoyingly), may be on track in this instance. Occasionally, even after an arthrogram or MRI you will remain puzzled and still suspect a displaced intra-articular fracture but cannot prove it. In such cases, it is usually wiser to err in favor of exploration than to rely on your small stock of undeserved miracles.

Consulting Senior Colleagues

When in doubt, discuss the case with a radiologist and consult a senior colleague (Fig. 2-23). One should not finalize a treatment plan until the diagnosis is clear. As noted previously, it is usually better to explore a puzzling physeal injury (open surgery) rather than cast, with hope that all will "turn out well."

Other Issues

Reduction should be early and gentle. These injuries unite quickly, so that attempts to correct malposition after 7-10 days are liable to do more damage than good to the physis. Repeated efforts at reduction may do nothing more than grate the plate away. If long-term problems are anticipated, whenever possible they should be communicated to the parents (without unduly alarming them) preoperatively.

Open or Closed Reduction?

It is usually possible to secure closed reduction of Type I and Type II injuries. Exact anatomic reduction, although desirable, may be unnecessary, because remodeling can correct many imperfections. Occasionally, soft tissue is interposed (e.g., at the ankle) or the part is so deeply placed (e.g., the radial head) that open reduction will be needed.

Open reduction is also required for significantly displaced separations of the medial epicondyle. Stability is sometimes achieved with a few periosteal sutures or more commonly a screw. Type III injuries commonly need open reduction in order to secure a smooth joint surface. Type IV injuries are commonly unstable, and accurate reduction is mandatory, both to ensure an anatomic joint and to ensure subsequent normal physeal growth.

This applies particularly to the lateral condyle of the humerus; it may be possible to reduce this injury, but it is difficult to be sure that it is stable and almost impossible to be sure (by examining radiographs of a flexed elbow taken

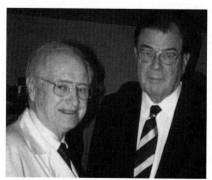

Figure 2-23   Before you go to surgery with a puzzling physeal fracture that you do not understand, you should consult a wise senior colleague (Dr. Sutherland, San Diego, and the late Dr. Heinz Wagner, Nuremburg).

through a cast) that the position is maintained. For these reasons, open reduction and internal fixation are much safer.

Infection—Chondrolysis

A growth plate may be destroyed by infection. This is a risk in all open fractures and to a lesser extent in any fracture in which open reduction is carried out. Kirschner wires used to maintain reduction often traverse joints and can lead to joint sepsis and chondrolysis as well as osteomyelitis (Fig. 2-24). For this reason, all K-wires should be either buried below the skin or removed early to minimize the risk.

Length of Immobilization

Various rules are invoked. The elbow may become stiff if immobilized for more than 3 to 4 weeks. For other joints, we allow 4 weeks for early union of an epiphyseal separation, and 6 weeks in a metaphyseal or diaphyseal fracture. Note the term "early union." The cast is removed well before solid structural union has occurred and the family must know this.

The child's activity level and temperament may require variations in advice [longer immobilization for dynamic athletes, attention deficit disorder (ADD) patients, and when parental control is an issue]. Children rarely get stiff joints, even if the cast immobilization extends a few weeks beyond what is usually advised. When the cast is removed, the fracture is only partially healed and patients must be advised of this ("healing"—not "healed"). Post-case splinting may decrease the chance for refracture in the dynamic child (most children fit this category).

Patient from "Elsewhere General Hospital"— Late Diagnosed Cases

Children presenting late with Type I and Type II injuries more than 7-10 days old, even though not adequately reduced, should be left with the displacement uncorrected, for fear of damaging the growth plate. Corrective osteotomy can be performed later if remodeling fails.

Open reduction of displaced Type III and Type IV injuries may be better undertaken late than never. Be careful not to devascularize the fragment at the time of replacement.

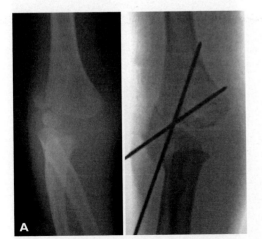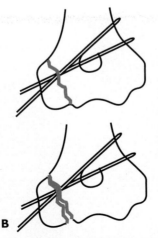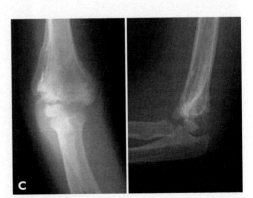

Figure 2-24 A) This child had a lateral condyle fracture with attempted K-wire reduction. B) The technique was suboptimal with the pins crossing at the fracture site. The child was very active and the fragment rotated on the cross pins. C) The films show malunion of the condyle, as well as probable AVN.

Bony Bridging (Physeal Closure Due to Trauma)

Growth stops when a significant bony bridge joins the epiphysis to the metaphysis. (note that a very small bridge can form and then be "broken" by the distractive power of a growing physis.) An early sign of a bony bridge may be a converging Harris line. In the early stage, the patient is free of deformity and complaints. In most patients, it takes many months to be sure that the bridge is real. Declaring physeal closure either too early or too late is inappropriate. A CT or MRI should be taken to confirm the diagnosis and to define the size of the bridge (Fig. 2-25).

Since Langenskiold, Bright, and Peterson described operative intervention that can allow resumption of growth after resection of the bridge, there has been much more reason to follow growth plate injuries carefully. Langenskiold replaced the bridge with autogenous fat, Bright with silicone rubber, and Peterson with methyl methacrylate. Silicon is no longer available, thus fat or methacrylate remain as the best choices. Careful delineation of the bridge size is made using a CT or MRI methods. The bridge is approached by making a window in the metaphysis.

Loops and a headlamp improve vision. The bridge is pale bone, in contrast to the red bone of the normal metaphysis. The bridge is removed with a curet or burr until the normal plate is seen. The bridge is usually more extensive than expected (Fig. 2-26). Image views during surgery may help to localize the bridge so that not too much and not too little is removed. The defect is then replaced with fat or methyl methacrylate.

Langenskiold reviewed 33 cases in 1978 with excellent results. A second operation for recurrence was indicated in three patients. Deformity has improved in most, but some have required osteotomy. Peterson has also reported promising results. Our experience suggests that his operation has only a 30%–50% chance for success. The surgery is technically demanding and surgeon experience benefits the patient. Even referral centers, with multiple orthopedic staff, should have one surgeon do all of these cases (so that the benefit of experience can be accumulated).

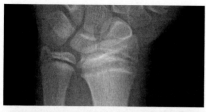
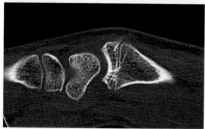

Figure 2-25 Plane films and CT study (lateral view) of a distal radius physeal bar (that followed a Salter-Harris II fracture).

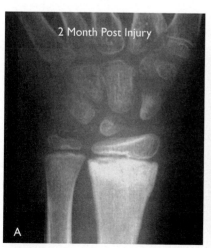
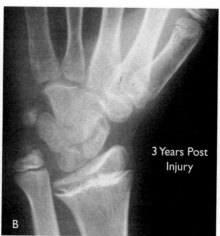
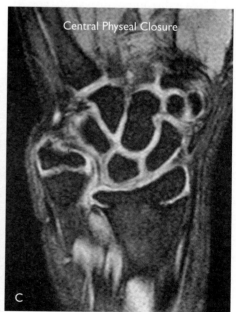

Figure 2-26 A) Salter-Harris I distal radius fracture. B) Three years following injury, note radial physeal closure and ulnar overgrowth. C) MRI confirms physeal arrest.

SUMMARY—PHYSEAL INJURY

Fortunately, the majority of growth plate injuries involve little risk of growth disturbance. In a few, simple surgical intervention can make a great deal of difference to the outcome of the injury. Happily, the number of children who have irretrievable damage is very small.

Suggested Readings

Bright RW: Operative correction of partial epiphyseal plate closure by osseous-bridge resection and silicone-rubber implant. J Bone Joint Surg 56A:655, 1974.

Bright RW, Burstein AH, Elmore SM: Epiphyseal-plate cartilage. A biomechanical and histological analysis of failure modes. J Bone Joint Surg 56A:688, 1974.

Bowler J, Mubarak S, Wenger D: The tibial physeal closure and genu recurvatum after femoral fracture. J Pedatr Orthop 10:653, 1990.

Brunner CH: Fracture in and around the knee joint. In Weber BG, Brunner C, Freuler F (eds): Treatment of Fractures in Children and Adolescents: New York, Springer-Verlag, 1979.

Carlson WO, Wenger DR: A mapping method to prepare for surgical excision of a partial physeal arrest. J Pediatr Orthop 4:232-238, 1984.

Dale GC, Harris WR: Prognosis in epiphyseal separation. An experimental study. J Bone Joint Surg 40B:115, 1958.

Godshall RW, Hansen CA, Rising DC: Stress fractures through the distal femoral epiphysis in athletes. Am J Sports Med 9:114, 1981.

Hresko M, Kasser J: Physeal arrest about the knee associated with non-physeal fractures in the lower extremity. J Bone Joint Surg (Am) 71:698 1989.

Johnston RM, Jones WW: Fractures through human growth plates. Orthopedic Transactions 4:295, 1980.

Langenskiold A: Surgical treatment of partial closure of the growth plate. J Pediatr Orthop 1:3, 1981.

Ogden JA: Skeletal injury in the child. Philadelphia: Lea and Febiger, 3rd Ed. 2000.

Peterson HA: Operative correction of post-fracture arrest of the epiphyseal plate: case report with ten-year follow-up. J Bone Joint Surg Am 1980;62:1018-1020.

Peterson HA: Partial growth plate arrest and its treatment. J Pediatr Orhtop 1984;4: 246-258.

Rigal WM: Diaphyseal aclasis. In Rang M (ed): The Growth Plate and its disorders. Baltimore, Williams and Wilkins, 1969.

Salter RB, Harris WR: Injuries involving the epiphyseal plate. J Bone Joint Surg 45A:587, 1963.

Salter RB, Simmonds DF, Malcolm BW et al: The biological effect of continuous passive movement on the healing of full-thickness defects on articular cartilage. J Bone Joint Surg 62A:1232, 1980.

3

Orthopedic Literacy: Fracture Description and Resource Utilization

Dennis Wenger

INTRODUCTION—TERMINOLOGY

Fracture language, which has evolved in a relatively standard manner throughout the world, makes medical communication more efficient. Learning fracture language, like learning a foreign language, requires time and exposure. In this chapter we will present common orthopedic terminology concepts that facilitate orthopedic communication and care.

Descriptive Planes

Describing fractures depends on first understanding the accepted terms used to describe the human body in three dimensions. The coronal plane (frontal plane) is at right angles to the sagittal plane, dividing a structure into anterior and pos-

> *"In a work of art the intellect asks the questions; it does not answer them"*
>
> —HERBEL

terior portions. The sagittal plane is a pure lateral view. The axial (transverse) plane is a cross section, as one might see on a CT or MRI study of the spine.

Also, orthopedic terminology is generally described as if one were visualizing a standing human with the upper extremities in extension and externally rotated (forearm supinated), thus the confusion in describing forearm and hand anatomy. With the forearm pronated, one would think of the thumb as being a medial structure yet by anatomic standard (forearm supinated) it is lateral. Thus the terms "radial" and "ulnar side" are best used for localizing forearm and hand conditions.

"Learning fracture language, like learning a foreign language, requires time and exposure"

FRACTURE LANGUAGE

Beginning orthopedic residents rapidly adopt the "tools of their trade," which include development of an "orthopedic language" as one of the most critical learned skills, both for the spoken and written word (letters, reports). Direction of displacement is commonly used to describe joint dislocation with wide acceptance that when one describes a posterior dislocation of the knee that one means the more distal member (tibia) is posteriorly positioned in its relationship to the femur.

The efficiency of "varus" and "valgus" rather than a full descriptive sentence quickly becomes apparent. Rather than stating that "the ankle fracture has healed in slight angulation with the heel in a more lateral position than would be normally expected" we simply state "the ankle is in valgus." What a triumph of efficiency! Once this "lingua franca" has been mastered, life becomes easy for the doctor but frustrating for patients, especially if their doctor does not understand the necessity of reverting to common language when speaking to children and their families.

Common Greek & Latin Terms used in Orthopedics

Cubitus = Elbow

Coxa = Hip

Genu = Knee

Hallux = Great toe

Pes = Foot

Carpus = Wrist

Tarsus = Ankle

Pronation = Forearm turned inward

Supination = Forearm turned outward

The Forearm—Pronation and Supination

Pronation (from Latin pronus): Turned or inclined forward.

The Roman scholar and husbandman M.T. Varro (116-27 B.C.) defined the prone position as lying on the belly with the hands above the head, such that the back projects away from the palms and the palms project toward the ground.

Supination (from Latin supinus): Turned or thrown backward, opposite of Latin pronus.

From Diab M. Lexicon of orthopaedic etymology, 1999

"Rather than stating that 'the fracture has healed in slight angulation with the heel in a more lateral position than would be normally expected' we simply state 'the ankle is in valgus'"

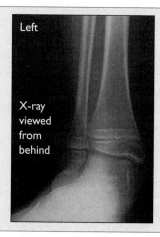

Left

X-ray viewed from behind

Valgus position – left ankle

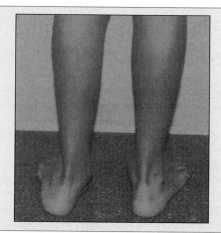

Standard Positions and Planes

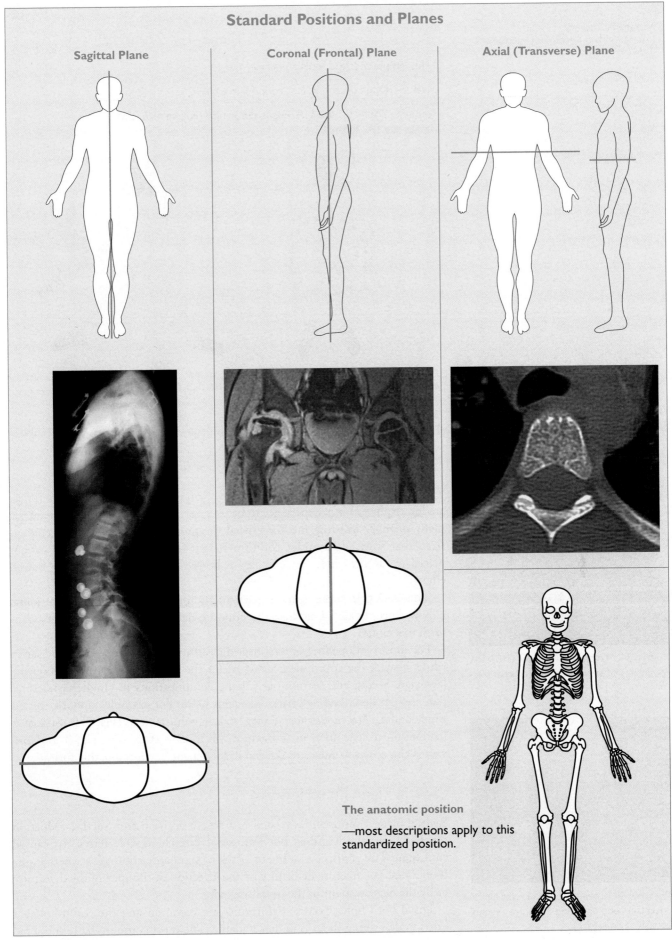

Sagittal Plane

Coronal (Frontal) Plane

Axial (Transverse) Plane

The anatomic position

—most descriptions apply to this standardized position.

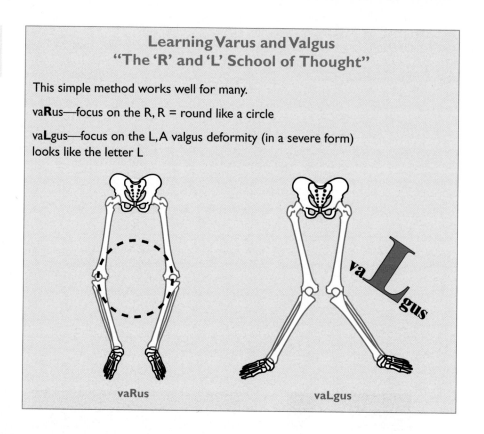

**Learning Varus and Valgus
"The 'R' and 'L' School of Thought"**

This simple method works well for many.

vaRus—focus on the R, R = round like a circle

vaLgus—focus on the L, A valgus deformity (in a severe form)
looks like the letter L

vaRus   vaLgus

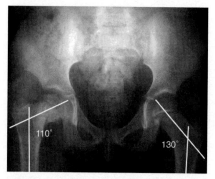

Figure 3-1. Cubitus varus, right elbow following a right supracondylar humerus fracture.

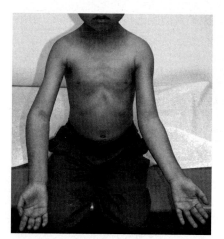

Figure 3-2. Coxa vara of the right hip of uncertain etiology (old fracture versus congenital coxa vara).

Frontal Plane Descriptions (Coronal)

The terms varus and valgus, easily learned on externally evident joints (knee, ankle), require a bit of experience to be used for the elbow and hip. None of the many memory assisting methods speed the process very much. Salter emphasized that varus deformities conform to an imaginary circle with a patient placed inside the circle (circular legs = bowed legs, cubitus varus = a bowed elbow).

This may help some learners, particularly for the externally apparent joints (elbow, knee, ankle). Logically, the opposite deformity (valgus) does not conform to a circle.

For most orthopedic learners, hearing and using the terms again and again while viewing the appropriate x-rays seems the best way to master orthopedic language. Seeing and learning about the complications in children's fractures that are best described by varus and valgus helps. For example, a poorly treated supracondylar fracture almost always heals in cubitus varus (Fig. 3-1). Similarly, inattention to a femoral neck fracture will lead to coxa vara (Fig. 3-2). Coxa vara is also seen secondary to skeletal dysplasia and in an idiopathic form.

Sagittal Plane Descriptions

Sagittal plane abnormalities related to fracture position and fracture reduction can be efficiently described but the use of interchangeable terms has caused confusion. The confusion is due to a lack of standardization as to whether one should describe fracture deformity by the direction of the apex of the deformity or by the displacement of the distal fragment.

Distal both bone fracture deformities are common and the confusion that exists in describing them is understandable. The most common pattern is a fall

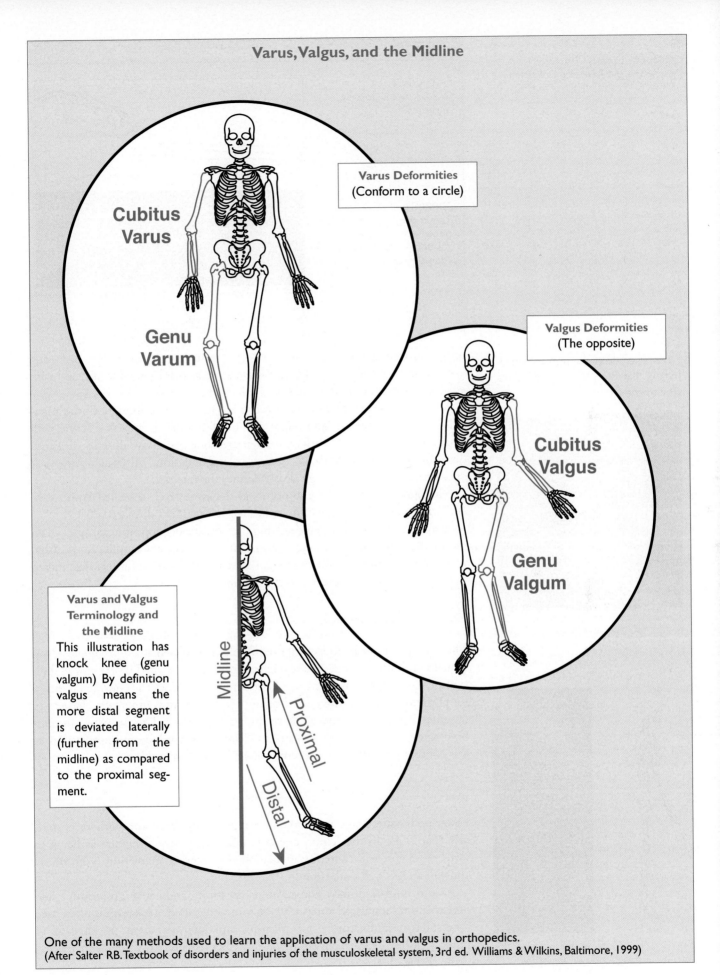

Varus Deformities
(Conform to a circle)

Cubitus Varus

Genu Varum

Valgus Deformities
(The opposite)

Cubitus Valgus

Genu Valgum

Varus and Valgus Terminology and the Midline

This illustration has knock knee (genu valgum) By definition valgus means the more distal segment is deviated laterally (further from the midline) as compared to the proximal segment.

Midline

Proximal

Distal

One of the many methods used to learn the application of varus and valgus in orthopedics.
(After Salter RB. Textbook of disorders and injuries of the musculoskeletal system, 3rd ed. Williams & Wilkins, Baltimore, 1999)

Table 3-1	How to Describe This Fracture?

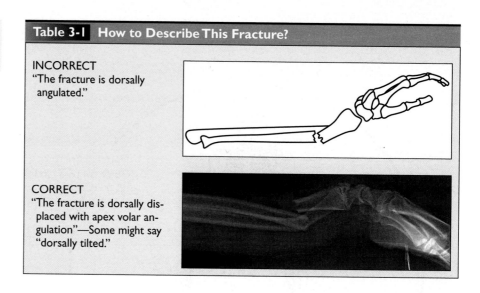

INCORRECT
"The fracture is dorsally
angulated."

CORRECT
"The fracture is dorsally displaced with apex volar angulation"—Some might say
"dorsally tilted."

"'Posterior dislocation of the knee'
means that the tibia is lying posterior to the femur"

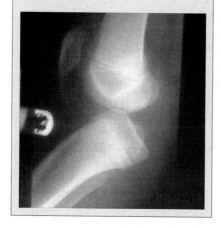

on an outstretched hand (so-called FOOSH injury) with the fracture occurring
3-4 cm above the physis, with the distal fragments displacing dorsally, and with
volar angulation at the fracture site (Table 3-1).

Most orthopedists like to describe this fracture by describing both the angulation and displacement and might say "displaced distal forearm fracture with
volar angulation of 45°." Perhaps even clearer, one could say "dorsally displaced
distal forearm fracture with 45° of apex volar angulation." Although some variance is accepted, the language clearly defines the fracture.

The opposite deformity also occurs at the same level (so-called Smith variant) with apex dorsal angulation and the distal fragment displaced volarly.

Also by convention, when describing a joint dislocation, for example, when
stating that "the knee is dislocated posteriorly"—"posterior" applies to the distal
member as compared to the proximal. "Posterior dislocation of the knee" means
that the tibia is lying posterior to the femur.

Other Descriptions

The concept of dorsal and ventral terminology is related to embryologic development and innervation. The segment of the leg innervated by the dorsal division of motor roots (back of leg; hamstrings, gastroceles) is considered dorsal
(or posterior), whereas the ventral division of motor roots innervates the ventral
(or anterior muscle groups—quadriceps, anterior tibial). Unfortunately the embryologic rotation of the limb makes clear understanding and application of
this concept difficult. Simpler terminology is therefore used.

Lower Extremity Descriptions

Lower limb issues relate to whether a fracture is angulated anteriorly or posteriorly (Fig. 3-3). In the femur, one commonly describes a fracture as being in
varus or valgus, with anterior angulation or posterior angulation (with dorsal
and ventral less well understood).

As one moves distally the term recurvatum (angulated posteriorly) and
procurvatum (angulated anteriorly) are sometimes used. This term is often used
for distal femoral fractures, tibial fractures, and deformity about the knee due to
physeal closure (e.g., recurvatum due to tibial tubercle fracture with physeal
closure) (Fig. 3-4).

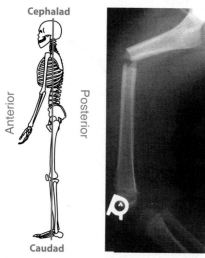
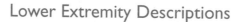

Cephalad

Anterior

Posterior

Caudad

Figure 3-3. Most would describe this
fracture as having anterior angulation.

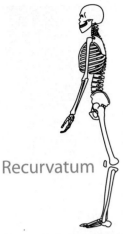
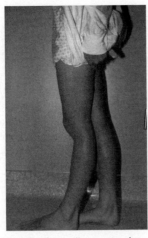
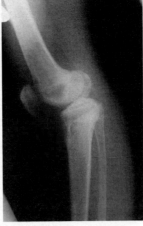

Recurvatum

Figure 3-4. This could be described as a "posterior bow at the knee" but is more commonly described as genu recurvatum in this case due to traumatic closure of the tibial tubercle (growth plate).

Thus "curvatum" terminology is more widely used in the lower extremity, likely because the terms dorsal and ventral are less well visualized in the biped (upright species), as compared to dorsal and volar in the forearm. In some parts of the world, an "apex ventral deformity" of the lower extremity might be easily understood as occurring on the anterior surface of the femur or the tibia; however, this terminology is not used in North America.

An example of how this language is used would be a distal tibial fracture, perhaps 4–5 cm above the ankle. If this fracture had an anterior angulation, it would be described as being in procurvatum (with apex anterior angulation). More commonly, this fracture has a posterior angulation (Fig. 3-5). If such fractures are casted with a neutral foot position, muscle and tendon forces tend to worsen the recurvatum or posterior angulation. Initial casting in equinus is advised (also see Chapter 15).

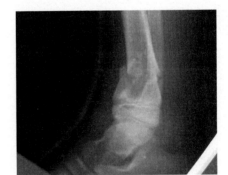

Figure 3-5. This tibial fracture has apex posterior angulation (recurvatum). Reduction plus casting in equinus will be required.

Foot Language

Language describing foot deformity leads to another level of confusion because the foot is generally perceived to be at right angles to the trunk and legs, thus the terms dorsal and ventral are hard to visualize. Do you visualize the bottom of your foot as being ventral or dorsal?

Angulation in the sagittal plane in the foot is sometimes described as apex dorsal or plantar angulation. Yet from a classic anatomic view point the bottom of the foot is its dorsal surface. Dorsal and plantar have been adopted as the most logical descriptions, although not anatomically correct. If humans only swam, dorsal and ventral would suffice (Fig. 3-6).

The term adduction and abduction are often used to describe forefoot position. Adduction implies that the distal segment is more toward the midline as compared to the proximal segment. Deviation away from the midline is called abduction.

A congenital deformity of the foot with medial deviation of the forefoot is referred to as either metatarsus varus or metatarsus adductus (Fig. 3-7). The varus term is applied because of the bowed deformity of the foot with the convexity appearing laterally (thus conforming to a circle). Adductus can also be used because the distal portion of the foot is more medial than the proximal segment. A first metatarsal fracture can produce an adduction deforming (or be described as in an adducted position Fig. 3-8).

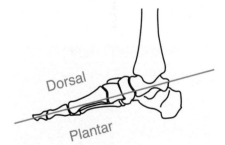

Figure 3-6. Dorsal and plantar describe the foot in stance phase.

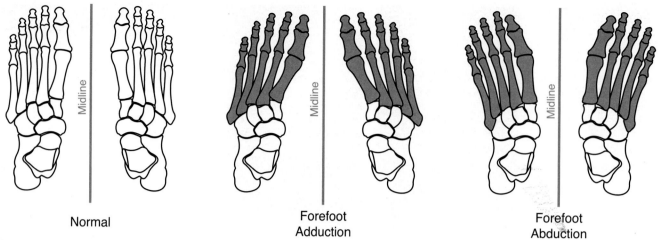

Normal

Forefoot
Adduction

Forefoot
Abduction

Figure 3-7. Common terms to describe the foot. Are these coronal or axial deviations? If the patient is standing, the axial plane prevails.

"Terms such as varus, valgus, procurvatum, recurvatum, etc. are confusing and instead should be defined in terms that most parents use in day to day conversation ('bowed', 'angled', etc.)"

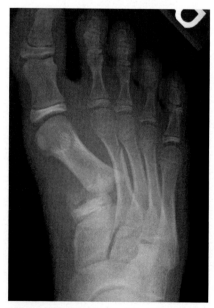

Figure 3-8. Adduction deformity in a first metatarsal fracture.

Deformity of the great toe with angulation of the metatarsal phalangeal joint (bunion deformity) is referred to as hallux valgus—the more distal segment (toe) deviates laterally making the metatarsal head translate medially (Fig. 3-9).

LANGUAGE AND FAMILIES

A growing area of orthopedic language application relates to discussions with patient, parents, and relatives. Sizing up the child and family you are treating includes assessing their knowledge base, allowing you to adopt terminology that is clear, descriptive, and appropriate for their level of understanding.

Internet savvy families often make special demands, mandating that you communicate at their newly attained level of communication. A gracious approach is required, acknowledging what they have learned and then adding your wisdom, gained through experience. Much can be learned by listening to (and briefly reviewing the hard copies) all that has been gathered by the Internet savvy parent. I usually make a copy for the chart.

On entering the consult room, one quickly determines whether the child and the parents should be communicated to in a more traditional method relying on lay terminology versus a more high tech "parental Internet knowledge" manner. As a general principle, it is usually best to use simple terms until the conversation leads elsewhere. For example, when describing a physeal injury it may be better to use the term "growth plate." Terms such as varus, valgus, procurvatum, recurvatum, etc. are confusing and instead should be defined in terms that most parents use in day-to-day conversation ('bowed', 'angled', etc.).

When discussing diagnostic studies such as MRIs or CTs, most patients light up since they have a relative who had such a study or they have seen a TV show that has presented the concept. Of course, everybody wants one (Fig. 3-10). To limit the voracious consumer demand for these studies, a brief explanation concerning the risk versus benefit issues of such a test (especially as concerns potential risks to the child—radiation for CT scan) is more effective than stating that the test is too expensive, which only leads to a feeding frenzy. When holding off on ordering a CT or MRI study you should assure the family that if the straightforward tests (exam, x-ray, complete blood count, sed rate, C-reactive protein) do not solve the problem that you will then order the special studies.

34

Language at Follow-Up

At follow-up for femoral fractures and other lower extremity physeal injuries, one commonly assesses limb length difference. I prefer the term "difference" rather than shortening. If one is describing limb length difference to an assistant, I find it better to state that one limb is longer than the other. "Short" has a negative connotation that can lengthen your explanatory day. Also with femoral fractures, the injured limb may in fact be the long one (due to growth stimulation).

Radiographic concepts such as angulation, bayonet apposition, and other issues plague the orthopedic surgeon-parent discussions. One must be cautious how and where one uses films to explain a child's orthopedic problem. In general, x-rays should be taken into the examination room because they greatly simplify your explanation. If fracture films show complete bayonet apposition and you choose to demonstrate them (in all their glory), you must be prepared for a lengthy explanation in many cases.

We keep a set of teaching films in our office and clinic so that we can quickly show an example of another patient who had a similar type of injury (and in which the fracture remodeled Fig. 3-11). On a busy day, you may decide that the art of children's orthopedics (on that day) includes not showing the bayonet apposition film on a fracture check visit, but it must be in hand if the parents request a review. (Usually they have already reviewed the films while returning from the x-ray department.)

The Modern Communication Era

The era of Internet image transmission has arrived and will revolutionize fracture language and communication. The future (really current) era allows a home, automobile, or satellite office positioned orthopedic surgeon to both listen to the history and review diagnostic x-ray images from a distance. This will radically improve analysis of cases and allocation of resources, allowing accurate decisions about "splint and send to clinic later this week" versus "splint and bring to clinic tomorrow" versus "needs to be admitted and go to the operating room."

As previously noted, this simultaneous discussion of the radiograph with the primary care physician who is analyzing the patient will greatly improve physician musculoskeletal education allowing the "orthopedic terminology" (dorsal and volar angulation, dorsal displacement, varus, valgus, antecurvatum, retrocurvatum, etc.) to be better understood by primary care colleagues.

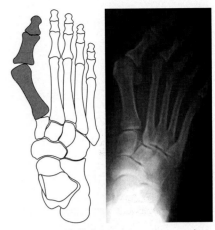

Figure 3-9. Hallux valgus—the toe deviates laterally in relation to the more proximal segment of the foot.

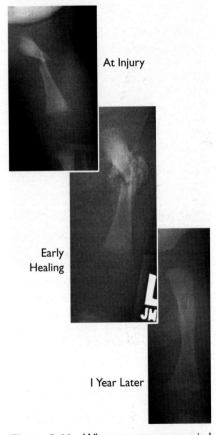

At Injury

Early Healing

I Year Later

Figure 3-11. When parents get worried about what we consider acceptable angulation or apposition, we show them films from our teaching file that demonstrate the child's ability to remodel. This case demonstrates how a femoral fracture in an infant will remodel.

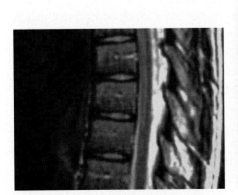
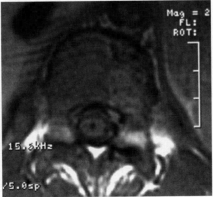

Figure 3-10. This child's parents insisted on a spine MRI (occasional backache). Amazingly a syrinx was found. The wide availability of sophisticated diagnostic methods sometimes produces more questions than answers.

"Consumer acceptance of the digital revolution will require education since many patients still prefer to 'see the orthopedic doctor' on the same day"

"This is a severe supracondylar fracture. You must see the child urgently in your ER"

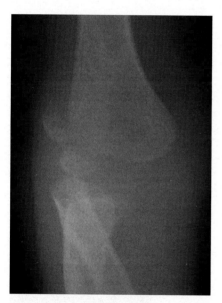

Figure 3-12. This was called in as an acute supracondylar fracture requiring emergent surgery. In fact this is a lateral condyle fracture and surgery could be done anytime in the next 4 to 5 days.

"The development of telecommunication methods, which allow transmission of digital x-ray images to an orthopedic surgeon's automobile, home, or offsite office will improve communication efficiency"

Consumer acceptance of the digital revolution will require education because many patients still prefer to "see the orthopedic doctor" on the same day. Economic and outcome studies will help correct this once the true cost of having a specialist see even a modest injury on the same day becomes apparent.

FRACTURE DESCRIPTION AND RESOURCE UTILIZATION—WHAT REQUIRES EMERGENCY REDUCTION?

"This is a severe supracondylar fracture. You must see the child urgently in your ER" (Fig. 3-12). As a consequence, the receiving surgeon's operating room (OR) staff is kept past their regular hours—sometimes on overtime pay—awaiting the urgent case only to find on the patient's arrival that the fracture was not severe or was a lateral condyle fracture, either of which could have been seen in the clinic the following day—saving thousands of dollars.

The growth of emergency medicine as a specialty as well as more prevalent urgent care centers, combined with the traditional pediatric trauma initially seen in the office of family practitioners and pediatricians, emphasizes the need for improved musculoskeletal communication skills among non-orthopedic surgeons.

Part of the problem relates to the limited musculoskeletal education provided to North American medical students. The crowded medical school curriculum, focused on basic science and molecular medicine, provides little time for musculoskeletal education, despite the fact that 30% or more of urgent medicine deals with musculoskeletal issues.

Orthopedic surgeons can help to improve this situation by encouraging increased attention to musculoskeletal disease education for the medical school curriculum and also by providing primary care, family practice, and pediatric residencies with the opportunity for clinic exposure and rotations on an orthopedic service. More practically, the orthopedist can take the time to discuss the clinical and x-ray findings with his/her colleagues when arriving to assess an emergency case.

As noted previously, accurate description of the fracture type and its severity has great economic consequence. Is the fracture open, thus requiring emergency débridement? As already noted, descriptions of deformity versus angulation are often confusing. Perhaps the best that one can expect is an accurate description of the degree of angulation of the fracture. Whether the displacement or angulation is dorsal or volar (upper extremity) or anterior or posterior (lower extremity) is likely less important for the initial discussion.

The development of telecommunication methods, which allow transmission of digital x-ray images to an orthopedic surgeon's automobile, home, or offsite office, will improve communication efficiency.

WHAT REQUIRES EMERGENCY REDUCTION?

The topic of orthopedic language and children's fracture treatment logically leads into efficient resource utilization. In this section I will present a few notes on treatment urgency, which will also be mentioned in Chapter 4.

Fracture Reduction Urgency

The urgency for fracture treatment in children has varied greatly. Often decisions about urgency are made according to the type of institution providing treatment and/or the social structure of the family. A commonly quoted system is that of John Royal Moore in Philadelphia who held a children's fracture reduction clinic every Thursday (see Chapter 4). Children injured throughout the week were consolidated and treated on a single day. Obviously, true emergencies were excepted.

Traditionally, orthopedic practices probably have provided same day reduction and treatment for many fractures, except for cases where swelling could not allow it. A child injured in school would hope to see an orthopedic surgeon that day with a cast applied and/or a reduction performed as needed. Splinting alone would be used only if swelling was extreme.

The development of large children's hospital treatment centers particularly with resident manpower available has led to an exaggerated sense of urgency regarding the need for acute reduction. Other factors have also contributed to this. These would include the development of emergency medicine as a specialty and also the use of emergency rooms (ERs) as urgent care centers by a large segment of the population, particularly the underinsured.

Patients arriving early in the evening are assessed by the emergency department attending and determined to need a reduction. With a resident available, it seemed only logical to get a consult and, if feasible, reduce the fracture on an urgent basis, using conscious sedation anesthesia. The problem lies with late arrivals, need for a certain length of nothing by mouth (NPO) status (4-6 hours), even for conscious sedation, and the 80-hour resident work week. Suddenly, one is faced with a child arriving at 9:00 p.m. who cannot be reduced until 3:00 a.m.

The pattern noted previously has led to an over-utilization of an institution's resources for fracture care and reductions. Clearly, nighttime care is more expensive than elective, daytime care and passing the load to residents is not the appropriate solution. Some of our solutions to this dilemma are presented in Chapter 4.

Open Fractures

A cardinal rule of fracture care at any age has been that an open fracture must be taken to the OR and débrided within 6-8 hours of the injury (Fig. 3-13). Classic literature suggested that if this time limit was not met, infection and even osteomyelitis were more likely. Skaggs et al. as well as Yang suggested a change in this protocol, particularly in Type I injuries. These publications suggest that if the patient has a clean wound, the wound is cleansed and sterilely dressed, and the patient is given intravenous antibiotics, the operative débridement of an open fracture can perhaps be done the next morning. This is highly controversial and should be applied only after careful study of the literature, one's experience, and the institutional standards.

Supracondylar Fractures

A second urgency issue concerns treatment of supracondylar fractures that can be quite severe and that, in very difficult cases, can have neurovascular complications. Accordingly, this fracture has been given a great deal of urgency and traditionally it has been advised that the child have urgent reduction plus pinning on arrival (Fig. 3-14).

Because large volumes of patients with supracondylar fractures have been concentrated in children's centers, it has been demonstrated that these patients can, in most cases, be splinted with reduction the next day.

The study by Gupta et al. from Los Angeles clarifies that most supracondylar fractures, even Type III injuries, providing they do not have a significant neurologic deficit or skin tenting on arrival, can be safely splinted and then treated

"The development of large children's hospital treatment centers particularly with resident manpower available has led to an exaggerated sense of urgency regarding the need for acute reduction"

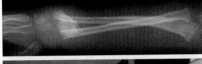
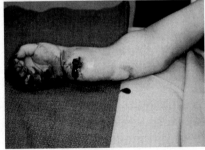

Figure 3-13. Open fracture requires urgent surgery for débridement as well as reduction and stabilization.

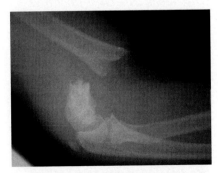

Figure 3-14. Severe Type III supracondylar fracture of the humerus. When must this be reduced as a super-emergency?

"Neither a practicing orthopedic surgeon nor an orthopedic resident will want to reduce a fracture at these hours if safe alternatives are available"

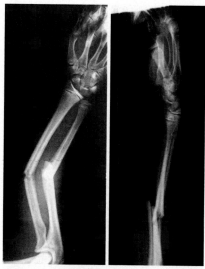

Figure 3-15. Does this fracture mandate urgent formal reduction at 3 a.m.? John Royal Moore would have suggested that it doesn't. If you ask your resident to do this reduction at 3 a.m. in the ER, he or she will not be available for surgery the next afternoon (and may miss doing an important case).

"...as the true cost of night and weekend care becomes apparent, and insurance schemes further involve families in sharing cost, it will become apparent that definitive treatment by a specialist in the middle of the night (or early in the morning) is not sustainable"

surgically within the next 24 hours, at a time that is more convenient for the surgeon (and economical for the hospital) while still producing good results.

Clearly, a careful assessment of the patient needs to be made and splinting needs to be done in relative extension to avoid increasing the tension on the elbow hematoma. Often about 30° of flexion is the ideal position of splinting. The child should be admitted to the hospital for monitoring.

Other Angulated Fractures

Because most supracondylar fractures can be splinted and treated within the next day; clearly moderately angulated forearm fractures do not require an immediate reduction at night. Our hospital has a very large number of such patients, and if the patient comes in early at night on an empty stomach, it is easy to give conscious sedation and reduce the fracture.

Because modern conscious sedation protocols (Chapter 4) are progressively geared toward making the child NPO for 6 hours prior to sedation, the child who arrives at 9:00 at night might not be able to have a reduction until 3:00 in the morning. Neither a practicing orthopedic surgeon nor an orthopedic resident will want to reduce a fracture at these hours if safer alternatives are available. A moderately angulated forearm fracture can simply be splinted and reduced and casted sometime within the next several days or even a week (Fig. 3-15).

Many private orthopedic practices and institutions have already had these more practical policies in place for some time. The 80-hour work week regulations for orthopedic residents will nudge training centers into this more realistic view of fracture reduction urgency. These less urgent policies allocate resources better and allow swelling to subside before the formal casting occurs. Another advantage in the North American resident training program setting is that the actual manipulative reduction can be carried out when senior staff are available, thus allowing proper supervision, as well as appropriate billing for rendering of services.

EDUCATING FAMILIES REGARDING URGENCY

Systems that are in the habit of providing overly urgent definitive care when it is not scientifically required or justified will take some time to reeducate their consumers when making the transition to a less urgent philosophy. The first task is to educate your emergency physician colleagues (both in your hospital and elsewhere). Giving an instructional course on how to splint makes a good start.

Often families believe that their child's fracture must be set immediately and are not happy unless their child is in a cast before the sun sets (or for late arrivals, the sun rises the next day). Families must be educated concerning the safety and value of delayed reduction and casting, and much of this instruction will come from the ER staff (Table 3-2). Also you must be certain that your office or clinic has readily available openings for appointments (and reductions) within the next few days.

The first advantage that can be pointed out to the family is that casting will be safer after swelling has receded. Careful splinting with casting in 48–72 hours allows the swelling to diminish, allowing a cast to be applied that often will not need to be split or bivalved. This in many cases will save an added visit to the orthopedic office.

A second advantage is that they will have definitive treatment during daytime hours by the most experienced team. This often includes the most experienced cast technicians and orthopedic surgeons.

Table 3-2	Advantages of Splinting Fractures (with formal reduction later)
Safer—allows swelling to decrease	
Definitive treatment in daytime hours—by experienced team	
Correct billing for reduction plus casting	

Finally, as the true cost of night and weekend care becomes apparent, and insurance schemes further involve families in sharing cost, it will become apparent that definitive treatment by a specialist in the middle of the night (or early in the morning) is not sustainable. Those who demand emergent reduction when it is not really required will need to bear the added cost.

SUMMARY

In summary, proper use of orthopedic language and technology makes children's fracture care more efficient. The transmission of digital images will allow the final decision makers to determine how severe the fracture is and whether or not urgent reduction is required, even if the treating surgeon is far from the hospital. Splinting protocols will be improved. Fracture reduction can then be performed during daytime hours. Late night and early morning hour care can be allocated to truly emergent injuries (severe open fractures, fractures with vascular compromise).

Suggested Readings

Diab, M. Lexicon of orthopedic etymology. Harwood Academic Publishers 1999.

Gupta N, Kay RM, Leitch K, Femino JD, Tolo VT, Skaggs DL. Effect of surgical delay on perioperative complications and need for open reduction in supracondylar humerus fractures in children. J Pediatr Orthop. 2004 May-Jun;24(3):245-8.

Gustilo RB, Anderson JT. Prevention of infection in the treatment of one thousand and twenty-five open fractures of long bones: retrospective and prospective analyses. J Bone Joint Surg AM. 1976 Jun;58(4):453-8.

Harley BJ, Beaupre LA, Jones CA, Dulai SK, Weber DW. The effect of time to definitive treatment on the rate of nonunion and infection in open fractures. J Orthop Trauma. 2002 Aug;16(7):484-90.

Salter RB. Textbook of disorders and injuries of the musculoskeletal system 3rd ed. Williams & Wilkins—Baltimore, 1999.

Skaggs DL, Kautz SM, Kay RM, Tolo VT. Effect of delay of surgical treatment on rate of infection in open fractures in children. J Pediatr Orthop. 2000 Jan-Feb;20(1):19-22.

Yang EC, Eisler J. Treatment of isolated type I open fractures: is emergent operative debridement necessary? Clin Orthop. 2003 May;(410):289-94.

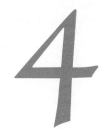

Emergency Fracture Reduction

Philip Stearns 🍂 *Dennis Wenger*

INTRODUCTION

Traditionally, simple minimally displaced or nondisplaced fractures in children were treated in the emergency room (ER) with minimal or no anesthesia. Moderately displaced fractures were sometimes treated in the ER with local anesthesia (hematoma block, IV lidocaine methods); however, most moderate and all severe fractures were treated in the operating room (OR) with general anesthesia. With the development of new methods for analgesia and the availability of compact digital imaging units, many significantly displaced and angulated children's fractures can now be treated in ERs, clinics, and office-based treatment centers. This has reduced the number of reductions performed in the OR, freeing those rooms for more severe cases.

This chapter will clarify how our hospital has developed and applied these new methods in a county of 3 million people and an emergency setting in which 4,000 new children's fractures are evaluated and treated annually. Key elements in this evolution include:

- A progressive orthopedic surgery group interested in safe, cost-effective fracture care that avoids OR use and hospitalization.
- In busier programs: residents, nurse practitioners (NP), and physician assistants (PA), trained in fracture care.

> *"Those who do not feel pain, seldom think that it is felt"*
> —DR. JOHNSON

- Internet digital transfer of images.
- Advanced Life Support (ALS) and Pediatric Advanced Life Support (PALS) certified doctors, nurses, and medical personnel—full-time ER medical staff.
- Development of safe, effective, conscious sedation anesthesia techniques (Fig. 4-1).
- Compact portable, low radiation, digital image intensifying machines to monitor reduction.
- Certified orthopedic technicians.

The combination of these factors has revolutionized fracture care efficiency in children.

Current Trends

Today, most children's fractures can be safely reduced in the ER ranging from forearm fractures to femur fractures. Initially, the treating orthopedic surgeon had the sole responsibility for analgesia, reduction, and casting. With newer methods, most ERs can provide an environment that allows a systematic "team approach" for fracture reduction. Conscious sedation can be administered, a nurse can monitor the patient, and a portable image intensifier allows one to monitor fracture reduction (Fig. 4-2).

Fracture Care Involving Orthopedic Residents in Training

In centers with resident training programs, the new methods have allowed residents to provide efficient fracture care, decreasing the need for staff orthopedic surgeons to be present for every reduction. Traditionally, most North American centers required a staff orthopedic surgeon to be present for all reductions performed in the OR. The presence of supervising, attending ER physicians (who provide overall supervision for the case) now allows resident fracture reduction in the ER with the on-call staff orthopedic surgeon in attendance only for problem cases.

"With the development of new methods for analgesia and the availability of compact digital imaging units, most significantly displaced and angulated children's fractures can now be treated in ERs, clinics, and office-based treatment centers"

ER or ED

Common emergency rooms have grown in size and complexity, they have often become departments. As such, they often ask that they be known as the "ED" (emergency department). Yet the common medical culture maintains "ER" (witness the popular television show). We try to use the language most commonly used in this text (which in our case is ER)

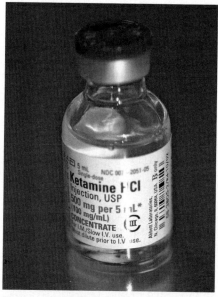

Figure 4-1. Ketalar (Ketamine) alone has proven to be a very safe agent for conscious sedation in children (see Green et al.—Suggested Readings).

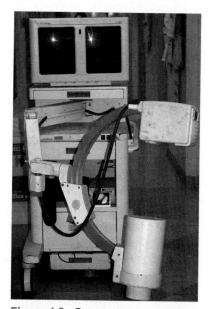

Figure 4-2. Compact image intensifiers allow accurate monitoring of reductions with minimal radiation exposure.

Internet transfer of digital x-ray images allows even more efficient off-site staff supervision of resident, NP, or PA activity.

Nurse Practitioners and Physician Assistants

The development of mid-level providers (NP, PA) in specialty care makes children's fracture care more efficient in centers with the volume to support such a system.

In our center, the orthopedic staff train not only orthopedic residents but also mid-level providers (NP/PA) in fracture management. This has helped us deal with new resident work requirements and with increased patient volume. Proper training and supervision allows mid-level providers to manage children's fractures safely and efficiently.

DEVELOPING A FRACTURE TREATMENT SYSTEM

To treat a high volume of fractures, an efficient system that coordinates care between the ER staff and the orthopedic team should be established. In this section, we will describe the methods that we have developed and use at Children's Hospital-San Diego. These methods can also be applied in a specialized fracture reduction clinic model, if appropriately trained personnel are available to manage conscious sedation (see Suggested Readings—Smith).

Efficient fracture care in a busy children's hospital requires a team that can focus on musculoskeletal problems. In our system, this team consists of an attending surgeon, an orthopedic resident, a mid-level provider (NP or PA), and an orthopedic technician.

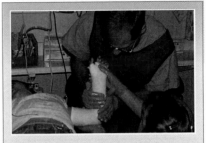

Mid-level Providers: Who Are They?

We use this odd term to describe physician assistants and nurse practitioners who have become experts in children's orthopedic care. Our service trains them as much as residents are trained. After about one year of training in the orthopedic clinics and observing in the ER, they become savvy enough to work in the ER eventually becoming experts in fracture reductions.

Photo courtesy of P. Stearns.

Arrival

Patients arrive to our ER through self-referral, by referral from an outside facility, or from their primary doctor. When a child is sent from an outside facility, a call has usually already been made notifying either the orthopedic team or the ER staff. In some cases, the team may decide, after talking with the referrer, that an expensive emergency visit is not required (Table 4-1).

Simple fractures (or suspected fractures) should be managed with a splint and sent to the outpatient clinic or office within a few days. Of course this is often hard to ascertain by telephone. We note errors weekly. A small puncture wound may not be recognized as an open fracture and a 1 a.m. transfer for a "severe supracondylar fracture" is often just a buckle fracture.

Not all fractures require reduction and not all patients need treatment in the middle of the night. Even in our very busy system, the full team is available only until 11 p.m. Fractures that are only modestly displaced or angulated do not require reduction at a very late hour. Such cases can be splinted by your ER staff and brought back for formal reduction in a few days.

This is sometimes difficult to implement because parents are anxious and concerned about their child's injured extremity. Although most parents want an immediate reduction, in almost every type of fracture, there is no scientific evidence that immediate reduction provides a better result (see insert about John Royal Moore in Philadelphia).

Once a patient has been accepted for treatment, both the orthopedic team and the ER staff should be notified so that triage can be started immediately on arrival. This ensures prompt treatment and limits unnecessary waiting time in an already busy ER.

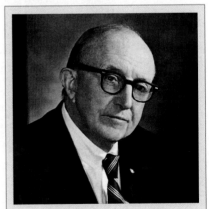

John Royal Moore

Moore, a prominent orthopedic surgeon from Philadelphia, created and implemented an effective fracture reduction clinic that met only once a week (every Tuesday). His method proved to be safe and effective and its principles are still used today. Splinting of small fractures with reduction (if needed) in 3 to 5 days allows swelling to subside, making casting safer.

Nurse Triage

On arrival, the emergency department triage nurse can assess the child and usually order the appropriate x-rays (sometimes after brief consultation with the ER staff or an orthopedic team member).

ER Physician Assessment

Because the child has entered the ER, most systems mandate that each child be briefly evaluated by the ER physician. The ER physician ensures that there is no underlying systemic injury and evaluates injury circumstances, social dynamics, and the child's overall health.

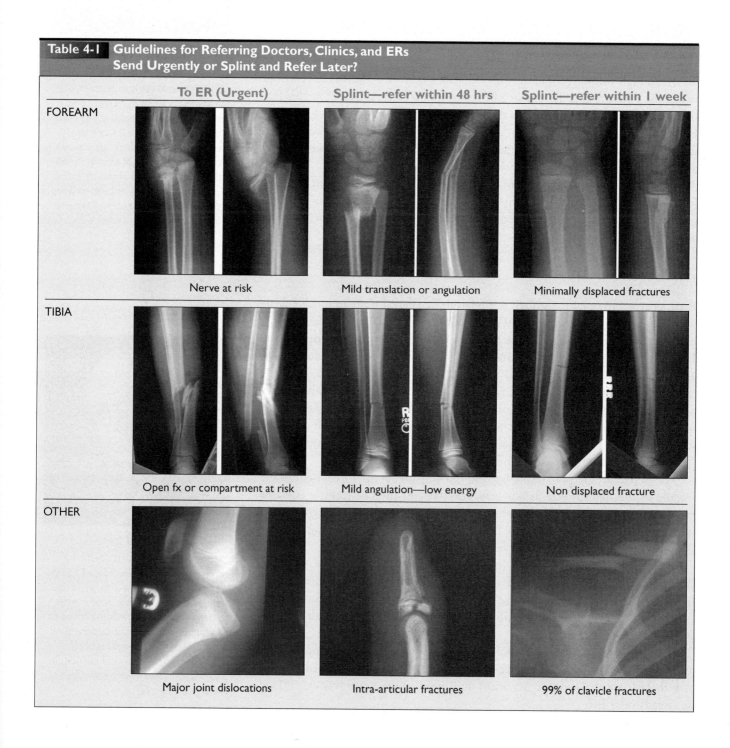

Table 4-1	Guidelines for Referring Doctors, Clinics, and ERs Send Urgently or Splint and Refer Later?		
	To ER (Urgent)	**Splint—refer within 48 hrs**	**Splint—refer within 1 week**
FOREARM	Nerve at risk	Mild translation or angulation	Minimally displaced fractures
TIBIA	Open fx or compartment at risk	Mild angulation—low energy	Non displaced fracture
OTHER	Major joint dislocations	Intra-articular fractures	99% of clavicle fractures

TECHNIQUE TIPS:
Pathway—Children's Fractures in the ER

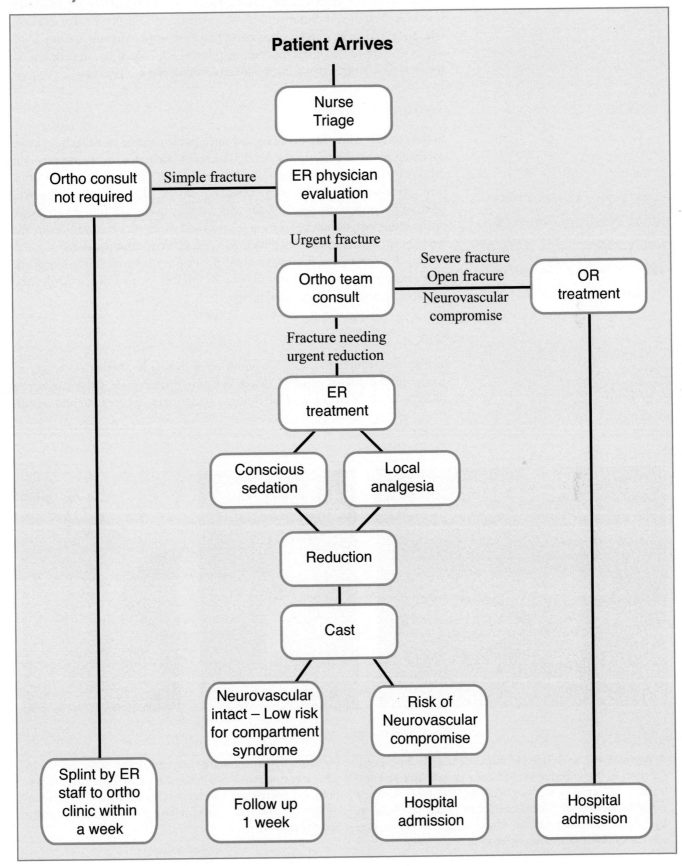

Orthopedic Assessment

With the patient now under orthopedic care, a history and physical are performed with special focus on issues such as neurovascular compromise and whether the fracture is open. A neurovascular assessment can be difficult in a young child who is in pain. You should document only that which is documentable. For example, in a 2-year-old child with no ulnar nerve function post-reduction, it is important not to have stated that it was functioning prior to reduction if you were uncertain; better to have written that accurate documentation was not possible.

Treatment Strategy

In busy centers where the attending surgeon and the resident are often busy in the operating room, the role of the NP/PA becomes important. In our hospital, the NP/PA is trained to reduce/treat children in the ER with straightforward problems, after discussing the case with the resident or staff. On a busy day, films can be taken to the orthopedic resident/staff who are busy in the OR (often transported by the orthopedic technician) for a quick read and advice on treatment (Splint and send home? Reduce in ER? Requires OR?—See technique tips pathway).

The treatment plan is implemented. All care is under the direction of the staff surgeon who is on call and may be in the ER, in the OR, or off-site and available by phone and/or e-mail image.

Fracture Reduction

In planning reduction, fracture location helps to decide whether conscious sedation in the ER is required. Most forearm fractures are good candidates whereas femur fractures in older children (older than age 5 or so) and signifi-

> *"One must recognize that not all 8 year olds have the same temperament; different children react differently to the same type of fracture"*

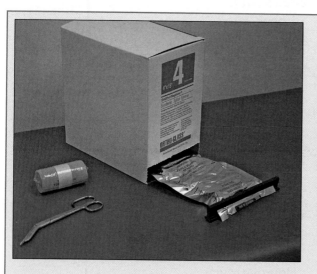 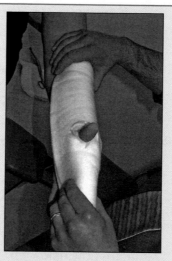 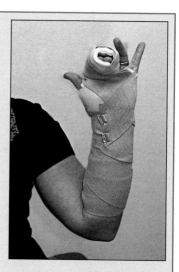

Splinting Fractures

A key element to a sensible musculoskeletal urgent care program is the widespread availability of safe and practical fracture splinting by outlying facilities. The more recently available fiberglass-felt-foam composite splints (available on bulk rolls) combined with an elastic wrap roll allows easy application for the trained orthopedist; ERs seem to do it well also. Training primary care doctors to splint safely is a great investment toward rational fracture care. Training sessions for referring practitioners provide a great community service that will save time, money, and frustration for you and the patient.

Table 4-2	Reduction in ER vs OR	
Good Candidates—ER Reduction	**OR Reduction Preferable**	
Wrist fractures	Complex tibia fractures (older child)	
Forearm fractures	Femur fractures (older child)	
Hand/foot fractures	Open fractures	
Infant femur fractures	Fractures with neurovascular compromise	

Table 4-3	Should Parents Be Present for Orthopedic Reductions? (In our center we ask the family to leave—Some of our reasons are listed below)
Grotesque maneuver required to lock fracture ends	
Audible noises (crunching of bone ends)	
Seemingly aggressive face or noises (suggests an "assault")	
Risk of fainting (parents)	
A tough reduction is like an operation (parents should not attend either)	
Focus on reduction better with no outside "audience"	

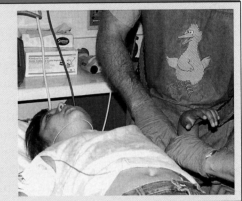

cantly angulated tibial fractures are often best treated in the OR with general anesthesia (Table 4-2). One must recognize that not all 8 year olds have the same temperament; different children react differently to the same type of fracture. Therefore, the decision about anesthesia methods should be adjusted according to the child's temperament and family dynamics.

Also, parental anxiety may determine where the fracture should be reduced (Table 4-3). We ask the parents to go to the waiting room while the actual reduction takes place (to avoid their exposure to the sounds and apparent aggression required to reduce a stubborn fracture). A few insist on staying; in such cases, OR reduction may be better and the treating surgeon should offer this option. We believe that the person who performs the actual manipulation deserves the degree of privacy that allows optimal performance. The patient's result may depend on this.

"We believe that the person who performs the actual manipulation deserves the degree of privacy which allows optimal performance"

ANALGESIA FOR REDUCTION

No Anesthesia

For fractures that require minimal manipulation, some children can tolerate casting and molding without anesthesia. The child and parent need to understand and be willing to accept that there will be mild pain with this technique. Often the child will agree and select this option once understood that formal analgesia requires needle sticks. After successful completion of this artful maneuver, the child is praised for cooperation in achieving good fracture position with no needles.

"Every treating orthopedist should develop local anesthesia skills and use them whenever possible"

Oral Medication

A second option for fractures that require minimal manipulation can include the combination of acetaminophen (Tylenol) with codeine (0.5-1 mg/kg) and oral midazolam (Versed) (0.3 mg/kg). This choice is sometimes selected for an anxious patient that in other circumstances would be casted without analgesia. The cast is placed with no preliminary manipulation and with the "gentle reduction force" applied as the cast sets.

Local Anesthesia

Despite the methods that we will describe in this chapter for conscious sedation, every treating orthopedist should develop local anesthesia skills and use them whenever possible. This is even more important because some centers apply very strict regulations regarding nothing by mouth (NPO) status (child must have empty stomach) before conscious sedation can be given. In many cases, deft local anesthesia skills will save you and your patient many hours and much frustration.

The most common local anesthetic method for fracture reduction is a hematoma block with 1% lidocaine (no epinephrine) solution directly injected into the hematoma at the fracture site (Table 4-4). The maximum recommended dose for lidocaine without epinephrine is 4.5 mg/kg (300 mg maximum). Withdrawing blood into the syringe, the so-called blood flash, indicates correct needle tip position and the lidocaine is then injected. Ideally, one should wait several minutes prior to fracture reduction to allow more effective analgesia.

Hematoma blocks can be used for many fractures and can be performed without the assistance of the ER staff (freeing them for more critical patients). These blocks work well for forearm fractures (especially in the distal 1/3 area) but are generally not used for larger bones such as the femur or humerus. Also, issues of maximum dosage come in to play (risk for seizures) if one attempts to use a hematoma block for a large bone fracture.

Lidocaine can also be used for digital nerve blocks, allowing one to reduce various fractures of the hand (metacarpal, phalanges, nail bed injuries, lacerations, MCP/IP dislocations) and foot (phalanges) (Table 4-5). One can block each nerve bundle separately or use a single midline injection (in line with the tendon sheath) that disperses and blocks both digital nerves.

Table 4-4	Reduction with Hematoma Block			
Preparation	**Superficial Block**	**Blood Flash**	**Reduction**	**Casting**
Prep with alcohol and povidone-iodine	Using 25-gauge needle, numb the skin around the fracture	Using 18-gauge needle, inject at fracture site (4-6 cc of 1% lidocaine)	Wait a few minutes and perform reduction	Apply well-molded cast

Table 4-5 Digital Block (Flexor Tendon Sheath)

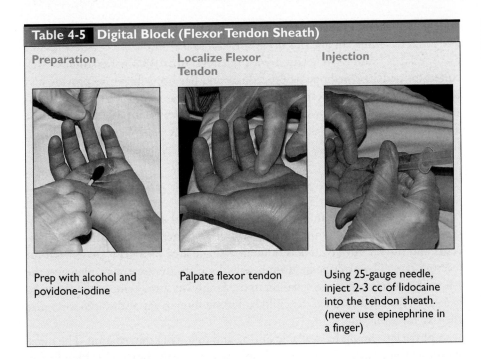

Preparation	Localize Flexor Tendon	Injection
Prep with alcohol and povidone-iodine	Palpate flexor tendon	Using 25-gauge needle, inject 2-3 cc of lidocaine into the tendon sheath. (never use epinephrine in a finger)

Regional Anesthesia

Intravenous lidocaine block (Bier block) can be very effective for reducing upper extremity fractures but requires special tourniquets and attention to detail. The Bier block, a technique of IV regional anesthesia originally described by August Bier in 1908, can be performed in an ER setting, office, or clinic, thereby avoiding the OR. The arm is elevated to exsanguinate it, a tourniquet is inflated, and dilute lidocaine is injected into a superficial hand vein. We rarely use this method in our hospital (due to custom) but others have found it to be highly effective in children.

Conscious Sedation

This method has revolutionized fracture care in emergency departments and specialized fracture reduction centers (Table 4-6). Ketamine (Ketalar), the most

Table 4-6 Medications Commonly Used for Sedation

Medication	Recommended Initial Dose/Max Dose	Side Effects	Contraindications Precautions
Ketamine (Ketalar)	1-2 mg/kg	Hypertension, hypotension, respiratory depression, laryngospasm, hallucinations	Increased intracranial pressure (ICP), seizures hypotension, CHF
Sublimaze (oral) (Fentanyl)	10-15 mcg/kg/dose max 400 mcg/dose	Respiratory depression, hypotension	Chronic pulmonary disease (CPD), head injury/increased ICP cardiac disease
Sublimaze (IV) (Fentanyl)	1-2 mcg/kg/dose q 30-60 minutes prn	Respiratory depression, hypotension	CPD, head injury/increased ICP cardiac disease
Morphine sulfate	0.1-0.2 mg/kg/dose q 2-4 hrs prn	Central nervous system (CNS) and respiratory depression, hypotension, increased ICP, nausea/vomiting	Upper airway obstruction, acute bronchial asthma, CPD, increased ICP
Midazolam (Versed)	0.05-0.1mg/kg over 2 minutes max total dose 0.2 mg/kg	Respiratory depression, hypotension, bradycardia	Existing CNS depression, glaucoma, shock

widely used agent, induces a state of catalepsy that provides sedation, analgesia, and amnesia. Interestingly, this drug is used illegally on the street and is known as "Special K" due to its relation with phencyclidine (PCP). Ketamine is well suited for pediatric orthopedic procedures and has been shown to provide better sedation with fewer respiratory complications [as compared to other commonly used agents such as sublimaze (Fentanyl)] because it preserves protective airway reflexes (Green et al.). Ketamine can be safely given between 1-2 mg/kg intravenously; the 2 mg/kg dose is favored by most centers.

Administration and Monitoring Sequence

Once the orthopedic team has determined the child should have conscious sedation, the process is then coordinated with the emergency department physicians and nurses. Ideally, this is done in a single area of the ER designated for fracture care. The orthopedic team briefly discusses the treatment plan and the ER staff explains conscious sedation to the family. In some centers, the analgesia is delayed for a few hours if the child had something to eat or drink to minimize the risk for aspiration.

A physician should be available during and following the sedation. The nurse monitors the patient. Ideally, the child's mental status, heart rate, blood pressure, respiratory rate, and oxygen saturation are monitored before, during, and after procedural sedation. Clearly, this ideal model of comprehensive monitoring is not be available in all parts of the world.

TECHNIQUE TIPS:
Patient Safety and Pediatric Conscious Sedation

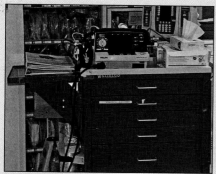

Emergency cart—Must be present in case of cardiac abnormalities induced by medication

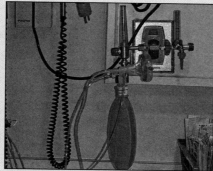

Oxygen and suction set-up present at bedside in case of respiratory emergency

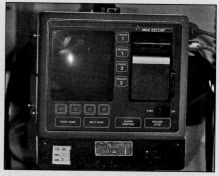

Monitor vital signs during sedation

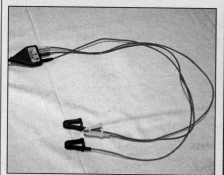

Leads to monitor ECG, heart rate, respiratory rate

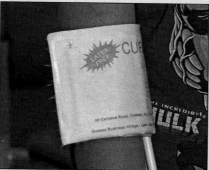

Blood pressure monitoring

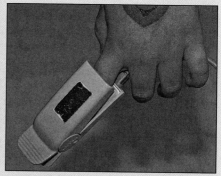

Oxygen saturation used to monitor patient oxygen levels

MANIPULATIVE REDUCTION

Once ready for reduction, the compact image intensifier is positioned and set up appropriately. The injury x-rays should be placed on a view box in the line of sight of the reducer to allow better visualization and pre-planning for the three-point reduction maneuver (we have seen fractures molded in "reverse" when this step is skipped!). The casting materials should be within reach.

The reduction maneuver is then performed. Alignment is assessed by imaging in both the AP and lateral plane, and if adequate reduction has been achieved, a carefully molded cast is applied.

Cast Application

A cast molded according to the fracture pattern maintains alignment and prevents loss of reduction.

Prior to the cast setting, alignment should again be assessed with the fluoroscan to ensure adequate reduction and molding. The finishing touches can then be applied to the cast. Finally the cast is "split" (univalved) to provide room for swelling (Fig. 4-3) (see Chapter 5). Finally, post-reduction, traditional x-rays are usually obtained to confirm alignment and to use as a comparison at the first clinic follow-up visit. This step is important because the compact image intensifier provides only a very focal view of the fracture.

Post-Reduction Events

Following reduction, another neurovascular assessment should be performed (when the child is alert) with any changes in status addressed and documented. Not every child should be sent home after closed reduction. For example, a child with a significant tibia fracture may need to be admitted overnight for observation to ensure that a compartment syndrome does not develop.

The parents are advised that the cast has been univalved (split) to allow for swelling. They should expect swelling within the next 24-48 hours and are advised to keep the limb elevated. We provide a typed instruction sheet outlining the diagnosis and treatment to the family. This sheet describes worrisome signs and symptoms and a contact number if there are problems. We also provide a

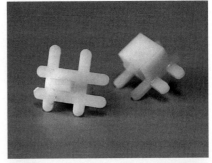

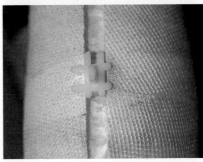

Figure 4-3. Multi-width, commercially available spacers used to hold the cast open once it has been univalved. This is especially important for synthetic material casts, which tend to spring closed after univalving and opening the cast.

Table 4-7 Reduction Under Conscious Sedation				
IV/Meds Given	**Reduction**	**Image View**	**Well-Molded Cast**	**Univalve**
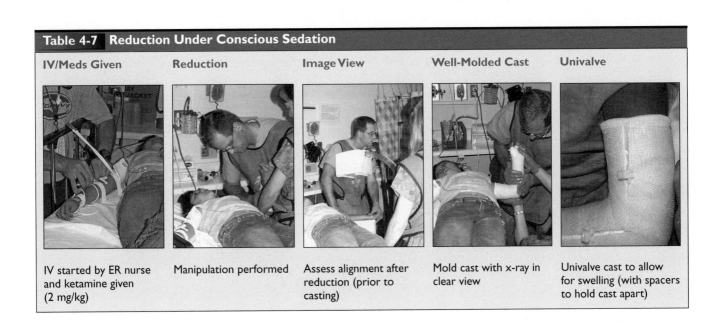				
IV started by ER nurse and ketamine given (2 mg/kg)	Manipulation performed	Assess alignment after reduction (prior to casting)	Mold cast with x-ray in clear view	Univalve cast to allow for swelling (with spacers to hold cast apart)

separate instruction sheet outlining the details of cast care. A prescription for oral pain medication is provided, usually a 3-day course of acetaminophen with codeine elixir for smaller children or tablets for older children.

Follow-up Protocol

Most patients are seen for a follow-up appointment within a week and typically fractures requiring manipulation are evaluated every week for 2-3 weeks. This allows early detection of reduction loss that can sometimes be salvaged by cast wedging.

SUMMARY

Modern ER manipulative reduction of children's fractures using conscious sedation has been a major orthopedic advance. Performed in an organized fashion, the method is safe, efficient, and economic and saves hospital beds for more severe cases. Furthermore, most children prefer to sleep in their own homes and in their own beds!

"Modern ER manipulative reduction of children's fractures using conscious sedation has been a major orthopedic advance"

Suggested Readings

American College of Emergency Physicians: Clinical policy for procedural sedation and analgesia in the emergency department. Ann Emerg Med 31:663-667, 1998.

Bell HM, Slater M, Harris WH. Regional anesthesia with intravenous lidocaine. JAMA 1963:186:544-9.

Bolte RG, Stevens PM, Scott SM, Schunk JE. Mini-dose Bier block intravenous regional anesthesia in the emergency department treatment of pediatric upper-extremity injuries. J Pediatr Orthop, 1994 Jul-Aug;14(4)534-7.

Furia Jp, Alioto RJ, Marquardt JD. The efficacy and safety of the hematoma block for fracture reduction in closed, isolated fractures. Orthopedics, 1997 May;20(5):423-6.

Green S, Nakamura R, Johnson N. Ketamine sedation for pediatric procedures: Part I, a prospective series. Ann Emerg Med 19:1025-1032, 1990.

Green S, Nakamura R, Johnson N. Ketamine sedation for pediatric procedures: Part II, review and implications. Ann Emerg Med 19:1033-1046, 1990.

Holmes C. Intravenous regional anesthesia: useful method of producing analgesia of the limbs. Lancet, 1963;1:245-7.

Jordan R, Rodriquez E. Contemporary trends in pediatric sedation and analgesia. Emergency medicine clinics of North America v20, #1. Feb 2002.

Smith J, Gollogly S, Clark N. Assuming the burden of pediatric fracture care in a children's medical center . . . Efficiently! A model for a pediatric fracture clinic. COMSS poster No. P489 - POSNA.

5

Casts for Children's Fractures

Dennis Wenger ❧ *Mercer Rang*

Predictable application and maintenance of complication-free casts in children is a slowly learned art and craft. In contrast to adult patients, in whom immobilization may produce osteopenia and joint stiffness, children rarely suffer long-term effects from typical periods of cast immobilization. Instead, children have a special set of complications, including poor application, poor fit, and loose casts that slide off. Physicians often fail to understand the effect that the carefree personality of a child has on the life, durability, and function of a cast. Also, children often do not complain if a cast is tight or produces ulceration with the damage noted only when the cast is removed.

This chapter is intended to present general principles for safe, predictable cast application for fractures in children and to demonstrate the many

"Show me your cast and I'll tell you what kind of orthopedist you are"
—CALOT

53

techniques we have developed at Children's Hospital—San Diego to make the use of synthetic cast materials safe and preditable.

HISTORY

Immobilization for fracture treatment can be traced to antiquity. Traditional methods included use of (a) muslin reinforced with egg whites or starches and (b) soft wood splints. Plaster of Paris was first used in the late 18th century by the Turks to immobilize limb fractures. The limb was placed in a box that was then filled with plaster—an awkward, bulky process.

Military surgeons were the first to push for less cumbersome methods of fracture immobilization with Mathijsen credited with the first use of plaster of Paris dressings in 1852. In his process, the plaster of Paris was applied to muslin

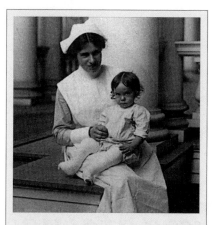

Casting in Children's Orthopaedics. This lovely photograph, taken in front of the Hospital for Sick Children (Toronto) in about 1915, demonstrates a child in corrective casts for clubfoot, attended to by her nurse. (Reproduced courtesy of Mercer Rang.)

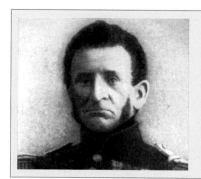

Anthonius Mathijsen

Anthonius Mathijsen (1805-1878), a Flemish army surgeon, was the first to use plaster of Paris impregnated in rolls of linen cloth that could be rolled onto the limb. In his first publication in 1852 he noted that his special bandages hardened rapidly, provided an exact fit to maintain reduction, and could be easily windowed or bivalved.

Casting Materials Timeline

From the beginning of time, sticks and mud and cloth have been used to stop fractures from moving about. We have knowledge only of recent events.

400 BCE	Hippocrates describes splints.
970 CE	In Persia, Muwaffak advises coating fractures with plaster.
1740	As a child Cheselden (Britain) has a fracture treated by a bonesetter with bandages dipped in egg white and starch. When Cheselden becomes a surgeon, he introduces the method for his patients. The bandages take a day to harden.
1799	A visiting diplomat reports that he saw a Turkish patient treated by holding the injured limb in a box that was then filled with plaster. He tried to interest European doctors in the method. The cast was big and heavy and prevented ambulation.
1814	Pieter Hendricks uses plaster bandages—but the idea does not catch on.
1824	Dominique Larrey, Napoleon's surgeon, uses egg white and lead powder.
1835	Louis Seutin: Starch bandages.
1852	Anthonius Mathijsen introduces plaster bandages in a medical book and has a friend who popularizes it. Soon, large numbers of people are putting plaster into bandages. Until the 1950s, it was a job for medical students on emergency call. Then machines led to commercial manufacture.
1903	Hoffa's belief that "the plaster bandage will remain the essence of orthopedics for all time" seems to be going the way of all predictions.
1970 to present	Development and widespread use of synthetic materials for casts.

Plaster did not enjoy universal popularity. Complete casts on fresh fractures can produce dreadful complications, and this led some influential leaders to ban casts. Thomas and Jones in Britain and Knight, founder of the first residency program in the United States, would have nothing to do with plaster. Knight fired one member of his staff for promoting its use.

Courtesy of Mercer Rang

or linen so that the resulting plaster dressing could be rolled onto the limb. This tedious process of rubbing the plaster into the muslin or linen was done manually, just prior to application, by the surgeon or his assistant and continued until about 50 years ago. Ready-to-use manufactured rolls of plaster of Paris were not commonly available until the mid-20th century.

Material Choices

Plaster of Paris has clearly been the standard material for cast construction over the last 150 years. Recently, synthetic materials have evolved to the point of being practical and safe for cast immobilization of fractures. Exponential improvement in the texture, "rollability," and "moldability" of synthetics has made them the cast material of choice for most modern orthopedic surgeons. Patients like them because they are lightweight and durable. We now use synthetics for all pediatric orthopedic casts, except for serial corrective foot casts used to treat clubfoot (Ponseti casts). However, some orthopedists still prefer the moldability of traditional plaster for reducing and maintaining acute fractures.

Synthetic cast materials are more expensive than plaster of Paris; however, in assessing overall cost one must consider the costs in time, labor, materials, and repetitive visits to cast rooms by children who have inadvertently soaked or damaged a plaster cast.

> ### Plaster of Paris
> *Plaster of Paris was named for the large gypsum deposit in the Paris basin. Gypsum is pulverized and heated to drive off the water to form anhydrous calcium sulfate. When water is added, the reaction reverses.*

Duration of Treatment

The issue of when and for how long cast immobilization should be used for fracture treatment has been historically controversial. Hugh Owen Thomas (prolonged immobilization) and Lucas-Championniére (early motion) developed diametrically opposing views in the late 19th century (see Chapter 2). The controversy remains but less for children's fractures.

GENERAL PRINCIPLES OF CAST APPLICATION

A great variety of cast types are used in children (body jackets, hip spicas, extremity fracture casts), and we will not attempt to describe them all. Instead, the focus will be on general principles of cast immobilization of extremity fractures, including hip spica casts (Figs. 5-1, 5-2).

Basic principles should be considered. For small children, you must decide who can best hold the child's arm or leg while the cast is applied. Although parents can assist, most casts are better applied with a trained assistant holding the

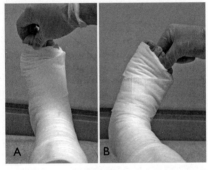

Figure 5-2. Toe holding for leg casts. A) If the foot holder holds the first and second toe, the foot will drift into undesired varus. B) Holding the third and fourth toe with the foot held in dorsiflexion ensures that the foot will end up in a desirable position of slight dorsiflexion, valgus, and eversion.

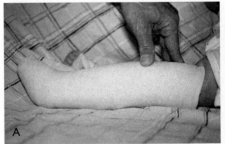
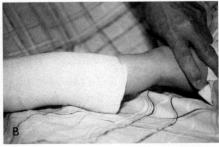
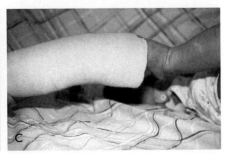

Figure 5-1. A) A poorly molded long leg cast in a young child. Note that the foot is left in equinus, which makes sliding off more likely. Also the heel is poorly molded. B) The cast was easily "slid" off in the clinic. C) The cast was entirely removed without splitting. These photographs illustrate the very common practice of applying poorly fitting casts in children. Because of their activity level, children require snug, well-molded casts.

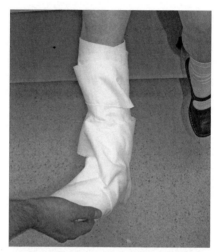

Figure 5-3. Excessive padding, often applied to prevent ulcerations, may actually increase the chance for skin irritation. Any advantage gained by excessive padding is usually lost because it leads to a loose, poorly fitting cast. The result is a cast that allows excessive movement of the limb (with potential for skin ulceration) or, in severe cases, one that slides off the limb.

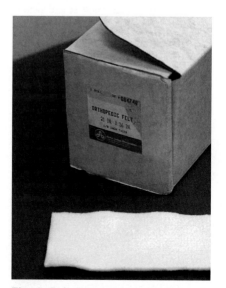

Figure 5-4. Felt at the junction (when the cast is applied in two parts) makes the transition safer. Felt at the end of the cast (proximal) makes it more comfortable.

limb. Special foot-holding stands designed to keep the ankle at a neutral position are useful for adolescents but are of little help in a young child.

Several steps increase your chances for a well-fitting cast. Whether or not stockinette should be used on the skin prior to soft-roll application (Fig. 5-3) depends on where and for what reason the cast is being applied. For elective casts applied in an office or an outpatient clinic, use of stockinette decreases "bunching" of soft-roll, allows a neat-appearing cast, stops the rough edge of the cast from abrading the skin, and makes cast removal easier and perhaps safer (less chance for cast-saw cuts or burns).

In postoperative casts applied in the operating room, the presence of surgical dressings, suction drains, percutaneous pins, etc., makes stockinette use difficult. Also, with difficult manipulative reductions performed in the office or clinic, application of stockinette is often an added step that impedes efficient, rapid application and molding of the cast.

Other cast application accessories include using a layer of felt proximally in the thigh, arm (humerus), or proximal calf. A 2- or 3-inch-wide band of felt padding provides comfort and decreases skin irritation (Fig. 5-4). In spica casts for thin children, we often use both (a) a complete layer of felt and (b) adhesive-backed foam padding for bony prominences (iliac crest, greater trochanter, and sacrum).

We advise that almost all casts applied in the operating room be immediately split or univalved while the child is still anesthetized to decrease the discomfort, aggravation, and fright involved in late-night cast splitting in the patient's room. This is particularly important in a children's hospital, where multiple-patient rooms are common and where not only the patient and family but also other patients and parents are present.

Rolling the Cast

Efficient rolling of the plaster or synthetic material requires experience. Appropriate rolling technique, including the placement of tucks to allow smooth wrapping over a conical structure, is a slowly learned art. This is most important for plaster casts in which the material will not stretch. Orthopedic residents need instruction in this art, followed by supervised practice. Often their opportunities for learning are blunted by the current trend toward having orthopedic technicians apply most casts in many training hospitals. The sad tradition of lumpy, formless, inefficient casts applied at "Elsewhere General" continues, applied by inadequately trained surgeons or technicians.

Great care must be taken to avoid making casts too tight. This is a particular problem with synthetic-material casts: They are often wrapped in the same manner that one applies an elastic (Ace) bandage, with stretching to accommodate limb shape change rather than placing tucks. This is possible because the underlying "cloth" is stretchable (in contrast to the muslin in plaster of Paris). The result is a cast that is often too tight, particularly when applied in the operating room following surgery. In circumstances where any swelling whatsoever is anticipated, synthetic cast materials should be applied with tucks, just as would be done with ordinary plaster. This makes a less restrictive cast.

Casts in the operating room should be applied after the tourniquet has been deflated to normalize limb volume. The cast is then applied, using the tuck technique. Then in most cases, the cast should be immediately split to allow further swelling, with the cast retightened 3-7 days later.

Cast Molding

Proper cast molding ensures good cast fit, thereby decreasing the chance for cast sores (Fig. 5-5). A cast should fit the limb contours and be thought of in the sculpting sense; that is, if the cast were removed and filled with plaster or wax, the result would be a casting identical to the patient's limb. Careful molding around bony prominences is required to achieve excellent fit. The calcaneus is at great risk in the lower extremities; the molding must be focused on the soft tissues above the tip of the calcaneus, leaving a recess for the heel prominence.

The concept of a well-molded cast contrasts with the terminology of applying a "plaster dressing" after surgery. Many surgeons prefer a bulky "Robert Jones" dressing after surgery, followed by application of a well-molded cast once the swelling has subsided. We rarely do this in children because we can achieve the same effect by splitting and spreading the cast immediately postoperatively, with later tightening. This avoids postoperative cast changes, which children detest.

Cast Ergonomics

Cast edge trimming is time-consuming, but it can be avoided by careful planning when the cast material is rolled. For instance, at the distal end of a leg cast,

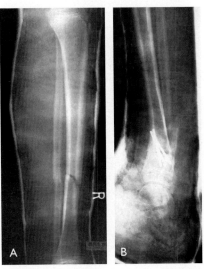

Figure 5-5. A) Example of a thin, well-molded cast applied to maintain reduction in a tibial fracture. The best casts have very little padding; skin irritation is avoided by careful contouring and molding. B) An extremely poorly molded cast. The posterior border is relatively straight, predisposing to heel ulceration. Failure to use a posterior splint has caused the anterior plaster to be nearly an inch thick. This makes cast removal difficult and dangerous. Plaster rolled around a right angle requires asymmetric application to have symmetrical thickness.

The Disappearing Toe Syndrome

The call is classic in children's orthopedics—"My child's toes are disappearing." Disappearing toes mean the poorly fitted cast is allowing the foot to pull up the cast. A skin ulcer will soon follow. In this case, there was an ulcer on the heel and on the dorsum of the foot.

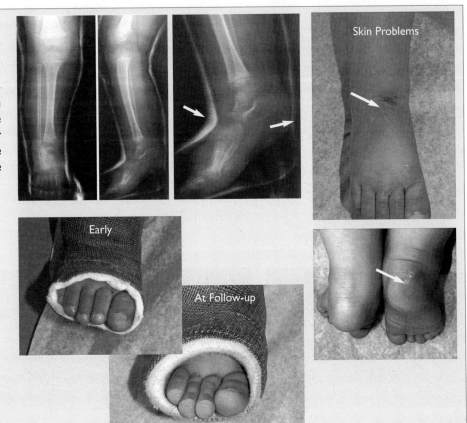

the plaster should be rolled at a 30° angle, keeping the lateral side short so that subsequent trimming in the area of the fifth metatarsal head is not required. I perhaps exaggerate by stating that no cast should ever end completely transversely. Whether in the foot, the popliteal fossa, the groin, or the proximal humeral area, casts predictably immobilize better, require less trimming, and fit better if they end obliquely. Learning to wrap casts with oblique ends greatly decreases the labor required to trim and finalize the cast. By avoiding trimming, few sharp edges remain (a particular problem with synthetics).

CAST SPLITTING (BIVALVE, UNIVALVE)

Traditional training suggested that any cast requiring splitting be split completely to the skin, including the soft-roll. We have no argument with the "always split to the skin" philosophy for hospitals with little supervision of patients casted following fracture reduction or operations. An edict issued by the "commanding officer" to split all casts to the skin is likely the best insurance against cast complications, compartment syndromes, etc., in these circumstances. Also, some orthopedists prefer a bivalve (double) split in all casts. With the use of spacers to maintain the separation, we have been able to use single splits in most cases—including synthetic casts (Fig. 5-6).

Although some insist on "always split to the skin" or "always bivalve," we advise a more refined approach for a private hospital or office or in a high-quality teaching hospital that provides close patient monitoring. This can be safe, economical, and, most importantly, less distressing to children.

Synthetic-material casts require special methods because even though the cast is split longitudinally (univalved), the resilience of the material will not allow the cast to stay separated. Special commercially available spacers are needed.

Graded splitting of casts following fracture reduction or orthopedic operations requires good orthopedic judgment. Limited splitting can provide great economic advantage to the hospital and surgeon without placing the patient at increased risk. Our policy of graded splitting according to risk is as follows:

Level 1. Only modest swelling anticipated (e.g., following simple limb surgery or reduction of simple distal radius fracture). Level 1 splitting includes a single longitudinal split in the cast, combined with spreading and placing a spacer but without cutting the underlying soft-roll. In our children's hospital environment, 95% of cast splits are level 1. This percentage must be interpreted within the context that we split nearly all postoperative casts and most fracture reduction casts. Note that synthetic cast splits will not remain open unless spacers are placed. Several manufacturers produce small plastic spacers of varying sizes that are inserted to keep the cast separated. These are removed in 4-7 days after swelling has subsided, with the cast then tightened with tape (upper limb) or another roll of cast material (lower limb).

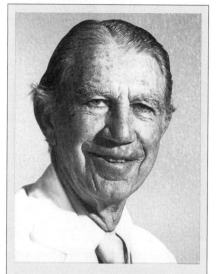

Brandon Carrell

Brandon Carrell 1910–1982. Chief of Staff at the Texas Scottish Rite Hospital, Dallas from 1945–1977. He emphasized the need for care in removing casts in children and was a strong advocate of splitting (univalve or bivalve) casts applied in the operating room.

"Although some insist on 'always split to the skin' or 'always bivalve,' we advise a more refined approach..."

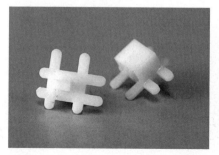
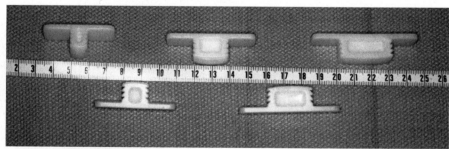

Figure 5-6. Spacers. A) Small commercially available spacers used for upper-extremity casts and for minimal spreading in lower-extremity casts. B) A variety of larger, commercially available spacers useful for leg casts and hip spicas as well as for corrective wedging.

TECHNIQUE TIPS:
Graded Cast Splitting According to Risk Severity

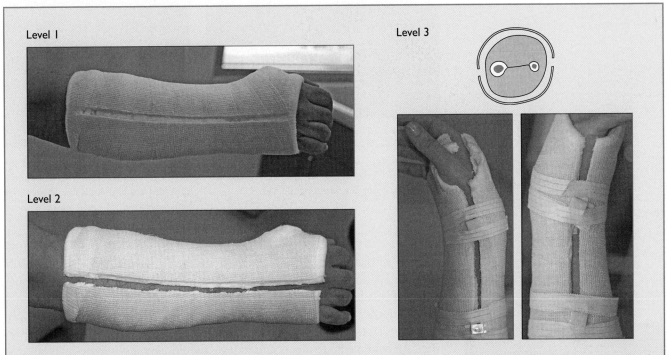

Level 1

Level 2

Level 3

Level 1. Cast split dorsally; soft-roll and underlying dressings not disturbed. For routine postoperative cases and simple fractures. A spacer must be placed to hold the cast open.

Level 2. Both cast material and underlying soft-roll split to skin. For more serious cases of swelling.

Level 3. Cast split medially and laterally, with soft-roll cut down to skin. Allows removal of entire anterior half of cast for inspection of skin and for palpation of compartments.

Level 2. For children with significant swelling anticipated (e.g., fracture with potential for vascular problems; postoperative triple arthrodesis; other similar cases). The single longitudinal split includes both the cast material and the underlying soft-roll down to the skin, allowing wide spreading of the cast. Once the soft-roll has been split, window edema can develop; therefore, thin strips of soft-roll should be packed longitudinally into the split and should be overwrapped with a gauze bandage. A cast with a level 2 split can still be repaired (pulled together) once swelling has subsided, although care must be taken to avoid "bunching" of the soft-roll (we rarely perform a level 2 split—most are level 1, a few level 3).

Level 3. Used for cases with marked swelling anticipated (e.g., tibial fracture in which compartment syndrome is suspected). This includes a medial and lateral complete split of both the cast material and the underlying soft-roll down to the skin. The anterior panel of the cast can then be removed for complete inspection of the limb and palpation of the compartments.

CAST REMOVAL

Cast removal problems are an important but under-emphasized topic in pediatric orthopedics. Traditional cast shears can be used for small casts (Fig. 5-7). Current cast-removal saws are loud, aggressive, somewhat dangerous, and terrifying to children. No amount of conversation or playful application of the vibrating cast blade to one's own hand to demonstrate that it "won't cut" will placate a

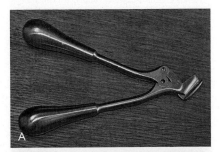

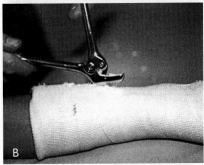

Figure 5-7. A) Stille cast shears. B) Use of Stille cast shears to remove a short arm cast. Developing skill with this instrument allows you to avoid noisy cast saws when removing certain casts. However, they work better for plaster than for synthetic materials.

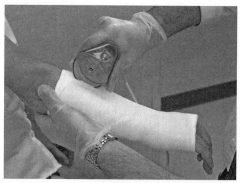

Figure 5-8. Proper technique is required to use a cast saw. Usually, the thumb is held against the cast and the blade itself is pushed in an "up and down" fashion against the cast material without dragging the saw longitudinally.

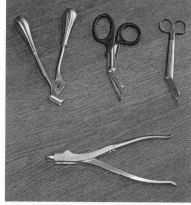

Figure 5-9. Accessories required for facile cast removal. Good scissors and a spreader are key. A plaster shears may allow removal of small casts without using the cast saw.

properly suspicious child. More compact, quiet saws have recently become available but are suitable only for small extremity casts. They are hopelessly outmatched by a hip spica.

Orthopedic technicians and orthopedists who deal with children can apply many special techniques to minimize cast-removal trauma. Empathy is the first step. All orthopedic residents and fellows should have a synthetic-material cast applied on their own limb and then removed by a fellow resident (see how they jump). This greatly increases sensitivity for the child's plight. We do a cast application-removal session with each new group of residents and fellows when they rotate through our hospital.

The correct mechanics of cast-saw use must be mastered. They include placing the thumb and/or fingers on the cast as a stabilizing guide, with careful reciprocal "up and down" movement (Fig. 5-8) rather than long dragging movements of the blade along the cast that increase the risk for skin injury (cut or burn). Avoid using the cast saw over bony prominences (medial malleolus, etc.) and pull the cast away from the skin as you begin the cut.

Many accessory tools aid with separating the cast, cutting the soft-roll, and getting the cast off (Fig. 5-9). Sophisticated plaster shears allow cast removal in children without use of a saw. Those made by Stille (Sweden) are particularly effective for removing clubfoot and other small casts. Orthopedists trained in the modern era are sometimes unaware of these special plaster shears that allow quiet, safe, cast removal.

UPPER EXTREMITY CASTS

Most of the principles that will be presented in the lower extremity section apply here. Application techniques are similar to those used for adults. We routinely use synthetic casts, even following acute fracture reduction. The cast is split immediately, with a spacer placed to hold the cast open until swelling subsides.

Application Principles

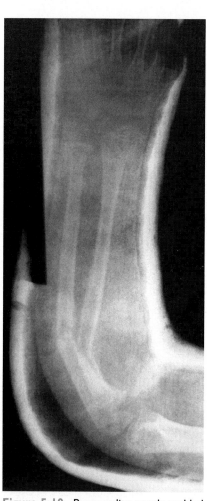

Figure 5-10. Poor-quality, poorly molded long arm cast. Note the space at the tip of the olecranon. Also note the thickness anteriorly in the antecubital fossa area. Reduction has been lost.

Precise three-point forearm molding technique is required both to maintain fracture reduction and to keep the cast from sliding off (Fig. 5-10). If only rolls of plaster are applied, the cast becomes excessively thick anteriorly at the elbow (antecubital area) and too thin over the olecranon. Charnley, in his classic fracture text, noted that if plaster is wrapped uniformly around a right angle, the cast will be four times as thick in the concavity as on the convexity.

Excess soft-roll and plaster in the concavity makes a cast ugly and increases the chance that it will slide off. We avoid this by using splints posteriorly over the olecranon area or by asymmetrically rolling the cast material with a back-and-forth motion over the convexity (olecranon) to minimize thickness anteriorly. Careful molding is then performed in the antecubital area to produce a beveled right angle. A properly applied long arm cast has a geometrically crisp look with (a) a sharp 90° (right) angle anteriorly in the antecubital fossa and (b) a sharp right angle posteriorly produced by a straight border molded along the ulna and humerus (Fig. 5-11). Such a cast is extremely unlikely to slide down or fall off, avoiding the shopping bag cast syndrome (mother brings the cast back in a shopping bag).

Forearm Molding

For reduction of forearm and wrist fractures, you will need to decide if you can apply a long arm (above-elbow) cast in a single phase or whether you will better hold the reduction and mold the cast if it is applied in two stages (first short arm, then extend to above elbow). In most circumstances, the latter is preferred. The junction must be carefully padded to avoid skin injury.

"Show me your plaster and I'll show you what kind of orthopedist you are"

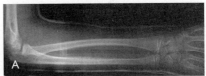
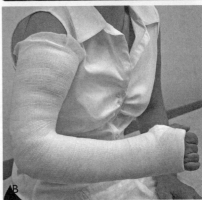

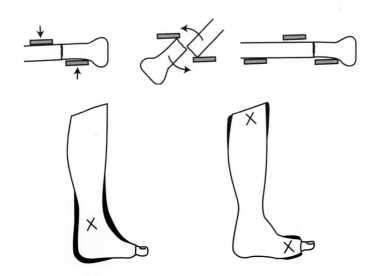

(Source: Charnley J. The closed treatment of common fractures. Edinburgh, Livingstone, 1980. [Figures reproduced with permission])

Figure 5-11. A properly applied long arm cast has a geometrically crisp look. A) The x-ray shows a sharp right angle anteriorly in the antecubital fossa. B) The ulnar border is straight as is the posterior humeral border.

Charnley, in his classic text, emphasized proper casting techniques: three-point molding is used to maintain reduction of fractures, and asymmetric plaster application avoids excess cast thickness in the concavity of joints.

TECHNIQUE TIPS:
Application of a Long Arm Cast to Reduce and Maintain an Unstable Distal Radius Fracture—Two-Stage Technique

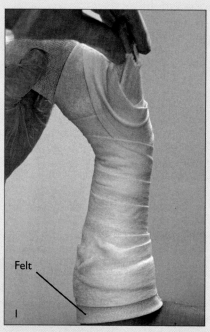

Felt

1

After reduction, padding is applied with the wrist ulnarly deviated and flexed—the circumferential felt allows safe extension of the cast.

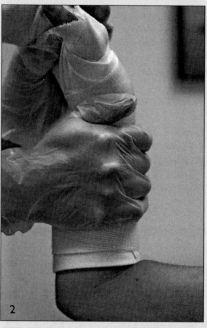

2

Synthetic cast applied—three-point molding.

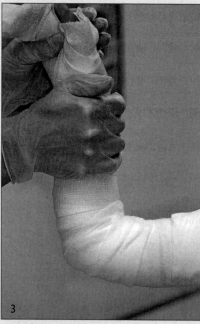

3

This cast is then extended above the elbow.

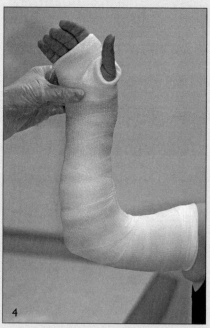

4

The final product—a cast of beauty and reliability.

Applying a cast to the forearm first and then extending it (elbow bent to 90°) carries a risk of producing a severe skin ulcer if the sharp proximal edge of the cast gouges into the antecubital fossa. A similar complication can occur if the entire cast is applied at once but in too little elbow flexion. As the cast sets, the elbow is "adjusted" to 90° with an ulcerogenic antecubital ridge produced (Fig. 5-12).

Hyndman et al. emphasized the need for careful forearm molding to maintain a reduction. The ratio of cast height to width as well as three-point molding are critical (Fig 5-13). If you get very good at this, you may be able to keep a distal radius fracture reduced with a short arm cast only, whereas others may need a long arm cast.

The final effect should be a cast that is thin, aesthetic, and biomechanically sound. Calot, the famous 19th-century French surgeon, stated: "Show me your plaster and I'll show you what kind of orthopaedist you are." We concur. I make a hobby of observing casts (in shopping malls, in restaurants, or on relatives of children in clinic) that have been applied by others, guessing who applied the cast (orthopedist, orthopedic technician, family practitioner, other). A well-trained orthopedist should apply functional, aesthetic casts that demonstrate a leadership role in caring for musculoskeletal problems.

Errors—Cast Too Short

Many people make their casts too short proximally. The long arm cast seen in Figure 5-14 was far too short (to just above the elbow) and reduction was lost despite pinning.

Conversion to Short Arm?

I rarely convert a long arm cast to a short arm cast simply to give the child early elbow motion. The cost of cast removal and placement of a new cast, particularly if synthetic materials and expensive labor are required (i.e., you or the cast technician), is prohibitive. Reimbursement is unpredictable. Also, children do not like their cast removed with a cast saw, as noted previously. For these reasons, in almost all long arm casts, we have the child wear the original cast until the fracture is healed (often 6 weeks).

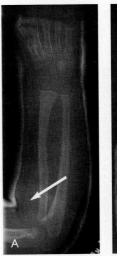
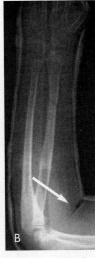

Figure 5-12. A) Long arm cast applied in a single phase, elbow flexed to 90° after fiberglass was applied. B) Long arm cast applied in a single phase with the elbow flexed after the padding was applied. The angle cannot be changed after application of any of the cast materials.

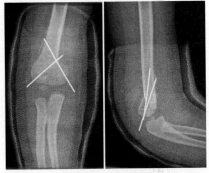

Figure 5-14. Cast too short. This child had a supracondylar fracture that was pinned anatomically but presented to us with loss of reduction, despite the pins. Her mini-cast is partially responsible, extending only a few centimeters above the fracture line.

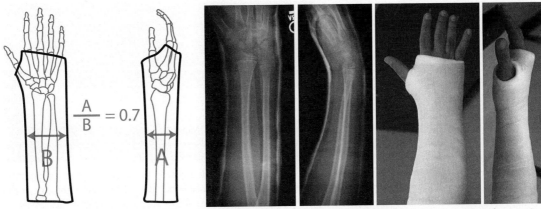

Figure 5-13. Hyndman's cast ratio. In his now classic paper, Hyndman noted that one needs not only a three-point mold but also a cast that is thin from top to bottom (as compared to width). The x-rays and cast shown here demonstrate this point.

$$\frac{A}{B} = 0.7$$

LOWER EXTREMITY CASTS

Principles—The cast should be molded with the foot in neutral position to avoid the development of equinus in the cast. Also, three-point molding and foot position help to maintain fracture reduction (Fig 5-15). To make a well-molded ankle joint, with the plaster thicker on the heel than anteriorly, a splint can be applied over the heel. Otherwise, as Charnley noted, the anterior area will be many times thicker than the heel (you will want to split the cast anteriorly, it should be thin here).

An ideal cast should be molded to demonstrate the calcaneal prominence and the malleoli. It is impossible to overemphasize the need for proper molding around the calcaneus, the most common area for skin irritation and ulceration in children's casts (Fig. 5-16). The depth of the sculpted inset above the calcaneus may need to be up to 2 cm, depending on the size of the child, to avoid pressure on the calcaneus (Fig. 5-17). Examining a basketball shoe demonstrates that manufacturers recognize the need for a deep recess for the heel, with a supportive "counter" above. With final heel molding, you should feel that the calcaneus is nested in a deeply molded "cup" that you have shaped. A cast with a straight posterior calf segment is much more likely to produce heel ulceration.

Similarly, the arch of the foot should be molded with a recess in the cast for the metatarsal heads. There is no place for a board or other rigid flat structure in molding the bottom of a cast. The modern cast should have a bottom shaped like the insole of a well-designed jogging shoe. With excellent molding, less cast padding is needed and the cast is less likely to slide off.

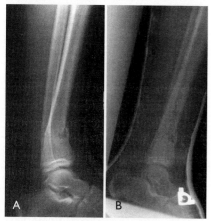

Figure 5-15. Clearly the biomechanics of fractures and their overlying muscles must be understood when applying casts. For example, in the so-called Gillespie fracture, if the foot is brought up to neutral position for casting, the distal tibial fracture will angulate (recurvatum) (Figure A). In this rare instance, the foot should be purposely casted in equinus (Figure B).

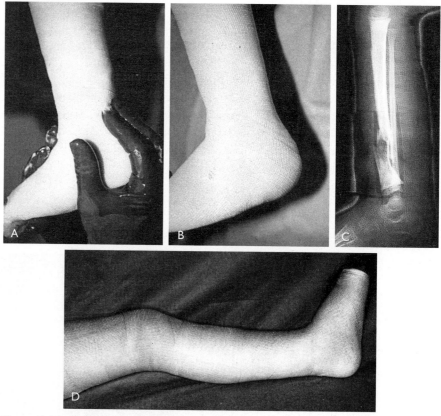

Figure 5-16. Molding around the calcaneus. A) With final molding, the tip of the calcaneus is palpated in the palm of your hand. There should be a deep cup in the cast at this area so that any pressure is taken on the soft tissues above the calcaneus rather than at the tip of the bone. B) The final product. C) A so-called stove pipe cast with a straight posterior border. This child is very likely to get a heel ulcer. The posterior border of a leg cast should never be straight. D) A properly molded long leg cast—note molded areas above ankle and behind knee.

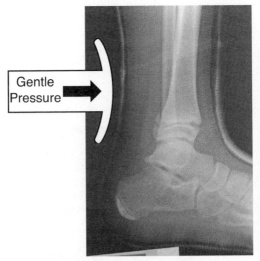

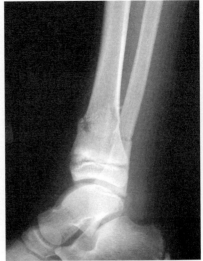

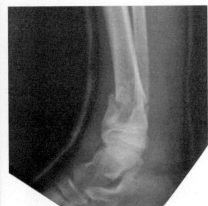

Figure 5-17. The ideal mold (lateral view) for a short leg cast. Note the beautiful relatively deep, but smooth, mold well above the calcaneous. This prevents heel ulcers. The area anterior to the ankle is very thin.

Figure 5-18. It requires experience and careful observation to avoid creating deformity with cast application. This fracture was made worse by the cast.

Long Leg Casts

A long leg cast requires careful molding about the knee with the knee kept at 10°-15° flexion to avoid posterior capsule strain. The decision regarding a long leg cast in one or two segments depends on the circumstances.

Sequence—Long Leg Cast for Tibial Fracture

For most tibial fractures that require reduction and casting, the cast is best applied in two segments, particularly in a larger child. Allow gravity to be your friend by applying and molding the below knee segment with the knee bent over the edge of the table (tibia vertical). The cast can then be extended for the above knee segment with the patient supine. Be very careful as the cast hardens to carefully attend to knee angle to avoid "late-stage hardening" buckles.

Creating Deformity with Casts

Each year we see fractures that come in with near anatomic alignment and after casting appear malreduced (Fig. 5-18). It requires experience and careful observation to avoid creating deformity with cast application, particularly in the tibia. The leg (calf) section is best applied first, with the leg in a vertical position to allow gravity to help as you mold the tibia section. Then after placing a circumferential felt band at the junction, the cast is converted to a long leg type.

Casts Applied in the Operating Room

Postoperative casts are particularly difficult to apply safely and correctly (Fig. 5-19). The surgical dressing should be thin to allow good cast fit. We commonly use suction drainage when bleeding is anticipated, rather than using a thick compressive dressing that leads to poor cast fitting.

Many surgeons prefer a bulky type of cast, a posterior and anterior splint, or even a Robert Jones bulky dressing following surgery, with the cast applied later. Again, sensitivity for the child and economics should be considered. If every child that you operate on requires a return for a complete cast change within a

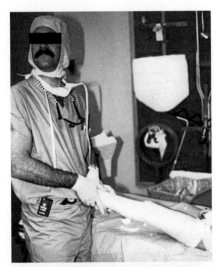

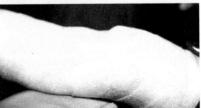

Figure 5-19. A) The assistant cannot be daydreaming when the cast is setting. If he does not pay rapt attention, the child is likely to develop a buckle in the plaster at the knee level. This is particularly a feature of synthetic casts. B) Buckle in cast in knee area. Such buckles are ulcerogenic.

TECHNIQUE TIPS:
Two-Stage Application of a Long Leg (Above Knee) Cast

(for reduction of tibia fracture in a larger patient—ensures that tibial segment, foot, and ankle are molded perfectly—then extended to proximal thigh)

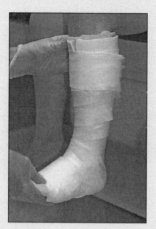

1) Leg vertical – padding applied plus circular felt at junction.

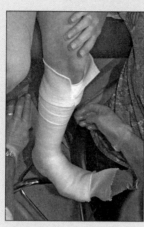

2) Synthetic material applied.

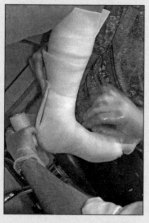

3) Splint over heel to make back thicker than front.

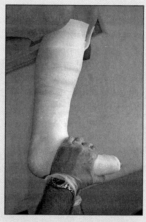

4) Very careful molding to contour of calcaneus—maintain fracture reduction.

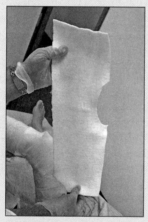

5) Circular felt to protect proximal thigh.

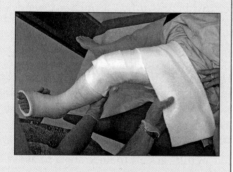

6) Padding extended plus apply felt in groin (for comfort).

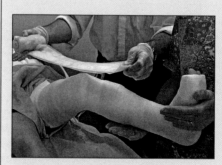

7) Patient now supine. Extend cast-splint over knee to strengthen.

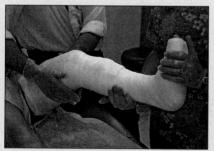

8) Molding long leg cast.

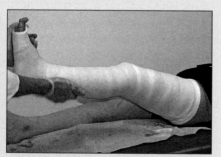

9) The final product. A few degrees less knee flexion might be better for subsequent walking.

week after surgery, the expense becomes significant. Also as already noted, children hate cast changes.

Posterior Splints in Children

Posterior splints, made of plaster or synthetics, are often used safely in adults as a temporary form of immobilization. Their use in children (especially in those younger than 5 years) is risky because they almost routinely pull their heel out of its intended spot, with a high risk for developing a heel ulcer (Fig. 5-20). Many experts advise that children younger than 6 years not be immobilized with a posterior splint. A cast is safer because it holds the ankle in its correct position.

CAST WEDGING

Careful planning and implementation of cast "wedges" to correct angular deformity can simplify the management of lower-extremity fractures in children. In the lower extremity, wedging can be used for femoral fractures (hip spica wedged—Fig. 5-21) as well as for tibial fractures. The correction is almost

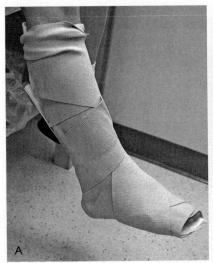
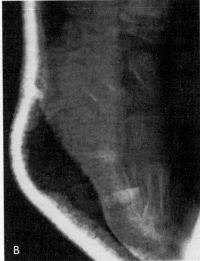

"Wedging techniques should be mastered by orthopaedists who care for children, since angular alignment is often all that is required for acceptable position and fracture healing."

Figure 5-20. A) Posterior splints are risky for use in young children because they routinely pull out of them, resulting in a risk for heel ulcer. B) Lateral x-ray of a child placed in a splint to temporarily immobilize for a distal tibial fracture. The child has pulled out of the splint and is a risk for developing a heel ulcer. If they are used, it should only be for a day or two. Better to use an anterior plus posterior splint or a temporary cast.

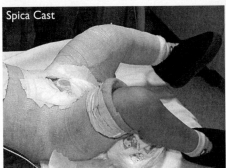
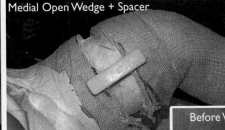

Figure 5-21. Young child with femur fracture that is drifting into varus angulation at the fracture site can be improved by wedging of the cast. Skill and experience are required to wedge casts safely.

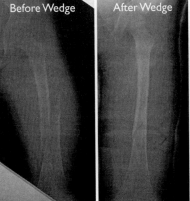
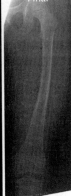

NOTE: Cast wedging requires skill and experience to avoid skin problems.

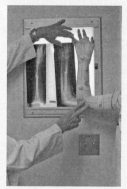

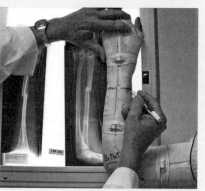

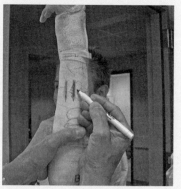

Look at cast and x-ray together. Determine level of fracture angulation (where you wish to correct).

Marking cast. (Cast had been univalved, this is a follow-up visit).

Hinge marked opposite side where cast will be opened.

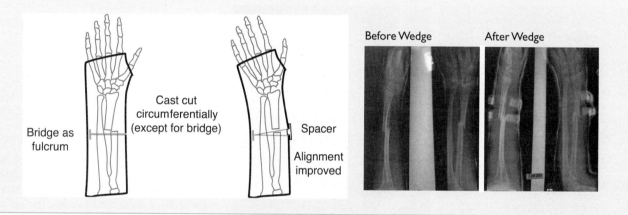

Bridge as fulcrum

Cast cut circumferentially (except for bridge)

Spacer

Alignment improved

Before Wedge   After Wedge

always an opening wedge formed by making a circular cut in the cast at the level of deformity, leaving about 1 cm of the cast uncut as a fulcrum. The cast is then levered open on the opposite side to correct the deformity. Care must be taken to make a smooth bend to avoid skin necrosis. Inspect the x-ray for a possible ridge, keep the patient around for 30 minutes to be sure the "post-wedge ache" subsides, and warn the patient to return if there is late pain.

Appropriate spacers are placed in the wedge, with image intensifier or x-ray views taken with the spacer temporarily taped in position. When the correction is adequate, the wedge and spacer are incorporated into the cast to maintain the new position. Artful cast room wedging has allowed us to avoid taking literally hundreds of children with loss of angular correction in femoral and tibial fractures back to the operating room.

Even in upper extremity fractures, opening wedges can be used to correct an angular deformity or "sag" in the mid-forearm following a bone fracture, sometimes avoiding re-manipulation and cast change under anesthesia. Wedging techniques should be mastered by orthopedists who care for children, because angular alignment is often all that is required for acceptable position and fracture healing.

HIP SPICA CASTS FOR FEMUR FRACTURES

A spica cast is the mainstay for treatment of femoral fractures in children. The use of femoral fracture hip spica casts can range from use in a 7-month-old victim of child abuse to an 8-year-old with a spiral midshaft fracture. Many variations of spica can be used, ranging from a simple one-and-one-half spica with the femur relatively extended to a complex, near 90°-90° hip-knee position to control shortening. We will present a few principles, focusing on a method that only moderately flexes the hip and knee. The more radical hip-knee flexion casts (so-called 90-90) can be used; however, because of increasingly common reports of nerve injury, skin slough, or calf compartment syndrome associated with their use, Frick has diminished our enthusiasm for the 90°-90° position (Fig. 5-22).

We use synthetic-material casts in all age groups because they are easier to apply, easier to wedge, and easier to maintain. For a child younger than the age of 2 years, with a simple oblique fracture of the femur, we will apply an early spica, usually without general anesthesia. If the fracture is a nondisplaced spiral fracture (the most common type at this age), a single hip spica can be used, making diapering and bathing easier.

In children aged 2-6 years, we sometimes place the children in skin traction for 24 or 48 hours, particularly if there are associated injuries. We then apply the hip spica with the child anesthetized. This variation of the early spica allows time for proper assessment of the child and to find a civilized operating-room time. Thus in our hospital the term "immediate spica" has been replaced with "early spica" and implies cast application within a few days of injury at a time that is safe and convenient for all parties. These children have a light general anesthesia with a one-and-one-half hip spica cast applied. Use of an image intensifier to confirm fracture position in the operating room (just prior to spica application) decreases the need for subsequent cast wedging. An immediate post-spica-application image intensifier view confirms the position, and, if wedge correction is required, it is done immediately while the child is still anesthetized.

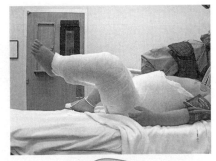

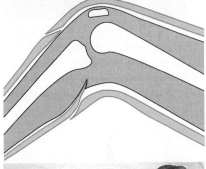

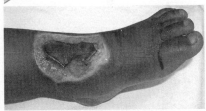

Figure 5-22. The risks in using a 90°-90° cast includes junctional problems (if traction applied to the leg cast, which is applied first. Reported problems include skin necrosis (behind knee), compartment syndrome (calf), and anterior skin loss (distal calf).

CAST COMPLICATIONS

All orthopedic surgeons are aware of the many complications related to cast immobilization. Some families do not understand cast care instructions but more often the child is uncooperative or not properly supervised. The resulting wet casts, damaged casts, destroyed casts, etc., are common to all age groups and will not be specifically addressed here. We emphasize, however, the importance of the orthopedic technician and/or surgeon giving the family a handout detailing cast care as well as providing clear and simple instructions.

The Veterinary Approach—Understanding Your Client

A perhaps slightly jaded, yet practical, approach to childhood behavior is to use what we call the veterinary approach when using a cast for an unstable lower limb (tibial, ankle) fracture. With certain families, rather than relying on instructions and handouts alone, we assume that they will not get the message (puppies do not read their "handouts"). Instead, we create a cast that keeps them from creating a problem. For example, in an unstable distal tibial (or medial malleolar) fracture, the cast would be a long leg type with the knee flexed to

TECHNIQUE TIPS:
Application of a Hip Spica for Child with Femur Fracture

(Cast in relative extension minimizes risk to skin and compartments)

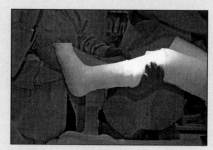

1) Short leg (below knee segment) applied first. To help hold the limb. Little traction or pressure can be used and the junction must be well padded (we use felt). (Many experts do not incorporate the foot and apply the calf segment last.)

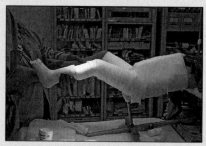

2) Limb positioned in relative extension. Cast padding added. Note temporary spacers under padding over abdomen (use towels or skin tape packs).

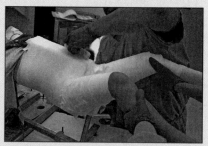

3) Synthetic material rolled on. Again note cast prominence over temporary abdominal protection spacers.

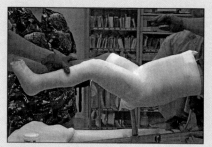

4) Spica completed.

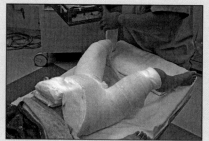

5) View from above—cast complete—note cast has been trimmed down to the umbilicus level to ensure easy abdominal expansion and breathing—The temporary pads will be removed once cast hardens.

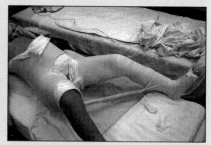

6) Spica cast complete abdominal pads removed. Wood is attached to opposite thigh for stability.

Pre-Spica film   After Spica

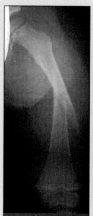 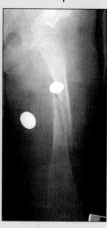

NOTE: We have changed to this more relaxed position, as compared to the 90,-90° position, which has a risk for skin and compartment problems in the calf. Some would not apply the calf segment first, nor incorporate the foot, to further minimize these risks.

90° (right angle) for the first 4 weeks. This position prevents weight-bearing, even in uncooperative patients or those who lack understanding.

Showering and Bathing

The issue of showering and bathing with a cast on remains controversial, even with synthetic-material casts. Children and adolescents seem to do poorly with the commonly prescribed method of taping a plastic bag over an upper- or lower-extremity cast for showering. The method commonly fails, leading to a wet cast that must be replaced—a process whose true cost may be several hundred dollars. Instead of showers, we suggest that the limb not be covered with any special plastic and that the child be bathed in a tub with the arm or leg cast left on the edge of the tub. A parent must be present to help the younger child with bathing.

On the other hand, newer types of special "shower in your cast" protective devices are coming on the market and may be considered. Issues, such as how well the patient applies the device (they often leak) and who pays for the new cast when they fail, remain.

Use of Gore-Tex cast material to produce a so-called swimming cast has gained popularity but has problems also (hard to mold for acute fracture reduction, expense—takes more time to apply and remove). The Gore-Tex option is a good one if your patient has the extra money for additional materials and technician time.

Foreign Bodies Under Casts

Cast instructions should emphasize that nothing be placed inside the cast. The need to scratch under a cast is common, with devices such as coat hangers or other sharp objects inserted for relief. Serious skin excoriation can result.

Despite your instructions, children will deposit all sorts of items under their cast either purposely or inadvertently (Figs. 5-23, 5-24). If a child complains of pain under a cast, you must be prepared to window or even remove the cast to evaluate for possible skin ulceration, which can be produced by foreign bodies under the cast.

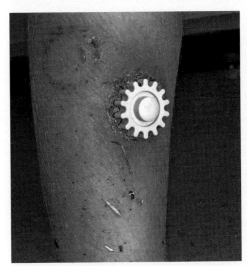 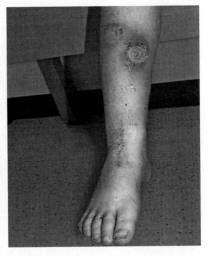

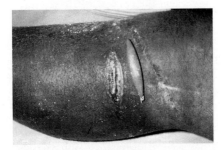

Figure 5-24. This child never complained of pain after surgery. Six weeks later, a significant ulceration produced by a hair barrette was noted. Apparently, the child had dropped it into the cast.

Figure 5-23. This child returned to clinic after 4 weeks in a short leg walking cast. A toy cog was found stuck to his skin.

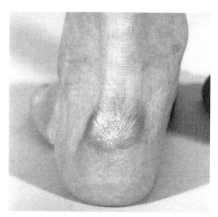

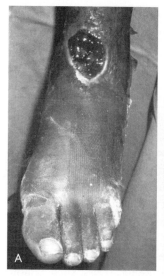

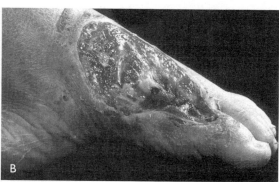

Figure 5-25. Typical old heel ulcer over the calcaneus in a patient who had a poorly applied long let cast.

Figure 5-26. Dorsal ulceration. A) Small ulceration in the area where anterior soft-roll and casting material was bunched. Likely the cast was further dorsiflexed after the casting materials had been applied, producing an ulcer. B) A more severe form of the same problem. The child sloughed the entire dorsum of the foot.

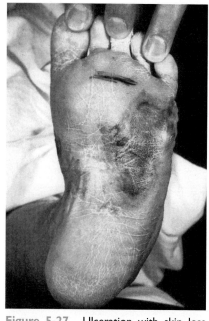

Figure 5-27. Ulceration with skin loss over the metatarsal heads in a child treated for fixed equinus. Postoperative casting with forced dorsiflexion led to this ulceration. The child never complained because he had a neurologic disorder.

Cast Ulcers Due to Poor Cast Design

Many cast problems are the result of inattention to detail by the applying surgeon or technician. Ulceration over the tip of calcaneus is the most common skin problem associated with leg casts (Fig. 5-25). Heel ulcers can be almost entirely avoided by understanding the normal contour and shape of the calcaneus and by careful cast molding about the calcaneus. Leg casts with an entirely straight posterior border are a set-up for heel ulceration. When detected, they should be corrected before skin ulceration develops. William T. Green, the famed Boston Children's Hospital surgeon, marked poorly applied casts with a black marker, an indication that they had to be changed before the sun had set.

Improperly applied leg casts can cause other types of skin ulceration. If the foot is left in equinus when the soft-roll and/or plaster is applied, with the foot subsequently dorsiflexed, the resulting dorsiflexion ridge in the cast anterior to the ankle will cause predictable skin ulceration. The entire dorsum of the foot can slough (Fig. 5-26).

Similarly, excessive pressure on the bottom of the foot can produce ulcerations over the metatarsal heads (Fig. 5-27). Careful molding of a metatarsal recess to accommodate the metatarsal heads is required to avoid this complication.

The juncture between the leg and thigh segments of a long leg cast that has been constructed sequentially (leg first, then thigh) is a common source of skin ulceration. If the posterior segment of the leg cast is left too long, with the knee then flexed to apply the thigh segment, the resulting ridge can produce a full-thickness ulceration in the hamstring area.

Unfortunately, children commonly do not experience any prolonged sense of pain when an improperly applied cast is producing skin ulcerations. It hurts only until the skin becomes numb and then stops. In many cases, you may not detect ulcerations or skin injury until the time of planned cast removal. It is thus imperative that orthopedists who treat children learn to apply postoperative casts that are extremely unlikely to produce skin pressure. Pressure of 30 mm Hg over 3 hours will produce skin necrosis.

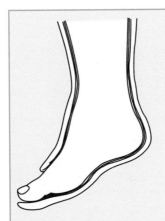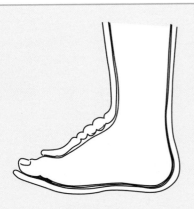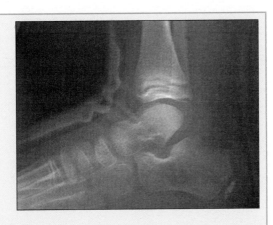

The Dorsiflexion "Crinkle"

This illustration for Albee's classic 1919 text *Orthopedic and Reconstruction Surgery* demonstrates the problems associated with dorsiflexing the foot after any material has been applied, either soft-roll or plaster. The dorsal bunching of the soft-roll and/or plaster often causes pain and sometimes causes ulceration. This is avoided by holding the foot dorsiflexed before any materials are applied.

Suggested Readings

Blount WP. Fractures in children. Baltimore: Williams & Wilkins, 1955.

Charnley J. The closed treatment of common fractures. Edinburgh: B & S Livingstone, 1950.

Chess DG, Hyndman JC, Leahey JL, Brown DCS, Sinclair AM: Short arm plaster cast for distal pediatric forearm fractures. J Ped Orthop 1994;14:211-213.

Czertak DJ, Hennrikus WL. The treatment of pediatric femur fractures with early 90-90 spica casting. J Pediatr Orthop. 1999 Mar-Apr;19(2):229-32.

Large TM, Frick SL. Compartment syndrome of the leg after treatment of a femoral fracture with an early sitting spica cast. A report of two cases. J Bone Joint Surg Am. 2003 Nov;85-A(11): 2207-10.

Wehbe, A: Plaster Uses and Misuses, Clinn Orthop. 167:242-249, 1982.

Weiss A et al. Peroneal nerve palsy after early cast application for femoral fractures in children. J Pediatr Orthop. 1992 Jan; 12(1):25-8.

Wenger D, Rang M: Casts in Children in the Art and Practice of Children's Orthopedics, Raven Press, 1993 (now Lippincott Williams & Wilkins).

Wu KK. Techniques in surgical casting and splinting. Philadelphia: Lea & Febiger, 1987.

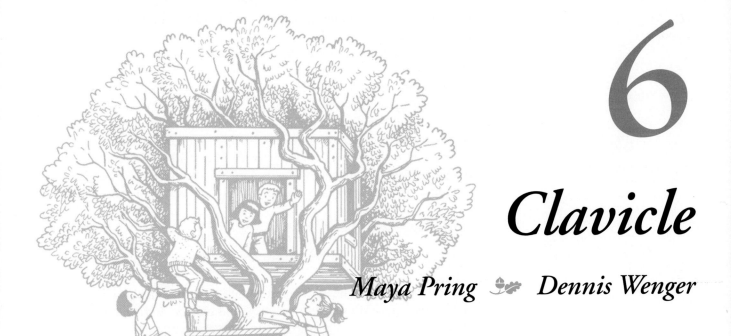

6
Clavicle

Maya Pring ❧ *Dennis Wenger*

INTRODUCTION

Sir Robert Peel, Prime Minister of Britain in 1834, would have been among the first to agree that the clavicle is a fragile bone. In 1850, he died after falling from his horse on Constitution Hill, having sustained a fracture of the clavicle, which probably penetrated the subclavian vessels.

The unique design of the clavicle allows dexterity and sophisticated use of the complex upper limb and serves as the only true skeletal attachment of the humerus and scapula to the axial skeleton. The small size of the clavicle and its relative fragility allow incredible dexterity but put it at risk for fracture, especially when bipeds suddenly become quadrupeds (falling down). Of course, children have such mishaps everyday; thus clavicle fractures are among the most common injuries in children.

Looking from above, the clavicle has an S shape from the sternum medially to the acromion laterally. In cross section, it changes from a round or prismatic

> *"Don't touch the patient—state first what you see"*
> —OSLER

"The small size of the clavicle and its relative fragility allow incredible dexterity but puts it at risk for fracture"

shape medially to a flattened shape along the lateral third, and when viewed from the front, it appears flat and straight (Fig. 6-1).

The unique double curve of the clavicle allows for motion of the shoulder in all directions and acts as a fulcrum to improve the effectiveness of the muscles that move the arm. The clavicle helps to suspend the upper extremity from the thorax while protecting the subclavian vessels beneath it. The deltoid, pectoralis major, and subclavius all have a significant portion of their origin on the clavicle; the sternocleidomastoid and trapezius insert onto this small bone.

The vast majority of pediatric clavicle fractures can be treated conservatively; however, one must recognize the rare fracture that requires surgical intervention as well as the very rare clavicle fracture that may be life threatening.

ASSESSING THE PATIENT

Infancy

Clavicle fractures are one of the most common injuries sustained during birth; children of large birth weight ($>$ 4,000g) and those with shoulder dystocia are at the highest risk. Infants who sustain a clavicle fracture may also sustain a brachial plexus injury due to nerve stretch (Erb's palsy). The neonate with a clavicle fracture may present with an asymmetric Moro reflex or an apparently flail upper extremity.

Differentiating a neurologic injury from a clavicle fracture during the first few weeks of life can be extremely difficult, and the child may have both. X-ray or ultrasound can diagnose the fracture, but clear neurologic assessment of the upper extremity may not be possible until the fracture has healed.

Children and Adolescents

Failure to palpate the fractured clavicle frequently leads to incorrect diagnosis (i.e., shoulder strain or AC separation). However, because the clavicle is subcutaneous for most of its length, fractures should be easy to identify in the older child and adolescent with a good physical exam. Clinical deformity, ecchymosis, swelling (Fig. 6-2) and point tenderness lead the physician to the diagnosis. Because of its subcutaneous nature, clavicle fractures can tent and erode

Lateral   Medial
AP view

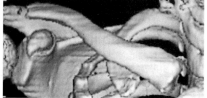

Superior view

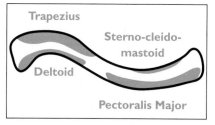

Inferior view

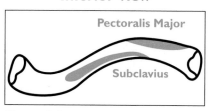

Figure 6-1. Anatomy of the clavicle.

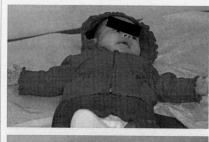

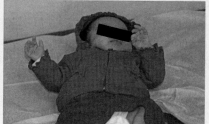

Ernst Moro (1874–1951)

German pediatrician born December 8, 1874 described a defensive reflex seen in the first 6 months of life. In response to a loud noise, an infant draws its arms across the chest in an embracing manner. An asymmetric Moro reflex may be secondary to neurologic injury or fracture.

through the skin if severely angulated. Carefully assess the fracture site so closed fractures do not become open fractures.

Limb-threatening concerns associated with clavicle fractures and dislocations that need to be identified immediately include vascular injury (subclavian vessels), neurologic injury (brachial plexus), and injury to the mediastinal structures (esophagus, trachea, pleura, lung) by angulated or displaced fragments.

RADIOGRAPHIC ISSUES

One of the first bones to ossify during the early weeks of gestation, the clavicle has three centers of ossification. There are two primary centers for the body (medial and a lateral), which appear during the fifth or sixth week of fetal life, and a secondary center for the sternal (medial) end, which appears in late teenage years. The shaft can be radiographically identified at birth; however, the medial epiphysis appears in the teenage years and does not fuse to the shaft of the clavicle until the early twenties. Salter-Harris fractures through the physis are often mistaken for medial clavicle dislocations in adolescents.

Almost all clavicle fractures can be adequately identified with a single AP view (Fig. 6-2). Problem fractures may require special views. The orientation of the clavicle makes it difficult to get two x-ray views at 90° to each other. Even with additional views, the medial portion of the clavicle is difficult to see because of the sternum and mediastinum. In addition to a straight AP view of the clavicle, an apical lordotic x-ray can help visualize the medial clavicle without overlap of the sternum (see Table 6-1). Any question about the nature of a clavicular injury should be futher investigated with a CT scan, which allows the best visualization of the clavicle. Concern for vascular injury mandates an arteriogram.

CLASSIFICATION

Fractures can be complete, or the clavicle can be plastically deformed with a greenstick type of fracture (Fig 6-3). The very thick layer of periosteum surrounding the pediatric clavicle tends to maintain the alignment of the fracture, which typically leads to early union in infants and children. As children become teenagers, the periosteum no longer acts as a strong supporting structure and nonunion becomes more common—especially in vigorous athletes and laborers.

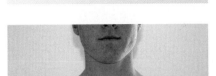
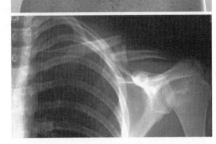

Figure 6-2. The clavicle is subcutaneous making deformity noticeable. This patient has a healing left clavicle fracture (healing in bayonet apposition). Patients need to be told about the size of callus that will appear (and later resorb).

At Injury

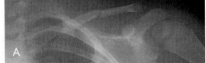

2 Weeks Later

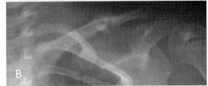

Figure 6-3. A) Greenstick clavicle fracture as frequently seen in young children. B) Healing with abundant callus.

Table 6-1	Radiographic Assessment of Clavicle Injuries	
AP View	**Apical Lordotic**
Allows good visualization of the superior/inferior displacement of shaft fractures	Allows better visualization of the medial clavicles without overlap of the sternum
Standard AP	Tube angled 40°–45°

Classification of Pediatric Clavicle Fractures

Basic types of clavicle fractures

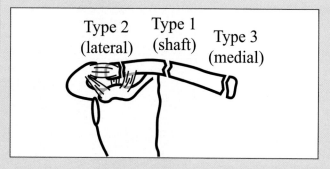

Type 2
(lateral) Type 1
(shaft) Type 3
(medial)

Type 1: Shaft fractures typically have shortening and superior angulation.

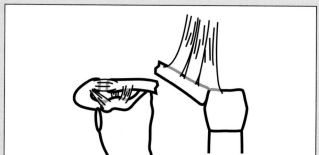

Type 2: Distal fractures (further subdivided by Dameron and Rockwood).
Note: The epiphysis and periosteum typically remain in place and the shaft displaces.

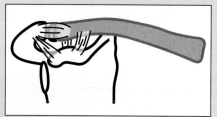

I Sprain of AC ligaments only

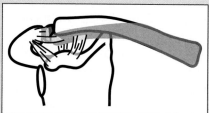

II Widening of AC joint

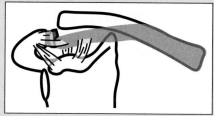

III Superior displacement 25-100%

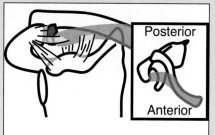

IV Posterior displacement

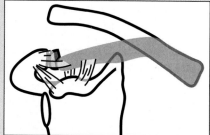

V Superior displacement >100%

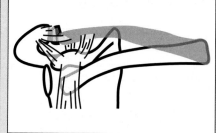

VI Inferior displacement

Type 3: Subdivision of medial clavicle fractures. The description of the fracture can be based on displacement of the shaft—anterior, posterior, superior, or inferior.

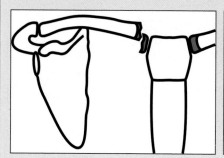

A. Physeal fracture

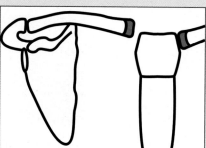

B. Sternoclavicular dislocation (rare)

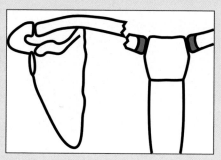

C. Medial shaft fracture

The basic types of fracture include medial, lateral, and shaft fractures. Medial and lateral fractures have been further subdivided based on location of the fracture and displacement of the shaft. (We believe that clavicle fractures have been overclassified in the literature. See "Classification of Pediatric Clavicle Fractures" for an overview of the subclassifications.)

TREATMENT

Shaft Fractures (Type 1)

Infant

Infant clavicular fractures can be treated by pinning the shirt sleeve to the shirt or elastic bandage wrapping the arm to the body for 2-3 weeks (Fig 6-4). This treatment provides some immoblization and pain relief and reminds people not to pick the baby up by the arm. Infantile fractures tend to heal well regardless of treatment. The associated injuries including brachial plexus palsy require more focused attention; however, these are difficult to evaluate until the fracture heals and motion can be better assessed.

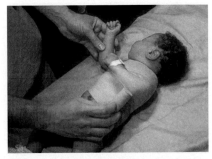

Figure 6-4. An infant with a clavicle fracture can be treated by pinning the sleeve (of the injured side) to the body of the garment. A second option (illustrated here): wrap the limb to the trunk gently with an ace bandage.

Children and Adolescents

It has been said that "if the two ends of the clavicle are in the same room they will heal and remodel adequately." Thus the typical case generally recieves little attention. The exception would be a fracture that severly tents the skin or risks the neurovascular bundle underneath.

A sling can be used for minimally displaced fractures. Many advocate a figure-of-8 brace to gently pull the shoulders back so as to minimize overlap of the fracture fragments; however, the pad of the brace must be soft to avoid undue pressure on a midshaft fracture, making the brace difficult to wear (see Table 6-2 and Fig. 6-5). In cases that are not markedly shortened, an imaginative approach is to provide both a sling and figure-of-8 brace to manage the fracture

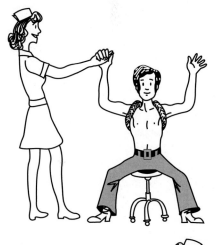

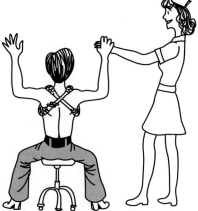

Figure 6-5. Perhaps the easiest way to apply a snug figure-of-8 brace without tears. Although commercial braces are available, a stockinet filled with cast padding and secured by two saftey pins can be used in a pinch.

Table 6-2	Classic Dilemma—Sling vs. Figure-of-8 Brace	
	Advantages	**Disadvantages**
SLING	Very inexpensive Easy to put on No pressure over fracture A few sizes fit all	No ability to pull fracture to length Hand is not free
FIGURE-OF-8 Photos courtesy of C. Farnsworth	Can hold fracture better reduced (in theory) Hands free for activities	Harder to put on Focal pressure over fracture site Need to keep multiple sizes in stock

At Injury

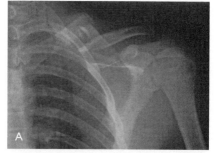

3 Months Later

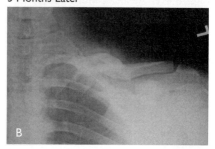

Figure 6-7. A) Significantly displaced and comminuted fracture in a teenager. B) Three months later—note remodeling

"Almost all medial clavicle fracture in patients under age 18 years appear to be sternoclavicluar dislocations but in fact are transphyseal injuries"

Anterior

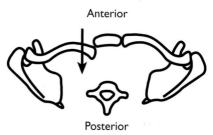

Posterior

Figure 6-8. Type 3A medial clavicle fracture with posterior displacement.

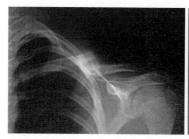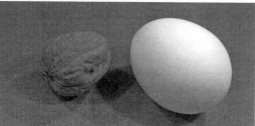

Figure 6-6. We warn parents that the resulting callus from a clavicle fracture may be the size of a walnut (or even an egg in a teenager).

symptomatically. The patient can use both initially (first 3-4 days when pain is greatest) and then one or the other according to which is most comfortable.

Protect the fracture for 3 weeks, with contact sports avoided for another 3 weeks. As in most simple injuries, half the treatment consists of educating the parents about the normal course: An unsightly lump will appear with fracture healing (callus) and will persist for at least a year while remodeling progresses (we tell parents that the lump may be the size of a walnut or an egg—Fig. 6-6). Although x-rays of a fracture healing in bayonet opposistion may frighten the parents, studies have shown that a significant amount of angulation and overlap can be accepted (Fig 6-7).

How should these patients be followed? Palpate the clavicle at each exam to assess for motion at the fracture site. One pushes on the medial or lateral segment to be sure the clavicle moves as a unit. Once the fracture is stable and non tender, the patient may slowly return to sports. Final x-rays are usually obtained at 6 weeks; if there are indications for nonunion, longer follow-up becomes necessary.

Lateral Fractures (Type 2)

Dameron and Rockwood suggest that type I, II, and III injuries will heal and remodel without intervention. Reduction and fixation of distal clavicle injuries is only necessary for types IV, V, and VI that have a severe and fixed deformity. Distal clavicle fractures in pediatric patients are usually trans-physeal and not true AC separations (as seen in adults). The intact periosteum allows children to heal and remodel with few complications without operative intervention.

Most lateral clavicle fractures are adequately treated with a sling or figure-of-8 brace for 3 weeks followed by an additional period in which contact sports are avoided. Early range of motion should be started as soon as pain allows. Complex harness brace devices designed to reduce clavicle fractures (Kenny Howard type harness) are rarely used in children.

Medial Fractures (Type 3)

Almost all medial clavicle fractures in patients younger than 18 years appear to be sternoclavicular dislocations but in fact are transphyseal injuries. As noted earlier the epiphyseal ossification center does not appear until age 18 years and may fuse as late as age 25 years. If the shaft displaces anteriorly, the chances of remodeling are excellent, with minimal risk to vital structures. These fractures are typically treated in a figure-of-8 brace.

If the clavicle displaces posteriorly, the mediastinal structures are at risk (Fig. 6-8). These fractures may be difficult to recognize (the patient may complain of medial clavicle or sternal pain with difficulty swallowing or breathing). In suspected cases, a CT scan is necessary for diagnosis. If the study shows any impingement or vascular compromise, the fracture should be reduced under general anesthesia with a vascular surgeon available.

Reduction of a posteriorly displaced medial fracture can usually be accomplished in a closed fashion. A bolster placed between the shoulder blades elevates the anterior chest. In thin patients, the surgeon can place his/her fingers behind the clavicle. Upward pressure while the arm is abducted, externally rotated, and extended can relocate the medial clavicle (Fig. 6-9).

If this fails, or the patient is too large for this maneuver, a carefully placed towel clip can be used to pull the clavicle anteriorly while an assistant applies lateral traction to the arm (Fig. 6-10). Towel clip application must be judicious because the subclavian vein lies just below the midshaft of the clavicle. After stable reduction, the patient is immobilized in a figure-of-8 brace. Open reduction should be performed if stable reduction cannot be achieved. The physeal fracture can be secured using a strong absorbable suture through the periosteum superiorly and/or anteriorly. Postoperative immobilization can be either a figure-of-8 brace or a shoulder spica.

The patient in Figure 6-10 had swallowing difficulties and his mother noted a prominent "shoulder blade" 1 month after a motorcycle accident where x-rays had been read as negative. His primary doctor diagnosed him as having a winged scapula. We confirmed the diagnosis of medial clavicle fracture with posterior displacement with a CT scan. The enitre shoulder girdle had rotated posteriorly causing the appearance of a prominent scapula from the back. The patient was taken to the operating room for closed reduction; this was not possible with manual manipulation and a towel clip was required to adequately reduce the clavicle. The reduction was unstable and went on to open reduction and suture fixation.

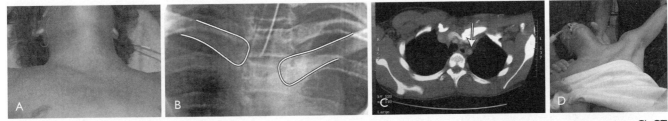

Figure 6-9. A) 14-year-old boy sustained a posteriorly displaced medial clavicle fracture. B) An apical oblique x-ray suggests injury. C) CT scan confirms posterior displacement (arrow). D) In thin patients, the clavicle can sometimes be reduced using manual manipulation with traction on the arm. Closed reduction was successful in this patient. He was then placed into a figure-of-8 brace.

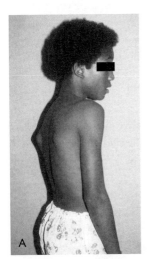
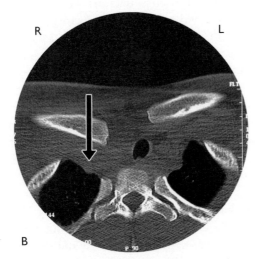
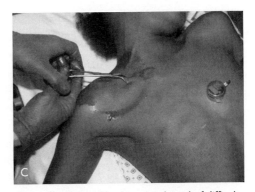

Figure 6-10. A) This 12-year-old boy was referred for a winged scapula 1 month after a motorcycle accident. He also complained of difficulty swallowing. B) CT scan confirmed a Type 3A clavicle fracture with posterior dislocation. C) He was taken to the OR for closed reduction, which required a towel clip to pull the clavicle anteriorly. The reduction was unstable and required open reduction and suture stabilization.

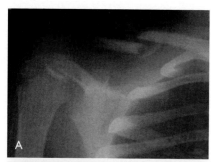

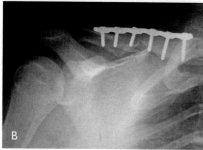

Figure 6-11. A) Some clavicle fractures create significant deformity and risk the overlying skin. B) This patient went on to open reduction and internal fixation to prevent skin erosion.

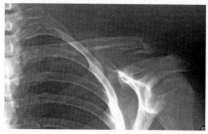

Figure 6-12. Lateral clavicle fractures may lead to a "double clavicle" deformity.

"Nonunion of the clavicle is supposedly rare in children but does occur particularly in muscular, vigorous male athletes"

Special Fractures

Fractures that compromise the skin, nerves, blood vessels, or mediastinal structures should be taken to the operating room for closed versus open reduction. The rare patient with possible subclavian artery injury requires a vascular study in the preparation for operative intervention. The thick periosteal sleeve makes suture fixation adequate to control both lateral and medial fractures, especially in the young child. However, sutures may not be adequate for shaft fractures; shaft fractures can be fixed with a contoured plate if necessary (Fig. 6-11). Typically, we use a contourable pelvic reconstruction plate. Smooth pin fixation should not be used, given the risk for pin migration.

Some centers are now using intramedullary stabilization with elastic nails. This method of treatment minimizes the unsightly scar that tends to result from open treatment and is reported to have few major complications. This method had been used in adults with good results and can be used in a small percentage of young patients with severely displaced clavicle fractures. Kubiak and Slongo have reported good results in five pediatric patients treated with intramedullary elastic nails and two treated with external fixation.

PROBLEMS—WHAT CAN BE EXPECTED?

In today's world of competitive sports and manual labor, there is some debate about the resultant function from clavicle malunions and nonunions. Wilkes and Hoffer studied clavicle fractures in head-injured children treated with no immobilization; the conclusion was that excellent results could be obtained with remodeling of up to 90° of angulation and up to 4 cm of overlap. However, other studies indicate that greater than 2 cm of overlap predisposes to nonunion (Wick) and that a "double clavicle" (Fig. 6-12) deformity can develop when nonoperative treatment is selected for more severe distal physeal injuries (Ogden).

Malunion/Nonunion of Clavicular Fractures

Nonunion of the clavicle is supposedly rare in children but does occur particularly in muscular, vigorous male athletes. This problem has become widely recognized in adult clavicular fractures with Hill et al. reporting a fifteen percent nonunion rate and a 31% "unsatisfactory result" rating in young adult males with midshaft clavicle fractures. Hill found that in adults, initial shortening of a clavicle fracture ≥ 20 mm had a highly significant association with nonunion (p < 0.0001) and the chance of an unsatisfactory result. Fifteen percent of the 52 patients in this study with midclavicle fractures had evidence of brachial plexus irritation, and 28 (54%) had cosmetic complaints. As children age, they are more likely to have unsatisfactory results from clavicle fractures; therefore teenagers with displaced fractures must be carefully treated and monitored. ORIF should be considered with markedly displaced fractures to prevent nonunion and cosmetic deformities.

Nonunion can lead to continued pain and discomfort with shoulder use. Ultrasound has been used to stimulate healing in some cases; the subcutaneous nature of the clavicle allows easy access for ultrasound or electric stimulation treatment. If alternative methods fail and the patient continues to have symptoms, open reduction should be performed with bone grafting and fixation with contoured plate (Fig. 6-13).

Nonunion

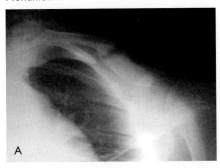

6 Weeks After Surgery

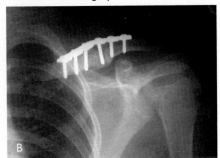

A

B

Figure 6-13. A) 14-year-old boy developed a painful nonunion of his midshaft clavicle fracture. B) Required open reduction and internal fixation with bone grafting. Six weeks after surgery he was pain free with full shoulder motion and returned to football 3 months after surgery.

Acceptable Results in the High Performance Era

The cosmetic deformity caused by angulation and callus formation accounts for the majority of complaints following a clavicle fracture. Armed Forces recruits with healed clavicle fractures commonly have discomfort when trying to carry a backpack, which turns the clavicle into a weight-bearing bone. These patients may require surgical recontouring of the clavicle malunion or osteotomy and ORIF in severe cases. Acceptable results tend to be determined by the patient and family. In this era of aggressive athletic performance with thousands of teenagers hoping to play college or professional sports that require hyper-performance of the upper limb (throwing sports), likely better studies will need to be done to assess what degree of clavicular malunion can lead to long-term functional compromise in such patients (Fig. 6-14).

SUMMARY

The vast majority of pediatric clavicle fractures can be treated conservatively, but the surgeon must know how to recognize the few fractures that are life or limb threatening and require operative intervention.

At Injury

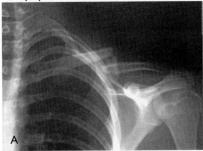

A

3 Months Later

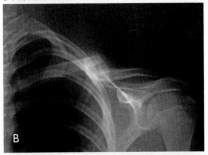

B

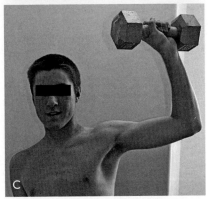

C

Figure 6-14. A) at injury. B) 3 months later. C) Full function. Following a clavicle fracture patients should be able to return to full activities and aggressive sports despite apparent deformity.

Suggested Readings

Caterini R, Farsetti P, Barletta V. Posttraumatic nonunion of the clavicle in a 7-year-old girl. Arch Orthop Trauma Surg. 1998;117(8):475-6.

Dameron TB. Rockwood CA. Fractures and dislocations of the shoulder. In Rockwood CA, Wilkins KE, King RE. (eds): Fractures in children. Philadelphia, J.B. Lippincott, 1984

Eidman DK, Siff SJ, Tullos HS. Acromioclavicular lesions in children. Am J Sports Med. 1981 May-Jun;9(3):150-4.

Goldfarb CA, Bassett GS, Sullivan S, Gordon JE. Retrosternal displacement after physeal fracture of the medial clavicle in children treatment by open reduction and internal fixation. J Bone Joint Surg Br. 2001 Nov;83(8):1168-72.

Hill JM, McGuire MH, Crosby LA. Closed treatment of displaced middle-third fractures of the clavicle gives poor results. J Bone Joint Surg Br. 1997 Jul;79(4):537-9.

Kocher MS, Waters PM, Micheli LJ. Upper extremity injuries in the paediatric athlete. Sports Med. 2000 Aug;30(2):117-35.

Kubiak R, Slongo T. Operative treatment of clavicle fractures in children: a review of 21 years. J Pediatr Orthop. 2002 Nov-Dec;22(6):736-9.

Leighton D, Oudjhane K, Ben Mohammed H. The sternoclavicular joint in trauma: retrosternal dislocation versus epiphyseal fracture. Pediatr Radiol. 1989;20(1-2):126-7.

Lyons, FA. Migration of pins used in operations around the shoulder. JBJS 72A: 1262-7

McKee M, Wild L, Schemitz E. Midshaft malunions of the clavicle. J Bone Joint Surg (Am). 2003 85A:790-797

Ogden, JA. Distal Clavicular physeal injury. Clin Orthop 1984; 188:68-73.

Waters PM et al. Short term outcomes after surgical treatment of traumatic posterior sternoclavicular fracture-dislocations in children and adolescents. JPO 23(4):464-69 2003.

Weinberg B, Seife B, Alonso P. The apical oblique view of the clavicle: its usefulness in neonatal and childhood trauma. Skeletal Radiol. 991;20(3):201-3.

Wick M, Muller EJ, Kollig E, Muhr G. Midshaft fractures of the clavicle with a shortening of more than 2 cm predispose to nonunion. Arch Orthop Trauma Surg. 2001;121(4):207-11.

Wilkes JA, Hoffer MM. Clavicle fractures in head-injured children. J Orthop Trauma. 1987;1(1):55-8.

7

Shoulder and Humeral Shaft

Maya Pring ❧ *Dennis Wenger*

INTRODUCTION

Fractures of the proximal humerus are common during birth and childhood. These fractures have an amazing potential to remodel as they heal; frequently little intervention is necessary. Of course, as children get older, their remodeling potential diminishes and more anatomic reduction is necessary.

Scapula fractures that do not involve the glenoid also heal with little help from a surgeon; however, the associated injuries must be recognized and treated.

ASSESSING THE PATIENT

Localization of a shoulder fracture especially in infants may be difficult. They may present with what appears to be a brachial plexus palsy because pain will keep them from moving the arm. You may not be able to determine whether there is a neurologic deficit until the fracture has healed.

"It is difficulties that show what men are"
—EPICTETUS

"Localization of a shoulder fracture especially in infants may be difficult. They may present with what appears to be a brachial plexus palsy as pain will keep them from moving the arm"

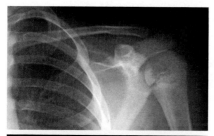
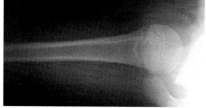

Figure 7-1. AP and axillary view of the proximal humerus. The triangular shape of the physis makes reading x-rays more difficult.

Older children are more cooperative with a neurologic exam. The brachial plexus may be disrupted or stretched by a shoulder injury. The axillary nerve is easily damaged by fractures or dislocations of the shoulder and can be checked by testing sensation over the deltoid. Rare cases may also have an arterial injury.

Scapula fractures are typically the result of great violence and associated injuries are common. Be sure to look for life-threatening injuries (closed head injury, thoracic trauma, spine fractures, etc.).

Anatomy

The proximal humeral ossification center appears at approximately 6 months of age. Those for the greater and lesser tuberosity appear around 2 years and 4-5 years, respectively.

The shoulder has a healthy blood supply from the axillary artery and avascular necrosis (AVN) is rarely a concern.

The shoulder does not have inherent bony stability as the hip does. The shoulder relies on the capsule and surrounding muscles to maintain its integrity.

It is important to understand the relationship of the bony anatomy to the brachial plexus.

RADIOGRAPHIC ISSUES

In most emergency departments, an injured shoulder is studied with an AP and axillary view of the shoulder (Fig. 7-1).

It is difficult to get orthogonal x-rays (two views at right angles) of an injured shoulder. Often an axillary view is not possible because the child is unable to elevate the arm, and moving the arm may further displace the fracture. In such cases, you should consider a transthoracic lateral or a scapular Y view in addition to the AP view to properly and safely evaluate shoulder fractures (Table 7-1). The transthoracic view is difficult to read because the ribs are in the way, but it gives the best information without moving the extremity.

If the joint is involved, either the glenoid or the humeral epiphysis, a CT scan will give a clearer picture, allowing you to better evaluate the joint surface.

Ultrasound of the shoulder girdle can help to identify fractures in infants without the risk of radiation and is a better study if you are concerned about epiphyseal separation when the head is not yet ossified.

Table 7-1 Views to Assess the Child's Shoulder				
AP w/ IR	AP w/ ER	Axillary	Transthoracic	Scapular-Y

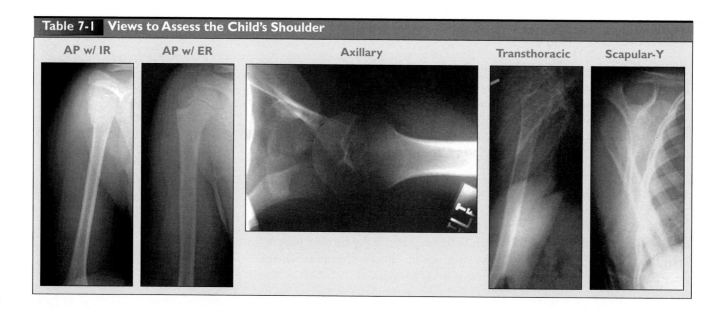

NEWBORN FRACTURES

Separation of the proximal humeral epiphysis frequently occurs during difficult deliveries when the shoulder becomes lodged in the pelvic outlet or when the arm is used to assist in extraction of the infant. The fracture is often difficult to localize and is frequently confused with a brachial plexus injury until abundant callus formation is palpable or noted on x-ray. Clinically, the infant may have an asymmetric Moro reflex as the only sign of injury or may refuse to move the arm at all. It is often impossible to sort out neurologic injury versus immobility secondary to the pain of an acute fracture ("pseudoparalysis").

The vast majority of shoulder girdle fractures sustained during delivery (Fig. 7-2) can be treated by simply pinning the infant's shirt sleeve to the shirt or using an elastic wrap around the body to immobilize the injured upper extremity for 2 to 3 weeks. Reduction and/or surgery are virtually never necessary in this age group. Birth fractures heal extremely quickly with abundant callus formation and remodel leaving little or no residual deformity. Once the fracture has healed, a better neurologic exam can be completed to evaluate for brachial plexus injury that may have occurred simultaneously.

SHOULDER DISLOCATION

Traumatic dislocation is typically seen in older adolescents after the epiphyses have closed (Fig. 7-3). This should be treated as an adult injury with relocation and immobilization followed by rehabilitation. Anterior dislocations should be immobilized in a shoulder immobilizer for 4-6 weeks, whereas posterior dislocations require a gunslinger splint or spica to maintain the shoulder in external rotation and abduction. Gunslinger splints are being used more frequently for anterior dislocations and proximal humerus fractures. The standard shoulder immobilizer holds the shoulder in internal rotation so the anterior structures scar down and prevent later external rotation.

Recurrent dislocation has been reported to be as high as 100% following traumatic dislocation in young patients (Rowe), and many articles report an incidence of 50%-90% regardless of treatment following the first dislocation.

Although many surgical interventions have been described for adults, there are very few reports of long-term outcomes following surgical intervention in children and adolescents. Any surgical intervention will require long-term rehabilitation with progressive physical therapy starting with gentle pendulum exercises and advancing to active motion and eventually strengthening.

Shoulder dislocations can result in a Hill Sachs lesion, which is an indentation of the articular surface of the humeral head (Fig. 7-4). They can also result in a Bankart lesion, which is an avulsion of the anterio-inferior glenoid labrum. This is the primary lesion in recurrent anterior instability.

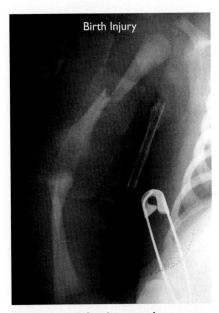

Figure 7-2. Infant humerus fractures are often sustained during difficult deliveries. They are easily treated with a few weeks of immobilization.

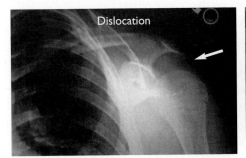
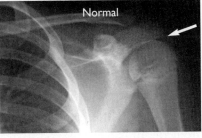

Figure 7-3. Traumatic dislocation is typically seen in older adolescents after the epiphyses have closed. This should be treated as an adult injury with relocation and immobilization followed by rehabilitation.

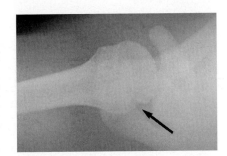

Figure 7-4. This is a patient with recurrent anterior dislocations. Note the anterior subluxation of the humeral head, and the Hill Sachs lesion (arrow).

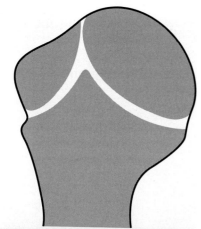

Normal X-ray

Figure 7-5. Tent-shaped physis of proximal humerus. This pattern often makes reading of x-rays difficult.

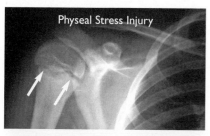

Physeal Stress Injury

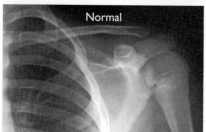

Normal

Figure 7-6. Pitchers may pull apart their proximal humeral physis—on this x-ray, note the widening of the physis and sclerosis signifying chronic stress. The same injury can also be seen in gymnasts.

"Party trick" dislocation or voluntary dislocation occurs in children with increased joint laxity and typically is not related to an injury. These patients are treated with strengthening exercises and surgical intervention should be avoided. Often, these loose-jointed children have difficulty with sports that stress the shoulder (swimming, throwing—overhead sports).

PROXIMAL HUMERUS

The proximal humerus has a tent-shaped growth plate and very thick posterior periosteum (Fig. 7-5). The proximal physis contributes 80% of the growth of the humerus. Force on the shoulder in pediatric patients typically produces a physeal fracture instead of dislocation as is seen in skeletally mature patients. A direct blow to the posterior shoulder or a fall on the outstretched hand frequently result in proximal humeral fracture; falls from horses are the most common mechanism resulting in this type of injury.

Classification

Proximal humerus fractures are broken down into physeal fractures (usually Salter-Harris I in patients up to age 5 years and Salter-Harris II in older patients), metaphyseal fractures, and fractures of the greater or lesser tuberosity.

Neer has classified the degree of displacement into four grades:

I.   Less than 5 mm displacement
II. One-third displacement
III. Two-thirds displacement
IV. More than two-thirds displacement

About 70% of patients have Grade-I or Grade-II displacement and require no more than a sling. Several methods of treatment have been advocated for the more severe grades of displacement.

Chronic proximal humerus separation has been reported in gymnasts, baseball pitchers, patients previously treated with radiation, and children with metabolic abnormalities. Repetitive motion with distractive forces can lead to physeal stress injuries or separation.

Treatment

Stress injuries to the physis (and the very rare slipped epiphysis) heal with rest in a sling or shoulder immobilizer for 4 weeks. The most important and most difficult part of the treatment is to stop the child from continuing the damaging activity (gymnastics or pitching) while the physis heals (Fig. 7-6).

Salter-Harris I fractures can be treated with gentle manipulation with traction, abduction, and flexion followed by short-term immobilization (3-4 weeks).

Adolescent Salter-Harris II injuries may be difficult to reduce and maintain; however, good results are the rule when these fractures are treated conservatively. About 70% of patients have mild to moderate displacement and require no more than a sling. Because 80% of the humeral growth comes from the proximal physis, this region has a great capacity for remodeling. The shoulder has a thick muscle cover and malunions tend not to be a cosmetic problem.

TECHNIQUE TIPS:
Immobilization Methods for Humeral Shaft Fractures and Shoulder Injuries

Hanging Arm Cast

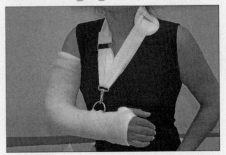

To supply traction to align humeral shaft fractures.

Shoulder Immobilizer

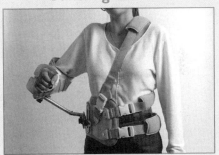

Most commonly used brace for shoulder and humerus injuries.

Sarmiento Brace

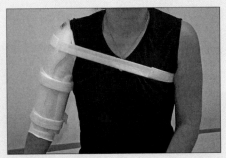

Custom brace for stabilization of humeral shaft fractures.
Brace courtesy of Bluebird Orthotics and Prosthetics—San Diego, CA.

Gunslinger Brace

Keeps the shoulder in external rotation to prevent contracture of the anterior capsule.
Photo courtesy of Seattle Systems.

Application of Velpeau Bandage (an inexpensive shoulder immobilizer)

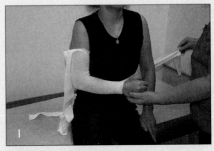

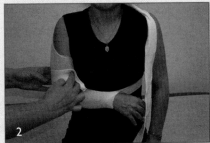

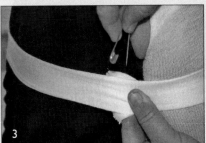

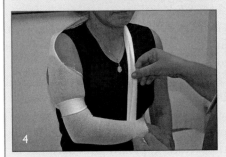

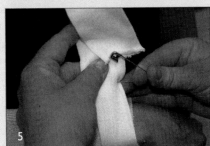

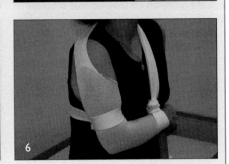

At Injury

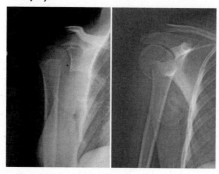

2 Weeks After Injury

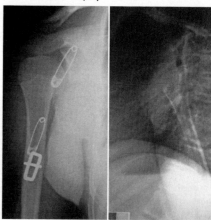

At Injury

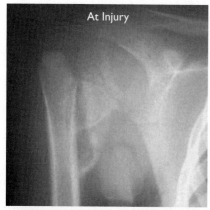

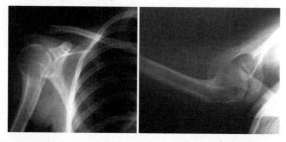

At Injury

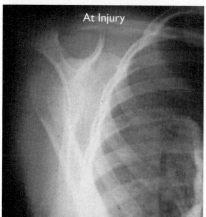

10 Months After Injury

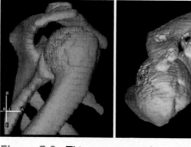
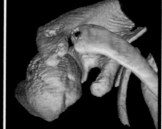

10 Months After Injury—
Malunion and limited motion

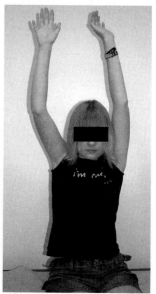

10 Months After Injury

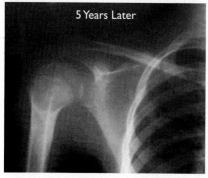

5 Years Later

Figure 7-7. This 6-year-old patient presented late with this severe Salter-Harris proximal humeral fracture. Over the next 5 years, the fracture completely remodeled and she went on to have normal shoulder function.

Figure 7-8. This teenager with a proximal humerus fracture and apparent mild displacement on x-ray healed with a malunion that slightly decreased her range of motion such that she was no longer able to play volleyball at a competitive level.

Amazingly, even severely displaced fractures can remodel in young children (Fig. 7-7).

Risk for Malunion—Need for Reduction

Although young children have excellent remodeling potential, less deformity can be accepted in a teenager. If the fracture heals with anterior bowing, shoulder flexion and abduction will be blocked. With little time remaining for remodeling, the patient will be left with a permanent loss of full shoulder motion.

Closed reduction followed by traction or casting with a Statue of Liberty cast has been described but is mainly of historical interest.

Closed reduction and percutaneous pinning permits the arm to be brought down to the side while reduction is maintained.

Open reduction is rarely necessary but can be used for fractures that are irreducible into an acceptable position secondary to interposed soft tissue (usually the biceps tendon) or periosteum. A deltopectoral approach gives adequate exposure for proximal humeral fractures; screw or pin fixation will then maintain the reduction. Intramedullary rodding can be used with distal insertion (at the

TECHNIQUE TIPS:
Closed Reduction and Pinning of Proximal Humerus Fractures

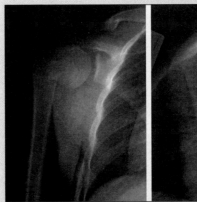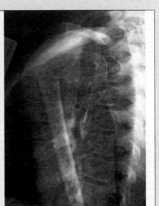

For significantly displaced proximal humeral fractures in patients with little remodeling potential (teenagers), closed reduction and percutaneous pinning is recommended.

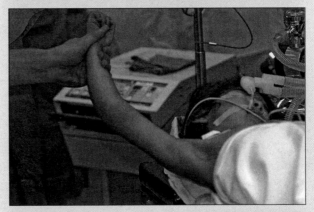

A sheet is placed around the body to provide counter traction. Care must be taken to protect the head and neck. While maintaining traction, the arm is brought out into abduction and flexion.

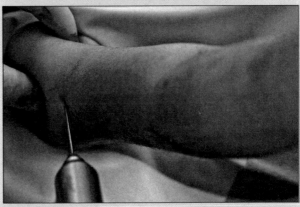

Flouroscopy can be used to check AP and axillary views. If the reduction is unstable, pins can be inserted from the lateral cortex (avoiding the axillary nerve) and into the humeral head.

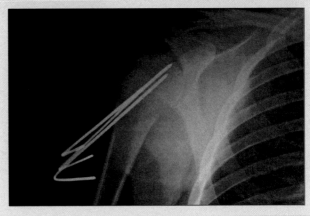

We often use K-wires or guide pins for cannulated screws as the treaded tip prevents early back out of the pins. The pins are bent and cut outside the skin. To be pulled out in 3 weeks.

lateral epicondyle). The 2-mm flexible rods can assist with reduction as well as maintenance of alignment.

Other Fractures of the Proximal Humerus

Greenstick fractures are common and can be treated symptomatically. Completely displaced metaphyseal fractures are more difficult than physeal injuries. The shaft may penetrate the deltoid to lie subcutaneously. A short incision may be required to disengage the distal fragment and push it back into place. This is typically a stable reduction in a sling without internal fixation.

Greater tuberosity fractures are almost never seen in children; on the rare occasion that one is encountered, it can be treated nonoperatively if minimally displaced. If there is marked displacement, open reduction and internal fixation should be considered as with adult fractures.

Lesser tuberosity fractures are also rare and can usually be treated symptomatically. Athletes that require significant subscapularis strength (competitive swimmers) may require open reduction and internal fixation to reattach the subscapularis insertion.

The majority of proximal humerus fractures should be treated nonoperatively because there is an amazing potential for remodeling and excellent outcome despite significant angulation and displacement (Figs. 7-9, 7-10). Surgery should not be the first line of treatment but is an option for some severe fractures and special situations as discussed in this chapter.

HUMERAL SHAFT

Transverse humeral shaft fractures are the result of a direct blow (Fig. 7-11). Spiral fractures are produced by a twist; even muscular violence will do this (Fig. 7-12). Spiral fractures are a common injury in soldiers learning to throw hand grenades.

These fractures are easily treated because they reduce themselves under the influence of gravity. The only important part of treatment is to maintain good public relations with the family. There are many ways of treating the fracture. A Velpeau bandage held in place with one roll of plaster or a stockinette Velpeau is simple for minimally displaced stable fractures. A U-slab provides better fixation. We often use a hanging arm cast to allow gravity to help reduce the fracture. Sarmiento braces are an excellent choice for midshaft fractures. We typically splint the patient when the swelling comes down and then the child is molded for a Sarmiento brace.

At Injury

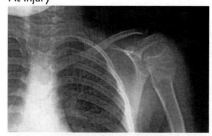

6 Months Later

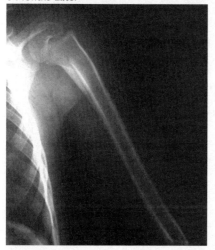

Figure 7-9. Minimally displaced metaphyseal fractures of the proximal humerus can be treated with a sling or shoulder immobilizer for comfort. They tend to remodel nicely.

At Injury   6 Months Later   1 Year Later

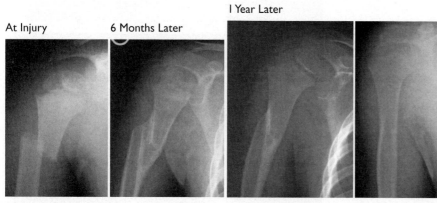

Figure 7-10. Fractures near the growth physis in a growing child have an amazing potential to remodel.

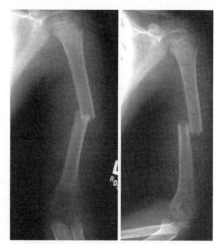

Figure 7-11. Transverse humeral shaft fractures are usually the result of a direct blow.

For a week, an attempt should be made to prop the child up at night for sleep. Bayonet apposition is satisfactory because overgrowth of about 1 cm can be expected. Varus angulation is common but should be kept at less than 20°. At the lower end, angular malunion may show and should be corrected; this is accomplished by manipulating the cast a bit. Immobilization for 3-4 weeks is sufficient.

Open fractures with bone loss at the lower end may not unite. Grafting and compression plating may be required and should be carried out before the elbow becomes stiff.

Pitfalls—Humeral Shaft Fractures

The radial nerve wraps around the humerus and may be injured by the fracture or the reduction. Radial nerve palsy is particularly likely to occur in fractures at the junction of the middle and lower thirds of the shaft. The nerve may become trapped between the fracture fragments. If a nerve palsy is present at presentation, watchful waiting is usually recommended. Spontaneous recovery can be expected; look for this first in the brachioradialis. If the fracture remains separated by soft tissue interposition, or if a radial nerve palsy follows manipulation, explore right away; otherwise, save exploration for the child with no signs of recovery after 3 months.

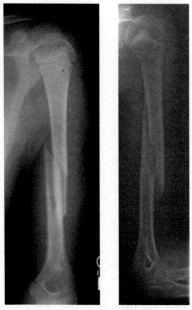

Figure 7-12. Spiral humeral fractures are often sustained after twisting or throwing.

SCAPULA

Classification

There are many classification schemes for scapula fractures; however, none are specific to pediatric patients. The important things to understand and describe are the location of the fracture within the scapula (body, neck, coracoid, acromion, or glenoid), associated fractures of the clavicle or AC joint that destabilize the shoulder, and amount of displacement.

Treatment

Fortunately, scapular fractures in children are rare and almost never require specific treatment. Scapular body fractures tend to heal in adequate alignment regardless of treatment as the muscular envelope maintains the shape of the scapula (Fig. 7-13). Isolated body fractures can be treated symptomatically with a sling or shoulder immobilizer.

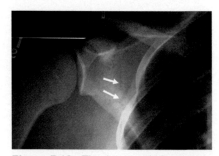

Figure 7-13. This 16-year-old boy was in a motorcross accident and sustained a scapular body fracture. Scapular fractures are typically nondisplaced and heal with little intervention, treatment is symptomatic.

Scapular neck fractures in isolation typically do not require anything beyond symptomatic treatment; however, if there is an associated clavicle fracture or AC dislocation, the shoulder joint becomes destabilized and may require intervention. In the case of unstable fractures, some recommend open reduction and fixation of the clavicle to maintain the suspensory function of the scapulo-clavicular complex. Others recommend ORIF of both the scapular neck and clavicle fracture.

Coracoid fractures with minimal displacement are treated conservatively. Again, if there is an associated clavicle fracture, some authors recommend ORIF of at least the clavicle fracture.

Acromial fractures are typically physeal fractures in the pediatric patient and the vast majority can be treated symptomatically with excellent results. Os acromionale can be a normal finding on x-ray and may be difficult to distinguish from a fracture. X-rays of the contralateral shoulder will help to differentiate fracture from a normal anatomic variant.

"Fortunately scapular fractures in children are rare and almost never require specific treatment"

Glenoid fractures are the scapular fractures most likely to lead to arthritis and disability later in life. As with most joints, a step-off greater than 2 mm is not well tolerated and every effort should be made to obtain anatomic alignment. The glenoid is very difficult to approach through an open incision and internal fixation is difficult given the anatomy of the scapula with its paper thin body; so many surgeons prefer nonoperative methods when possible. Skeletal traction can be used or early range of motion to attempt to recontour the glenoid during the early healing process. If the equipment and expertise are available, glenoid fractures can be reduced and fixed arthroscopically.

Suggested Readings

Beringer DC, Weiner DS, Noble JS, Bell RH. Severely displaced proximal humeral epiphyseal fractures: a follow-up study. J Pediatr Orthop. 1998 Jan-Feb;18(1):31-7.

Dameron TB, Reibel DB: Fractures involving the proximal humeral epiphyseal plate. J Bone Joint Surg 51A:289, 1969.

Deitch J, Mehlman CT, Foad SL, Obbehat A, Mallory M. Traumatic anterior shoulder dislocation in adolescents. Am J Sports Med. 2003 Sep-Oct;31(5):758-63.

Dobbs MB, Luhmann SL, Gordon JE, Strecker WB, Schoenecker PL. Severely displaced proximal humeral epiphyseal fractures. J Pediatr Orthop. 2003 Mar-Apr;23(2):208-15.

Goldberg BJ, Nirschl RP, McConnell JP, Petttrone FA. Arthroscopic transglenoid suture capsulolabral repairs: preliminary results. Am J Sports Med. 1993 Sep-Oct;21(5):656-64; discussion 664-5.

Lawton RL, Choudhury S, Mansat P, Cofield RH, Stans AA. Pediatric shoulder instability: presentation, findings, treatment, and outcomes. J Pediatr Orthop. 2002 Jan-Feb;22(1):52-61.

Moore EM: Epiphyseal fractures of the superior extremity of the humerus. Trans Am Med Assoc 25:296,1974.

Neer CS, Horwitz BS: Fractures of the proximal epiphyseal plate. Clin Orthop 41:24, 1965.

Rowe CR, Pierce DS, Clark JG: Voluntary dislocation of the shoulder. J Bone Joint Surg 55A:445, 1973.

Smith FM: Fracture - separation of the proximal humeral epiphysis. Am J Surg 91:627, 1956.

Visser CP, Coene LN, Brand R, Tavy DL. Nerve lesions in proximal humeral fractures. J Shoulder Elbow Surg. 2001 Sep-Oct;10(5):421-7.

Williams DJ: The mechanisms producing fracture—separation of the proximal humeral epiphysis. J Bone Joint Surg 63B:102, 1981.

Elbow—Distal Humerus

Maya Pring ❧ Mercer Rang ❧ Dennis Wenger

INTRODUCTION

The last edition of this book started the elbow chapter with "Pity the young surgeon whose first case is a fracture around the elbow…at every stage these fractures present difficulties: difficulties of diagnosis and reduction, vascular and neurologic problems, slippage in the cast, malunion, and stiffness."

However, in 1995, Rang and Gillingham revised the statement to "it is no longer necessary to pity the young surgeon whose first case is a child's elbow fracture. Current education will have prepared him or her for it. Save pity for the old surgeon unacquainted with the advances that have taken place in the diagnosis and treatment of elbow fractures. Modern methods have improved outcome but are more technical. Technical skills, once mastered, are inclined to rust without use. The gap between those who can pin an elbow and those who cannot continues to widen."

> *"We retain from our studies only that which we practically apply"*
> —GOETHE

"It is no longer necessary to pity the young surgeon whose first case is a child's elbow fracture"

"The elbow, more than most other joints, can readily become stiff following injury or surgery"

Although they are not simple fractures, the goal of this chapter is to help you recognize and treat pediatric elbow fractures while avoiding the complications that are abundant in the older literature.

Anatomy

The elbow is a sophisticated joint composed of three separate articulations: radiocapitelar, proximal radioulnar, and ulnohumeral. The spiral orientation of the trochlea allows flexion and extension about an oblique axis; this brings the forearm from a position parallel to the humerus in full flexion to a valgus carrying angle of 15° in extension (Fig 8-1).

The carrying angle has evolutionary significance, allowing the upper extremity to carry an item with clearance of the pelvis as the arm swings. Females have a slightly greater carrying angle because the pelvis is wider.

The elbow also allows pronation and supination about the long axis of the forearm (Fig. 8-2). These complex motions require maintenance of an anatomic relationship between all three articulations. Fracture management requires an understanding as to what degree of angle change or displacement requires surgical intervention. Unfortunately, anatomic reduction and union do not guarantee good postinjury motion.

The elbow, more than most other joints, can readily become stiff following injury or surgery. Often, the surgeon must make the difficult decision of early motion (and risk for non-union) versus cast immobilization (and possible stiffness). In addition to complex design issues, there are multiple growth plates near the elbow that fractures often traverse. If not properly treated, this can lead to nonunion or growth arrest.

ASSESSING THE PATIENT

In the busy season, we may see 50 injured and/or swollen elbows each week. As a note of precaution, on initial exam, it may be very difficult to distinguish between an injured and an infected elbow in a young child. At least twice a year, we see a child with a history of trauma and a swollen elbow who turns out to have a septic

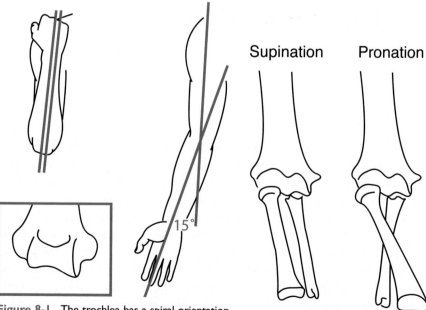

Figure 8-1. The trochlea has a spiral orientation that brings the forearm from in-line with the humerus in flexion to a carrying angle of 15°, valgus in extension.

Figure 8-2. In addition to flexion and extension, the elbow allows ~90° of supination and pronation.

joint. Never let the history of trauma lead you away from suspecting infection, especially in a young child with a "soft" history (a soft history often consists of "she has a sore elbow since yesterday. Her six-year-old sister says she "fell down""). The questions regarding who observed the injury must be precise. Did the child scream with pain immediately? Who observed this? If the picture is not clear, order a complete blood count (CBC), sedimentation rate, and C-reactive protein to rule out infection.

Once the area of concern is identified, gentle palpation may help with fracture localization, but this is often difficult in an uncomfortable young child with a painful elbow. Carefully examine the skin to rule out an open fracture. Check areas where the skin is tented or at-risk; the sharp bone ends of a displaced supracondylar fracture can easily penetrate the skin; a closed fracture may be only a cell layer or two from an open fracture.

The contralateral elbow should be examined to determine the normal carrying angle and the child's natural ligamentous laxity or ability to hyperextend.

Next, the examiner proceeds with vascular assessment; radial pulses should be symmetric and capillary refill less than 2 seconds. If pulses are not palpable, a Doppler can be used to check for blood flow to the hand. A dysvascular hand is an emergency and should be taken to the operating room (OR) for immediate reduction. A compartment syndrome can also impede blood flow and must be addressed immediately (see Chapter 19).

Older children can comply with your neurologic exam: test the radial nerve by asking the child to extend the thumb (Table 8-1). Anterior interosseous nerve testing includes flexion of the distal interphalangeal joint of the index finger and the interphalangeal joint of the thumb. The ability to grasp indicates median nerve function, and finger spread and ability to cross the fingers indicates that the ulnar nerve is functioning. Test sensation to light touch and/or 2-point discrimination on the radial and ulnar sides of each digit and over the dorsum of the thenar web.

Unfortunately, young injured children are not capable of complying with this neurologic exam; avoid documenting that the patient is "neurovascularly intact" (NVI) unless each test has been successfully performed. Document only what you can effectively test; if the patient has a nerve palsy postoperatively and you have written NVI on the initial exam sheet, it may be difficult to prove that the nerve injury was not caused by the reduction (or surgery).

The neurovascular status of the upper extremity must be monitored carefully until definitive treatment is completed and for at least 24 hours following treat-

"The questions regarding who observed the injury must be precise. Did the child scream with pain immediately? Who observed this? If the picture is not clear order a CBC, sed rate, and CRP to rule out infection"

Table 8-1	Quick Motor Nerve Testing for the Upper Extremity
"Thumbs up"	"OK"

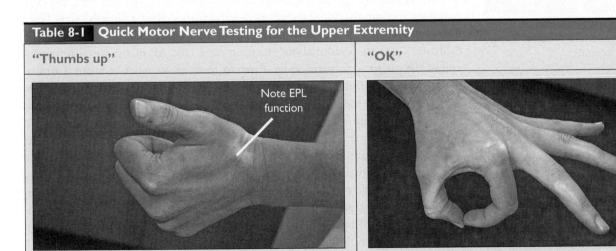

Note EPL function

| Radial nerve—Extension of wrist and thumb | Unlar nerve—Abduction of digits 3-5 |
| Median nerve—Flexion of digits 2-3 | Anterior interosseous nerve—Flexion of index and thumb DIP |

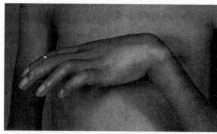

Figure 8-3. Volkmann's ischmic contracture, a dreaded complication of a supracondylar fracture, is much less common in the era of percutaneous pinning.

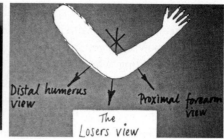

Figure 8-4. "Loser's view"—with the elbow flexed. It may be difficult to get a true AP of the distal humerus or proximal forearm.

AP	Lateral	Oblique

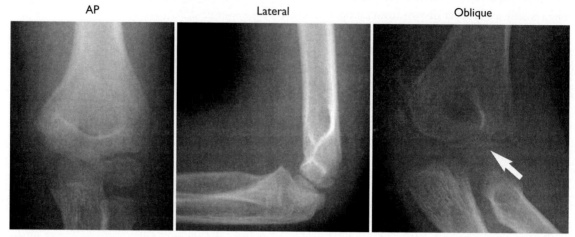

Figure 8-5. Lateral condyle fractures may be difficult to see on AP and lateral x-rays—oblique x-rays show the true displacement of the fracture (arrow).

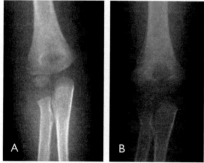

Figure 8-6. A) The occult fracture B) was better understood once callus formed after 3 weeks of casting.

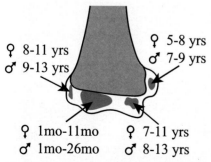

Figure 8-7. Age at ossification of the distal humerus growth centers for males and females. (Adapted from Haraldsson.)

♀ 8-11 yrs
♂ 9-13 yrs

♀ 5-8 yrs
♂ 7-9 yrs

♀ 1mo-11mo
♂ 1mo-26mo

♀ 7-11 yrs
♂ 8-13 yrs

ment. The risk of compartment syndrome and Volkmann's contracture (Fig. 8-3) is increased by casting and by elbow flexion of more than 90°. For arms that are at risk of developing compartment syndrome following difficult reductions, it is better to use a posterior splint with the elbow in less than 80° of flexion until the swelling has resolved.

RADIOGRAPHIC ISSUES

Obtaining true AP and lateral x-rays in the injured child can test even the best radiology technician. Some radiology departments deliver a "loser's" view (Fig. 8-4)—an AP view of an elbow flexed about 90°, which makes diagnosis more difficult. Don't be bashful about insisting on a true AP of the distal humerus and of the proximal forearm, even if two or more views must be taken. Correct diagnosis is everything. Sometimes only the conviction that there must be a fracture will drive the clinician to obtain oblique films of the joint, radiographs of the normal elbow, or even stress films.

Although many fractures are obvious on the AP and lateral x-ray, some are not. Occult fractures may be detected only by clinical suspicion and a careful study of the soft tissue on x-ray. The displacement of lateral condyle fractures may only be visible on oblique x-rays (Fig. 8-5); if there is any question about the direction or amount of displacement, four views (AP, lateral, and two oblique views) will help. The fracture is sometimes only visualized when callus begins to form after 3 weeks of immobilization (Fig. 8-6).

Growth plates cause much confusion for those who do not regularly treat children's fractures. Fortunately, the opposite elbow can be radiographed as a control, which is extremely useful in determining the normal anatomy for a particular child. Understanding the timing of growth center ossification and fusion helps the orthopedic surgeon in evaluating an elbow injury, but it is generally not part of a primary doctor's training (Fig. 8-7).

Even for the experienced pediatric orthopedist, there are times when the exact diagnosis remains elusive. Some cases may require an arthrogram, CT, or MRI to further clarify the fracture. This is most likely in young children in whom much of the elbow remains as radiolucent cartilage.

X-ray Landmarks

Several x-ray landmarks help in evaluating an injured elbow:

Baumann's angle on the standard AP x-ray assesses the angulation of the physeal line (of the lateral condyle) in relation to the long axis of the humeral shaft (Fig. 8-8). A normal Baumann's angle is approximately 20°. A decrease in Baumann's angle (0° for example) suggests cubitus varus.

The **anterior humeral line** on the lateral view should pass through the middle third of the ossification center of the capitellum. The anterior humeral line of an extension type supracondylar fracture will intersect the capitellum more anteriorly or may not intersect it at all (Fig. 8-9).

On the lateral x-ray, the **shaft-condylar angle** should be about 40°. A decrease in this angle suggests hyperextension through the fracture site (Fig. 8-10).

Fat pad sign (often referred to as a sail sign) is a small amount of fat that overlies the elbow joint both anteriorly and posteriorly. With injury (or sepsis) and elbow swelling, the fat is pushed away from the bone and may be visible on a high-quality lateral x-ray. An anterior fat pad is a normal finding on many pedi-

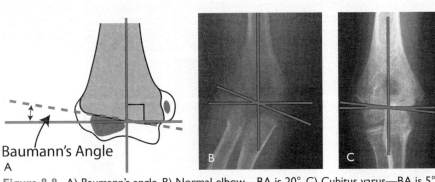

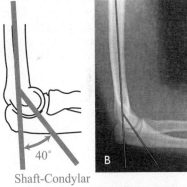

Figure 8-8. A) Baumann's angle. B) Normal elbow—BA is 20°. C) Cubitus varus—BA is 5°.

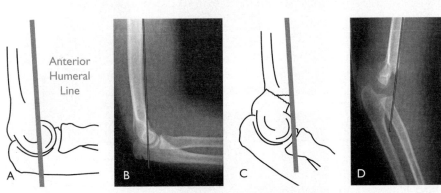

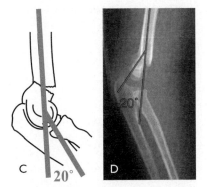

Figure 8-9. A-B) The anterior humeral line should intersect the middle third of the capitellum. C-D) If the anterior humeral line is anterior to the capitellum, the extension supracondylar fracture needs to be reduced.

Figure 8-10. A-B) A normal shaft-condylar angle is ~ 40°. C-D) This angle decreases with extension of a supracondylar fracture.

atric elbow x-rays; a posterior fat pad on x-ray often indicates an occult fracture about the elbow (Table 8-2).

With a posterior fat pad sign and no obvious fracture, oblique x-rays should be obtained to help rule out medial or lateral condyle fractures. Skaggs and Mirzayan prospectively examined a group of children with acute elbow trauma and a posterior fat pad sign without a visible fracture on AP and lateral x-rays. At 3 weeks, new radiographs were taken and were evaluated for signs of fracture healing; they found that 34 out of 45 patients (76%) had evidence of an elbow fracture. These included:

- Supracondylar fractures—53%
- Proximal ulna fractures—26%
- Lateral condyle fractures—12%
- Radial neck fractures—9%

FRACTURE TYPES:

TRANSPHYSEAL DISTAL HUMERUS FRACTURES

Separation of the distal humeral epiphysis in an infant with an unossified epiphysis looks like a dislocation (Fig. 8-11). Remember that dislocation of the elbow without an associated fracture is very rare in children. Transphyseal distal humerus fractures are frequently associated with child abuse and warrant further investigation. They occur only in young children.

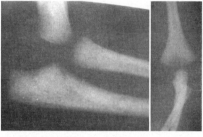

Figure 8-11. Transphyseal fractures may be confused with an elbow dislocation on x-ray. Remember that elbow dislocations in children are rare without an associated fracture.

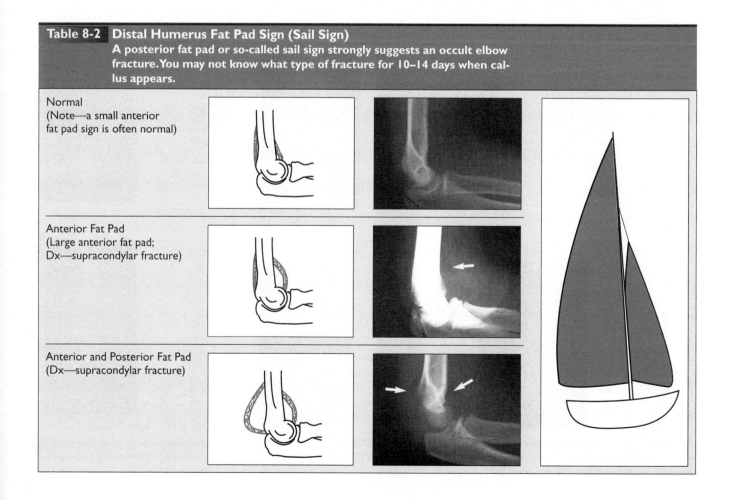

Table 8-2	Distal Humerus Fat Pad Sign (Sail Sign)
	A posterior fat pad or so-called sail sign strongly suggests an occult elbow fracture. You may not know what type of fracture for 10–14 days when callus appears.

Normal (Note—a small anterior fat pad sign is often normal)			
Anterior Fat Pad (Large anterior fat pad; Dx—supracondylar fracture)			
Anterior and Posterior Fat Pad (Dx—supracondylar fracture)			

Typically the distal fragment is displaced posteriorly and medially, so the alignment of the proximal radius and ulna are no longer in line with the distal humerus. In comparison (although extremely rare in young children), elbow dislocations usually have posterolateral displacement of the proximal radius and ulna. If there is inadequate ossification to evaluate the fracture on plain films, an ultrasound study or arthrogram can help to classify the diagnosis.

Many of these injuries have a small piece of the distal metaphyseal bone attached to the physis and are thus technically a Salter-Harris II fracture pattern. Radiographic evidence of this small Thurston-Holland triangular fragment plus posteromedial displacement of the proximal radius and ulna helps to confirm the diagnosis.

"Transphyseal distal humerus fractures are frequently associated with child abuse and warrant further investigation"

Classification—Transphyseal Fractures

Delee classified transphyseal fractures into three groups (Table 8-3) based on the degree of ossification of the lateral condylar epiphysis (lateral condyle begins to ossify around 1 year of age). Group A fractures are Salter-Harris type I. Group B fractures can be Salter-Harris I or II. Group C fractures are classified as Salter-Harris II and are identified by the metaphyseal fragment (also know as a Thurston-Holland fragment) that remains with the epiphysis (see Chapter 14 for further description of the Thurston-Holland fragment).

Treatment—Transphyseal Fractures

If the fracture is diagnosed early (less than 5 days), closed reduction plus cast immobilization is recommended for transphyseal fractures (Fig. 8-12). Keeping the arm flexed and pronated assists with maintaining the reduction, allowing casting in this position as treatment for infants.

Older children have a greater risk for cubitus varus and usually require percutaneous pinning following closed reduction; two lateral pins are adequate with the pins left in place to maintain alignment for 3 weeks until healing is complete. An arthrogram can be used to confirm the reduction if there is insufficient ossified bone to confirm fragment position.

Frequently, children are brought in late with transphyseal fractures (particularly if they are secondary to child abuse); if the fracture is more than 5 days old, or there is periosteal new bone noted on x-ray, the fracture should probably not be reduced because the reduction maneuver may cause further damage to

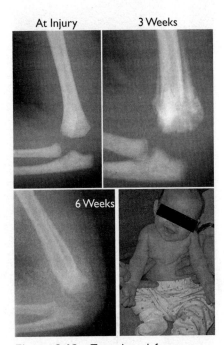

Figure 8-12. Transphyseal fracture sustained during delivery healed with significant callus at 3 weeks. At follow-up the patient had full range of motion at the elbow.

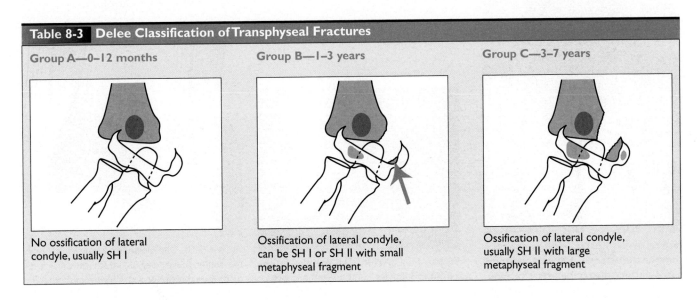

Table 8-3	Delee Classification of Transphyseal Fractures	
Group A—0–12 months	**Group B—1–3 years**	**Group C—3–7 years**
No ossification of lateral condyle, usually SH I	Ossification of lateral condyle, can be SH I or SH II with small metaphyseal fragment	Ossification of lateral condyle, usually SH II with large metaphyseal fragment

the physis. Such fractures should be splinted or casted for comfort and often adequate remodeling occurs in infants. If there is not sufficient remodeling, an osteotomy can be done to correct alignment when the patient is older.

Pitfalls—Transphyseal Fractures

Recognizing the injury as a "classic sign" of child abuse and completing a social workup prior to discharge may be may be the most important issue for future safety of the child. Failure to identify transphyseal fractures is a common pitfall (Fig. 8-13), with cubitus varus the most common deformity following undertreated transphyseal fractures (Fig. 8-14).

The vascular supply to the medial crista of the trochlea travels through the physis and injury to this blood supply can cause avascular necrosis (AVN) of the trochlea. Yoo reported 8 patients who developed AVN of the trochlea following transphyseal distal humerus fractures. This appears as a "fishtail" defect on x-rays (Fig. 8-15).

SUPRACONDYLAR FRACTURES

Supracondylar fractures are produced by forcibly hyperextending the elbow. The level of the fracture is determined by the olecranon forming a fulcrum in the supracondylar region (Fig. 8-16); the collateral ligaments of the elbow attached to the metaphysis usually prevent dislocation.

These fractures are more common in children with naturally hyperextendible joints, likely because a 10°-20° normal hyperextension makes the lever arm more efficient. Traditionally, boys were reported to be at higher risk of sustaining supracondylar fractures, but our series showed a slight preponderance for girls to sustain this injury. Females more commonly have natural joint hyperextensibility as compared to their male counterparts, which may increase their risk. Also in our area, females lead a very rigorous sporting life, earning the honor of a supracondylar fracture incidence equal to or greater then their male counter parts.

In experiments, the periosteum remains intact so long as the force is pure hyperextension. When the fracture is forcibly rotated, the sharp corner of the proximal fragment tears the periosteum, permitting gross displacement (Fig. 8-17). With progressively more force, the sharp edge will first tear the brachialis and then the skin. It also puts the neurovascular structures at risk.

At Injury

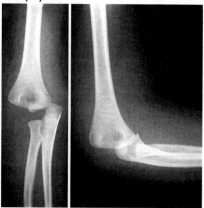

After Treatment

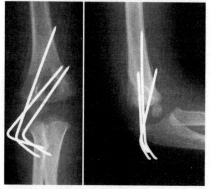

Figure 8-13. Transphyseal fracture of distal humerus in a child. One must think of child abuse in such a case. A) At injury. B) After reduction plus K-wire fixation.

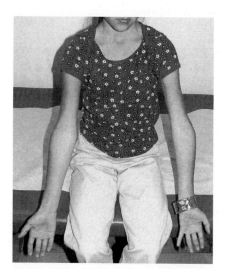

Figure 8-14. Cubitus varus is the most common late deformity following an undiagnosed and untreated transphyseal fracture.

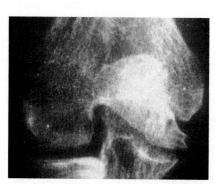

Figure 8-15. AVN of the trochlea causes a fish-tail deformity of the distal humerus.

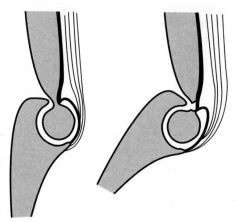

Figure 8-16. The olecranon forms a fulcrum in the supracondylar region, which causes a fracture when the elbow is forcibly hyperextended.

Nerve injuries are usually transient stretch injuries and are relatively common in displaced supracondylar fractures, Campbell reported a 49% incidence of neurovascular compromise in patients evaluated for type III supracondylar fractures. Fifty-two percent of the injuries were to the median nerve (usually with posterolateral displacement) and 28% to the radial nerve (all from posteromedial displacement).

Classification—Supracondylar Fractures

The standard classification of supracondylar humerus fractures includes extension and flexion types; flexion type fractures are much less common with the distal fragment anterior to the shaft on the lateral x-ray. The more common extension fractures are classified as types I through III. Type I are minimally displaced, type II are extended but have a posterior hinge, and type III are completely displaced. Extension fractures can be further subdivided as described in Table 8-4.

Treatment—Supracondylar Fractures

Prior to definitive management, the elbow should be splinted in about 30° of flexion. Flexing a displaced supracondylar fracture in a splint tends to compress the neurovascular structures. Also, splinting in full extension may increase pressure in the neurovascular structures (by spicules of the fractured distal humerus). It is foolish to have a child waiting for radiographs with an ischemic limb. Put the splint on before the radiographs are taken to keep the technician from twisting the arm through the fracture.

Specific treatment of this injury has two goals:
1. Avoiding neurologic and vascular problems
2. Preventing long-term angular (usually cubitus varus) and extension deformity

Cubitus varus used to be thought of as a "cosmetic deformity" but is now recognized as a condition that places the child at risk for later fractures, specifically lateral condyle fractures (Davids et al.).

TYPE I SUPRACONDYLAR FRACTURES

Most type I supracondylar fractures can be treated with cast immobilization (for about 3 weeks). Prior to deciding on conservative management, the contralateral elbow should be checked for hyperextension. If the patient naturally has significant laxity and hyperextension (as determined by examining the normal elbow), even a mild increase in this extension due to a slightly extended supracondylar fracture can lead to significant deformity (Fig. 8-18). Thus the

"Traditionally, boys were reported to be at higher risk of sustaining supracondylar fractures, but our series showed a slight preponderance for girls to sustain this injury."

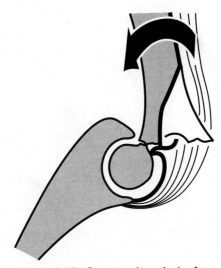

Figure 8-17. Rotation through the fracture may cause the sharp anterior spike to tear through the brachialis and skin.

"Cubitus varus used to be thought of as a 'cosmetic deformity' but is now recognized as a condition that places the child at risk for later fractures (specifically lateral condyle fractures)"

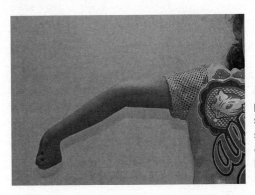

Figure 8-18. Patients with natural hyperextension may be at increased risk of supracondylar fractures. Allowing a supracondylar fracture to heal slightly extended may cause gross deformity in a hyperlax child (and put them at risk for re-fracture).

more naturally lax the child, the greater the indication for reduction. During the period of cast immobilization, it is important to monitor with radiographs to ensure that the fracture does not displace into further extension or varus.

Type IA are typically very stable fractures, but type IB may slowly collapse into varus because of the medial cortical buckle. Failure to recognize a IB fracture may

Table 8-4	Classification of Supracondylar Fractures	
Extension Fractures	**Displacement**	
TYPE IA	Nondisplaced, no varus or valgus, capitellum, anterior humeral line on lateral x-ray	
TYPE IB	Minimally displaced with medial cortex buckle, capitellum intersected by anterior humeral line	
TYPE IIA	Extended, posterior cortex intact, capitellum posterior to anterior humeral line—no rotation	
TYPE IIB	Straight or rotatory displacement, still some fracture contact	
TYPE IIIA	Completely displaced posteriorly, no cortical contact. Most common posteromedial displacement	
TYPE IIIB	Wide displacement with soft tissue gap between bone ends, and significant overlap and/or rotatory displacement with no fracture contact	
FLEXION-TYPE FRACTURES	Displaced anteriorly (rare)	

lead to a poor result and cubitus varus if conservative management is chosen and the patient is not followed closely. The cast should be appropriately molded to try to counteract the varus collapse, and a gentle thumb-print in the olecranon fossa can help to prevent further extension of a supracondylar fracture (Fig. 8-19).

TYPE II SUPRACONDYLAR FRACTURES

Type II fractures need to be reduced to prevent hyperextension and angular deformity of the elbow. These injuries often appear to be in a single plane; however, it is also important to evaluate and correct any varus angulation or rotation. Although closed reduction can be maintained with casting or splinting in hyperflexion, this significantly increases the risk of neurovascular compromise to the extremity and is no longer recommended in centers where the skills and equipment are available for percutaneous pinning.

Type IIA fractures are in only one plane and some advocate treating them in a cast; we prefer to reduce and pin all type II fractures. Type IIB fractures have a rotational component that make reduction and maintenance of reduction more difficult; no one argues that these fractures require pinning.

Percutaneous pinning maintains the fracture reduction while allowing a safe casting position (flexion of <90°). The majority of supracondylar fractures have a posteromedial hinge of the periosteum that aids in the reduction process (Fig. 8-20).

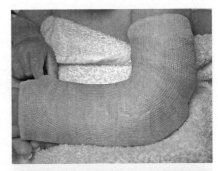

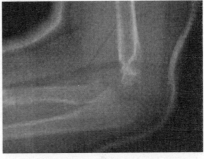

Figure 8-19. For type I supracondylar fractures the cast can be molded gently with your thumb to prevent extension of the fragment. Be careful not to overmold and create skin necrosis. (Method of Klaus Parsch—Stuttgart, Germany.)

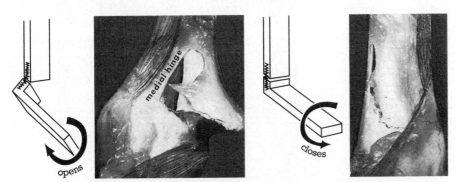

Figure 8-20. The periosteum usually remains intact on one side of the fracture allowing it to act as a hinge for reduction. In most supracondylar fractures, the distal fragment displaces medially and the medial hinge is intact. This allows a repeatable sequence for reduction with the elbow extended and supinated, then gentle flexion and pronation typically reduces the fracture.

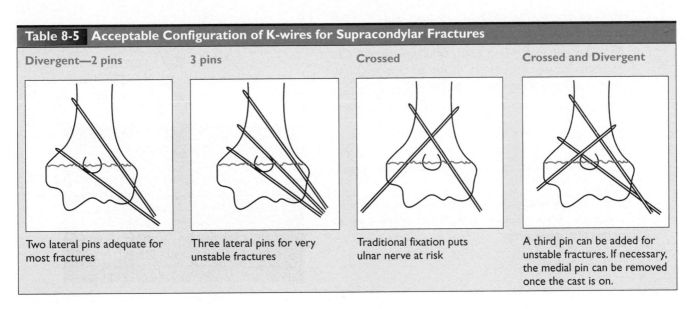

Table 8-5	Acceptable Configuration of K-wires for Supracondylar Fractures		
Divergent—2 pins	**3 pins**	**Crossed**	**Crossed and Divergent**
Two lateral pins adequate for most fractures	Three lateral pins for very unstable fractures	Traditional fixation puts ulnar nerve at risk	A third pin can be added for unstable fractures. If necessary, the medial pin can be removed once the cast is on.

TECHNIQUE TIPS:
Reducing Supracondylar Fractures

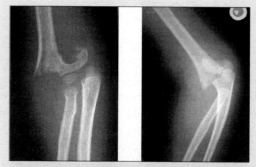

The majority of supracondylar fractures displace in a postero-medial direction and can be reduced in a reproducible fashion.

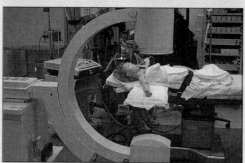

Position patient supine with armboard.

Fluoro (from head of bed and paralled to bed).

Monitor (easy for surgeon to see without turning head).

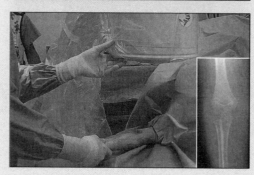

Milk soft tissue out of fracture.

Initially, keep the elbow extended and supinated.

Under image control, align the fracture on AP with traction and varus or valgus pressure.

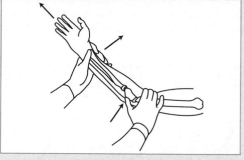

Only after the AP view is aligned should flexion be attempted.

Maintain traction (anesthesia can help with a sheet around the chest for counter traction).

Flex elbow up with thumb gently behind olecranon. (Do not over-reduce and convert to flexion-type fracture!) Gradually pronate the arm as you flex it.

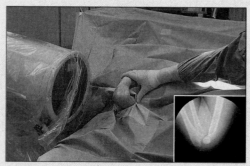

The elbow is flexed to ~130° with full forearm pronation.

If fracture is unstable the fluoro should be rotated while maintaining elbow position to avoid loss of reduction to obtain the lateral x-ray.

TECHNIQUE TIPS:
Pinning Supracondylar Fractures

Following reduction, hold the humerus parallel to the floor with the elbow flexed to 130°.

Start the first pin just lateral to the olecranon through the capitellum.

Aim at ~ 45° toward the medial metaphyseal cortex.

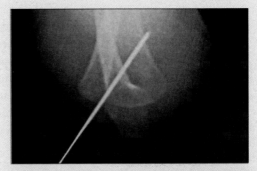

Start the second pin more proximally and diverge from the first.

Aim toward the medial diaphyseal cortex.

Make sure all pins penetrate the medial cortex.

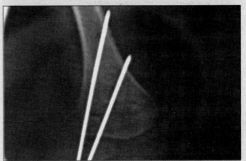

If reduction is not stable, consider a third lateral or medial pin.

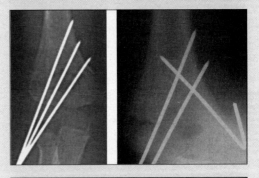

For medial pin, palpate the ulnar nerve with thumb and push nerve posteriorly.

Extend the elbow and insert pin anterior to thumb.

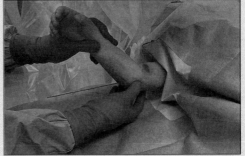

Bend the pins to a 90° angle as close to skin as possible.

Cut the pins ~ 2 cm distal to bend.

Place felt over the pins to protect the skin.

Cast the elbow with < 80° of flexion and split the cast to allow for swelling.

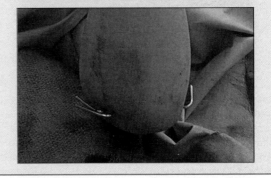

Pinning Patterns

There is debate as to the optimal number and configuration of K-wires; two or three pins can be used to stabilize most supracondylar fractures. Traditionally, cross pinning (one pin from medial and one from lateral) was performed. Currently, for typical supracondylar fractures, most centers use two or three pins from the lateral side to avoid ulnar nerve injury. Typically, two pins are adequate for type II fractures and three pins are frequently used to stabilize type III fractures.

Pins should diverge to create maximum space between them at the fracture site; they should not cross at the fracture site because this creates a rotationally unstable configuration (Table 8-5). When using a medial pin, one must avoid the ulnar nerve. This pin should not be placed with the elbow flexed, because flexion moves the ulnar nerve anteriorly putting it closer to the entry site of the K-wire.

For a typical fracture, two lateral divergent pins are adequate fixation. We recommend placing two lateral pins, and, if the reduction is felt to be unstable, a third lateral or medial pin can be added. If the fracture line exits far distally on the lateral side, a medial pin may be necessary for stabilization (Figs. 8-21, 8-22).

For medial pin placement, extend the elbow to allow the nerve to fall posteriorly. The ulnar nerve can be palpated and pushed more posteriorly with your thumb allowing safe medial pin entry. With a three-pin technique, if two lateral pins are in place and the patient wakes up with an ulnar nerve palsy, the medial pin can be removed through a window in the cast and the fracture will likely remain stable. If there is only a single lateral pin, this is not usually enough to maintain the reduction if the medial pin has to be removed.

TYPE III SUPRACONDYLAR FRACTURES

All type III fractures require reduction and internal fixation (there is often a rotational component that when added to the complete displacement can make reduction very difficult). In parts of the world where technology for safe percutaneus pinning is not available, traction methods (Fig. 8-23, Fig. 8-24) can be

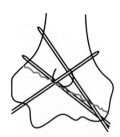

Figure 8-21. Fractures that exit very distally on the lateral side are difficult to stabilize with only lateral pins. A medial pin is frequently necessary.

Error—Not Stable

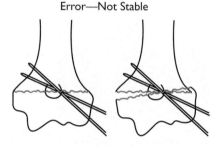

Figure 8-22. Pins that cross at the fracture line are rotationally unstable and should be avoided.

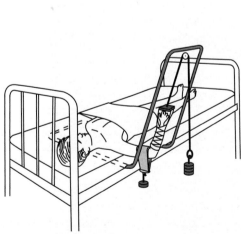

Figure 8-23. Bed traction can be used to align a supracondylar fracture but is not commonly used if equipment and skills for pinning are available. Accurate reduction is less likely; however, this simple method may be the only choice in certain parts of the world.
(Adapted from Blount. Fractures in children.)

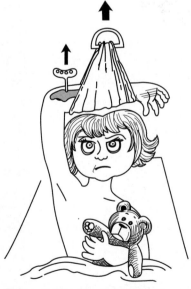

Figure 8-24. Overhead skeletal traction can be used to align a severe supracondylar fracture, again, results are inferior to closed reduction and percutaneus pinning.

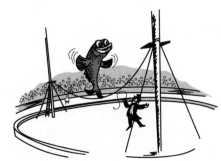

Figure 8-25. The humerus at the level of a supracondylar fracture is shaped like a fish tail: its narrowness can turn a stable reduction into a balancing act.

used but are not as effective, with residual cubitus varus common. At the level of a supracondylar fracture, the bone is extremely narrow and shaped like a fish tail—turning a stable reduction into a balancing act (Fig 8-25).

Frequently reduction can be done in a closed fashion with associated percutaneous pinning, but the fracture on occasion needs to be opened if soft tissue interposition prevents anatomic reduction or if there has been injury to the brachial artery. An ischemic hand is a surgical emergency, which will be addressed later in this section. The absence of a radial pulse is not an indication for exploration if the fingers are pink and can be painlessly extended; the brachial artery is likely in spasm and circulation can be monitored following reduction if the extremity is still adequately perfused.

Prior to attempting reduction of a type III fracture, one can "milk" the soft tissues down the arm; this may pop the interposed tissue out of the fracture site. Puckered skin on the anterior aspect of the elbow indicates soft tissue and on occasion brachial artery entrapment (Fig. 8-26).

We have had several cases where the ulnar nerve was entrapped in the fracture site and prevented anatomic reduction (Fig. 8-27). If persistent medial fracture gap remains, the surgeon should consider making an incision rather than repeatedly grinding the bone ends against a nerve, vessel, or other interposed soft tissue.

The incision for opening supracondylar fractures depends on the fracture; the most direct approach is usually directly over the prominent bony fragment whether it is anterior, medial, or lateral. Care needs to be taken to protect the brachial artery and median and radial nerves during the exposure and reduction.

Postoperative Care

Following closed reduction and percutaneous pinning of a supracondylar fracture, the type of immobilization will depend on the amount of soft tissue injury and risk of swelling. Type 2 fractures with moderate swelling and a single reduction maneuver can be placed in a cast flexed to about 80° at the elbow, as long as the cast is split (univalved). The cast can be tightened and overwrapped in 1 week.

Type III fractures should generally not be immediately casted unless the cast is bivalved and the web-roll split to allow for swelling. A better choice is a long posterior splint for the first week, which can then be converted to an above elbow cast. We recommend monitoring patients in the hospital overnight following percutaneous pinning of a supracondylar fractures to ensure that any neurovascular compromise is recognized and treated early.

Three weeks following surgery, the cast can be removed and the percutaneous pins can be removed in the clinic—sedation is almost never used. Pins should not be left in longer than 3 weeks given the risk of infection and the tendency for supracondylar fractures to heal quickly. In the majority of cases, there is adequate healing to begin motion at this time. A few fractures will remain clearly visible with little callus and require a second cast or splint for 2-3 weeks. However, it should be noted that supracondylar fractures rarely displace after 3 weeks, and the risk for stiffness increases if the elbow is immobilized in flexion longer than 3 weeks. This is in contrast to lateral condyle fractures that need the pins maintained for 4 weeks and occasionally longer to avoid nonunion. Physical therapy is rarely needed to regain elbow motion (Fig. 8-28).

The Pulseless Arm

Few cases raise the new-to-practice orthopedists stress titer more than a severe supracondylar fracture with vascular compromise. Concerns remain, although the incidence of vascular complications has decreased with early recognition, ad-

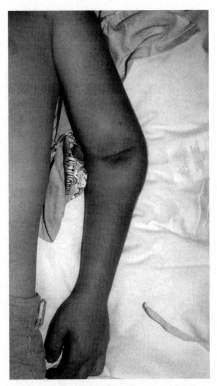

Figure 8-26. "Puckered" skin on the anterior aspect of the elbow indicates soft tissue entrapment.

After Closed Reduction Attempt   After Open Reduction

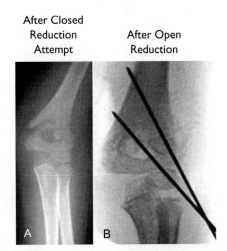

Figure 8-27. A) This was the best reduction that could be obtained closed; there was concern about the medial fracture gap. B) The fracture was opened and the ulnar nerve was found in the fracture, blocking reduction. Once the nerve was removed from the fracture, anatomic reduction could be obtained.

"Few cases raise the new-to-practice orthopaedists stress titer more than a severe supracondylar fracture with vascular compromise"

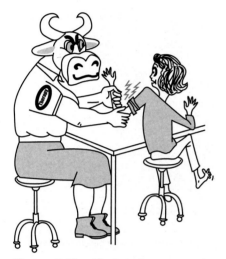

Figure 8-28. Physical therapy may be painful and is unlikely to improve motion following malunion of a supracondylar fracture. (Adapted from Blount. Fractures in children.)

vanced techniques for closed reduction and percutaneous pinning, and avoidance of hyperflexion. Over the last 10 years, a gradual consensus has evolved that allows effective treatment of the pulseless arm (see Technique Tips).

Historically, the "5 Ps" (pain, pallor, paresthesias, paralysis, pulselessness) were considered the most important signs of ischemia; however, these are late signs and a surgeon should never wait to treat a compromised arm if these symptoms are not present. Copley et al. reviewed a large series of patients with type III supracondylar fractures and found that the absence of a pulse was the earliest and most reliable indicator of ischemia. Several studies have shown that early reduction and pinning of type III supracondylar fractures in children with diminished or absent pulses will restore the blood flow in the majority of cases. There is a small percent that do not recover the pulse following reduction, and knowing when to get an arteriogram or return to the OR for exploration is critical.

Following closed reduction and pinning, immediately reassess the vascular status. If there is no pulse by palpation or Doppler, you need to determine if the hand has adequate blood flow. The artery may be in spasm that will resolve with time; there is a rich collateral circulation that can maintain the viability of the hand. If there is brisk capillary refill and the hand remains pink and warm, most surgeons choose to monitor the arm carefully with frequent neurovascular exams postoperatively.

If the neurovascular status worsens (signs of compartment syndrome, hand is no longer pink, slowed capillary refill, decreased sensation), immediate intervention should ensue. Initially, this may include angiogram and/or compartment pressure measurements followed by fasciotomy or open exploration with arterial mobilization (for artery trapped in the fracture site), vessel repair, reconstruction, or thrombectomy depending on the findings. In the case of isolated thrombus, urokinase can be attempted for thrombolysis.

Sabharwal recommends angiogram if the pulse does not return within 8-12 hours of appropriate reduction and fixation.

Pitfalls—Supracondylar Fractures

The goal of treatment is safe anatomic reduction and avoidance of residual varus and extension that are common complications following supracondylar fractures.

Severe malunion of a supracondylar fracture may lead to a so-called gunstock deformity, which consists of varus, medial rotation, and extension; (Fig. 8-29) best visualized by having the patient extend the arms fully and parallel to the ground. The bony deformity causes a block to motion that cannot be regained with physical therapy.

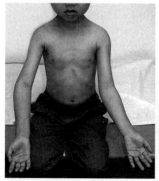
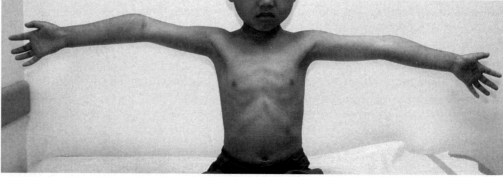

Figure 8-29. Gunstock deformity: This boy has residual varus and extension of the right elbow following nonoperative treatment of a supracondylar fracture.

TECHNIQUE TIPS:
Vascular Assessment and Management

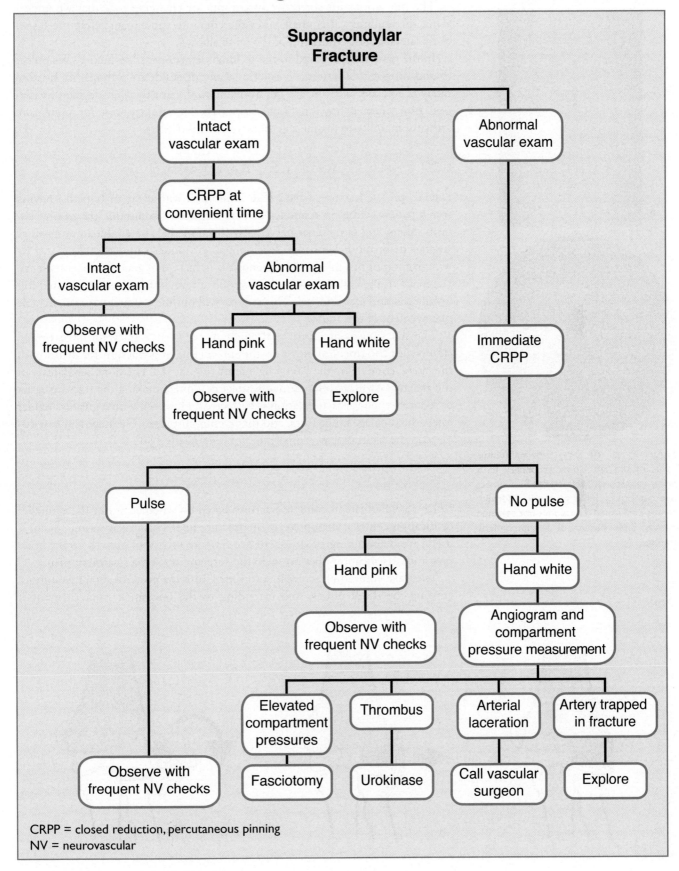

CRPP = closed reduction, percutaneous pinning
NV = neurovascular

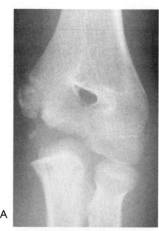

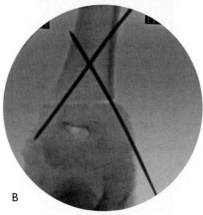

Figure 8-30. A) X-ray showing cubitus varus of the left elbow secondary to a prior supracondylar fracture. B) Corrective osteotomy for a gunstock deformity can be performed if motion is not regained 1 year after healing of a suprcondylar frature.

Corrective osteotomy (Fig. 8-30) for cubitus varus is hard to do well and should be done only after the elbow has regained mobility, usually at least 1 year after the original fracture. Malunion is obviously more difficult to correct than to prevent.

The indications for corrective osteotomy are changing now that we understand that cubitus varus predisposes the elbow to subsequent refracture (especially lateral condyle fractures of the same elbow).

In the past, some referred to the residual deformity as "cosmetic." We object to and do not use the term cosmetic in any of children's orthopedics because rarely if ever are scientific studies available to document what degree of variation from normal has functional risks (risk for reinjury, risk for premature arthritis, inability to pursue a certain type of sport, etc.).

LATERAL CONDYLE FRACTURES

Lateral condyle fractures have a bad reputation with every orthopedist having seen a patient, either in residency or practice, with a nonunion, progressive cubitus valgus, and tardy ulnar nerve palsy (from medial stretch due to progressive angular deformity). With the development of modern understanding and K-wire fixation of this injury, the prognosis is in fact quite good for most patients. For many of the children we treat now, only a few clinic visists are required following pin and cast removal. This section will outline a strategy for predictable management of this injury.

The mechanism of injury is thought to be a varus force on an extended elbow with the trochlear ridge on the ulna acting as a fulcrum for avulsion of the lateral condyle by the lateral ligaments (Fig. 8-31). The bone separates, but the articular cartilage often remains intact as a hinge making the fracture easier to reduce (when varus angulation is corrected). However, with a greater angular force, the cartilage hinge tears, and the fracture displaces. The fragment can displace in the sagittal plane, sometimes rotating nearly 180°.

Classification—Lateral Condyle Fractures

Milch classified lateral condyle fractures based on whether or not the capitellar ossification center is disrupted by the fracture line. This classification system is useful for determining prognosis of the fracture or risk of growth arrest; however, this classification does not help the surgeon develop a treatment plan.

The most common fracture line traverses from the posterolateral metaphysis, crossing the distal physis, and extending to the unossified trochlea without

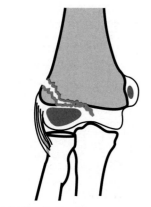
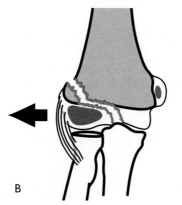
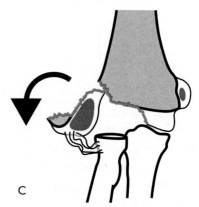

Figure 8-31. A) Cartilage hinge intact. B) Articular surface disrupted. C) Complete displacement of lateral condyle.

interrupting the capitellar ossification center. This fracture is referred to as a Milch Type II fracture. Milch Type I fractures are much less common, typically the fracture begins in the metaphysis, crosses the physis in an oblique fashion, then traverses the capitellar ossification center. This fracture has a higher risk of growth arrest as the ossification center is disrupted (Fig. 8-32).

Treatment—Lateral Condyle Fractures

Lateral condyle fractures are intra-articular and cross the distal humeral physis; they require anatomic reduction both for good joint function and to ensure normal distal humeral growth. For this reason, most fractures are treated with open reduction (Fig. 8-33) and K-wire fixation. Some have referred to this as an "A-O" (always open) fracture. With time and experience, a few minimally displaced fractures can safely be treated with casting only.

Minimally displaced fractures are occasionally seen and can be treated in a long arm cast providing two oblique distal humerus x-rays (in addition to the AP and lateral views) confirm 2 mm or less of displacement. This rule is of course a bit arbitrary because x-ray magnification can make one doctor's 2-mm measurement seem like 4 mm to another measurer. If non-operative treatment is chosen, we recommend removing the cast and obtaining AP, lateral, and two oblique x-rays every week for 3 weeks to ensure that the fracture does not displace in the cast (Fig. 8-34). Once one discovers the tension, time, and energy required to ensure healing with non-operative treatment, many surgeons choose k-wire fixation for the borderline case.

Joint surface disruption by a lateral condyle fracture should be anatomically reduced and fixed with K-wires; this typically requires open reduction for good visualization of the joint surface to ensure there is no joint step off or incongruity. Some lateral condyle fractures are displaced on the lateral side but have a cartilage hinge at the joint surface. Confirmation of intact articular cartilage can be made with an arthrogram at the time of surgery. If the joint surface is intact, the reduction can sometimes be obtained in a closed fashion by pushing the fragment back into place, relying on the hinge for anatomic reduction. The exact candidates for this variation of treatment are hard to define. Likely the less experienced surgeon should open and pin all borderline cases until the experience/judgement titer is optimized.

Whether obtained in an open or closed fashion, the reduction should be maintained with percutaneous smooth K-wires. In all cases, K-wires should be left in

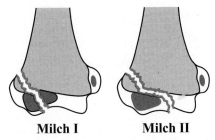

Milch I   Milch II

Figure 8-32. Milch classification of lateral condyle fractures (Type II are the most common).

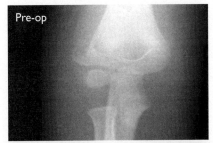

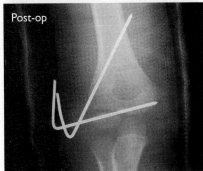

Pre-op

Post-op

Figure 8-33. Lateral condyle fracture before and following open reduction and pin fixation.

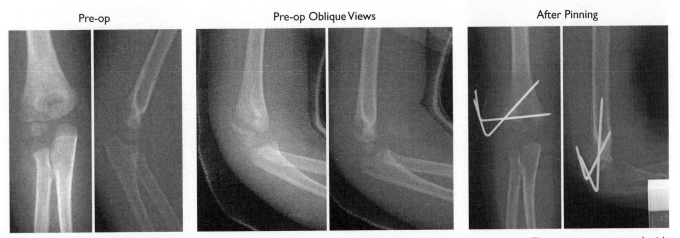

Pre-op   Pre-op Oblique Views   After Pinning

Figure 8-34. Displaced lateral condyle fractures are frequently more clearly visualized on the oblique x-rays. This patient was treated with open reduction and pin fixation.

"Likely the less experienced surgeon should open and pin all borderline cases until the experience/judgement titer is optimized"

longer than those used for supracondylar fractures because lateral condyle fractures are usually bathed in synovial fluid, which can delay union and may lead to non-union. We recommend 4 weeks of immobilization with pins in place followed by an additional 2-4 weeks of casting or splinting (until callus is visible crossing the fracture site). Every year we see two or three lateral condyle fractures where the original treating surgeon (from the infamous "Elsewhere General Hospital") correctly diagnosed, reduced, and pinned a lateral condyle fracture but then removed the pins at 2 or 3 weeks and allowed early motion with subsequent nonunion.

Pitfalls—Lateral Condyle Fractures

The classic severe complication of non-union with late severe cubitus valgus and tardy ulnar nerve palsy is now almost never seen in developed parts of the world where early diagnosis and pin stabilization are standard. The most common problems in advanced centers are now more subtle.

Delayed union (Fig. 8-35) can occur if any gap remains at the fracture site, allowing synovial fluid to track into the fracture line from the joint surface, which interferes with healing. If the joint line is not well visualized at the time of surgery, or closed treatment plus pinning is attempted, an immediate arthrogram can be performed to confirm that there is no tracking of dye into the fracture.

Wadsworth has observed that premature growth plate closure may occur, even in undisplaced fractures. This can lead to a valgus deformity of the elbow joint requiring later supracondylar osteotomy. Another common problem is cubitus varus due to growth stimulation of the lateral portion of the physis, likely secondary to increased blood flow in the area of the fracture. This mild deformity is not progressive. Another rare outcome is cubitus varus secondary to focal physeal closure in the medial one third of the physis (in the fracture type that extends very medially), despite proper reduction and pinning.

Because the lateral condyle is directly subcutaneous, even with perfect reduction, the healed lateral condyle fracture commonly results in a "bump" on the lateral aspect of the elbow. This can be minimized by careful closure of the fascia-muscle layers laterally. This is not a functional problem but some patients and parents are bothered by the prominence.

The trochlear notch may appear deepened on the AP x-ray following adequate reduction and union, due to focal AVN. The pattern must be recognized but is rarely treated.

Initial Injury—Minimal Displacement

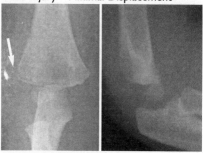

After 4 weeks in cast

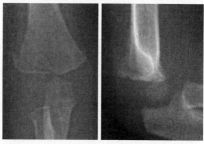

Figure 8-35. Lateral condyle fractures may displace while in a good cast. It is important to check x-rays weekly for 3 weeks to ensure alignment is not lost. This patient seemed to have only a few millimeters of displacement (arrow) at the time of injury. She had late displacement and required open reduction.

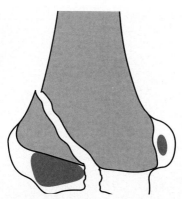

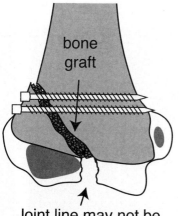

bone graft

Joint line may not be anatomically aligned

Figure 8-36. Flynn method of treating a lateral condyle nonunion.

Delayed diagnosis cases occur occasionally—a child presents after several weeks with a displaced fracture of the lateral condyle. Should this be accepted or surgically reduced? The results of surgery are less satisfactory because of the risk for stiffness and AVN. However, in most cases even up to 6 weeks post injury, we would carefully open the fracture, remove the evolving callus, and pin the fracture. In cases of significant delay with established nonunion, we advise Flynn's method of metaphysis to metaphysis screw fixation above the physis, which may leave the joint malreduced (Fig. 8-36). This prevents proximal migration of the condylar fragment and cubitus valgus. The results are not ideal but are often satisfactory.

In summary, the long-term sequelae of a severely displaced, untreated lateral condyle fracture is so severe that we usually proceed with surgical stabilization, no matter how long beyond the original injury. The procedure selected differs according to the delay (as noted) with the outcome less predictable than in acutely treated cases.

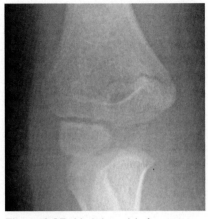

Figure 8-37. Medial condyle fractures are rare in children, this fracture was non-displaced and treated with a cast.

MEDIAL CONDYLE FRACTURES

Medial condyle fractures (Table 8-6) are very rare (Fig. 8-37). Because it is an intra-articular fracture, a neglected fracture of the medial condyle has the same poor prognosis as a neglected fracture of the lateral condyle. The medial condyle or trochlea ossifies between the ages of 7-11 for girls and 8-13 for boys. The unossified medial condyle in a young child casts no shadow and avulsion is a matter of conjecture. A common mistake is to confuse a condylar fracture with an epicondylar fracture because the epicondyle ossifies earlier (between 5 and 9 years). It may be possible to avoid this mistake in children who have soft tissue swelling on the medial aspect of the joint by examining the elbow under anesthesia and/or with arthrogram. A condylar fracture is often associated with valgus instability of the elbow and posteromedial subluxation of the elbow.

If non-operative treatment is chosen, it is important to check x-rays regularly during the healing process to ensure the fragment does not displace. Similar to lateral condyle fractures, union may be slow if the fracture is bathed in synovial fluid, so pins should be left in place 4 weeks, and the elbow casted until good callus is noted on x-ray.

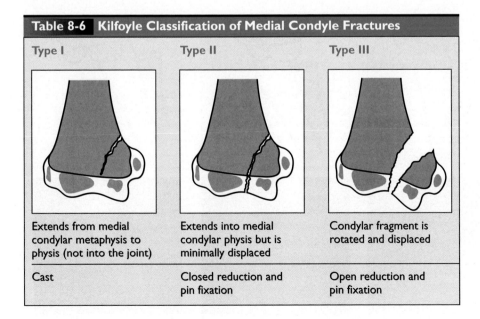

Table 8-6	Kilfoyle Classification of Medial Condyle Fractures	
Type I	**Type II**	**Type III**
Extends from medial condylar metaphysis to physis (not into the joint)	Extends into medial condylar physis but is minimally displaced	Condylar fragment is rotated and displaced
Cast	Closed reduction and pin fixation	Open reduction and pin fixation

Pitfalls—Medial Condyle Fractures

Failure to recognize a displaced medial condyle fracture can lead to nonunion and cubitus varus. AVN can occur if the blood supply to the trochlea is disrupted either by dissection or by the original trauma.

MEDIAL EPICONDYLE FRACTURES

The medial epicondyle of the distal humerus ossifies between the ages of 5 and 9 years and can be avulsed by valgus stress and contraction of the flexor muscles (Table 8-7). We frequently see this injury in young gymnasts and baseball pitchers; this can be an acute on chronic injury or a single acute injury. Traumatic elbow dislocation is often accompanied by medial epicondyle fracture; the bony fragment can become entrapped in the joint. In children younger than the age of 9, the clinical signs of hematoma may be more obvious than the radiographic ones. If the epicondyle is ossified, a film of the opposite elbow may help to clarify the normal position of the epicondyle. The degree of displacement should be assessed and the presence of other injuries noted, such as fracture of the radial neck and injury of the ulnar nerve that lies close by.

Treatment—Medial Epicondyle Fractures

Indications for displaced fractures remain empiric because there have been no good studies comparing long-term outcome of operative and non-operative treatment of medial epicondyle fractures. If the fracture has minimal displacement (less than 5 mm in any plane) and minimal soft tissue swelling, cast im-

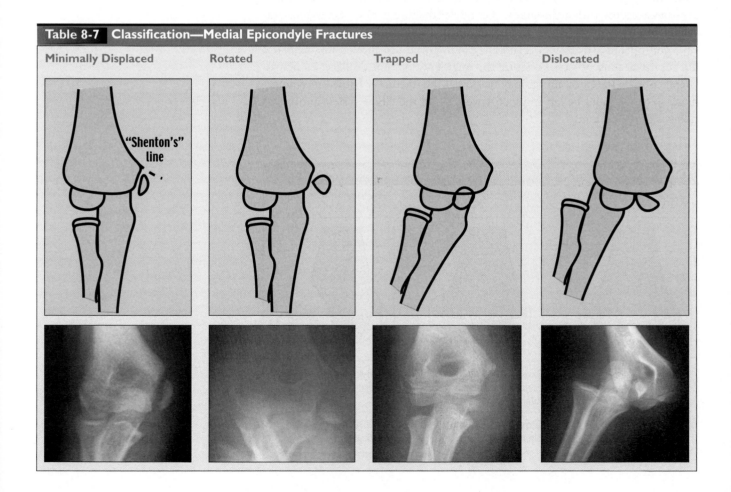

Table 8-7 Classification—Medial Epicondyle Fractures

| Minimally Displaced | Rotated | Trapped | Dislocated |

mobilization alone can be considered. X-rays should be checked during early healing to ensure that there has been no further displacement.

If a medial epicondyle fracture is allowed to heal in a significantly displaced position, the flexor-pronator origin is moved distally and laterally. Theoretically, this may lead to elbow weakness or valgus instabilty; therefore many surgeons now advise anatomic reduction and internal fixation of displaced fractures.

It is often difficult to establish the true fragment displacement on plain radiographs, and there is significant debate as to the amount of displacement that is acceptable for normal elbow function with a medial epicondyle fracture. If there is any question, the elbow can be tested under anesthesia. If the elbow is found to be unstable, open reduction and fixation is preferred. In general, if the fracture fragment is displaced more than 5 mm, we perform surgical reduction especially in athletic patients (Fig. 8-38).

If the child presents with a dislocated elbow and a medial epicondyle fracture, the elbow should be emergently reduced to assist the circulation and relieve pain. If the medial epicondyle remains trapped in the joint during the reduction, it can sometimes be extricated by applying a valgus stress and supinating the elbow; however, the fragment rarely returns to its bed. Open reduction should be performed in these cases.

For open reduction, the patient can be positioned supine with the arm externally rotated on an arm board or prone with the arm in a half-Nelson position (behind the back). A small incision is centered at the level of the bed of the epicondyle in line with the posterior border of the humerus (remember that the medial epicondyle is posterior on the humerus). Hematoma is usually encountered just under the subcutaneous fat and leads to the fracture bed.

The ulnar nerve must be identified through the posterior periosteum and protected. The nerve does not need to be dissected out; temporary nerve palsy can result from overelaborate display of the nerve, but it should be palpated and identified.

The fragment with the flexor-pronator origin can then be milked proximally up into the incision with the forearm pronated to relax the volar musculature. Now the orientation can be visually determined and the fragment replaced into its anatomic position. A towel clip will secure the reduction while fixation is placed.

In younger children, a smooth K-wire can maintain the reduction with a few sutures in the periosteum. In older children (>6 years), the medial epicondyle can be fixed with a single cancellous screw starting in the fragment and continuing up the medial column of the distal humerus. Postoperatively, the patient is casted at 90° of elbow flexion and pronation to relax the flexor-pronator group for 3-4 weeks and then range of motion is begun.

At Injury

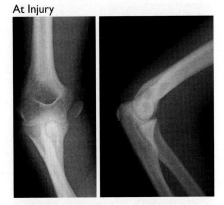

After Open Reduction

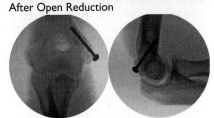

Figure 8-38. Medial epicondyle fractures that are significantly displaced are typically treated with open reduction and internal fixation.

"There is significant debate as to the amount of displacement that is acceptable for normal elbow function with a medial epicondyle fracture"

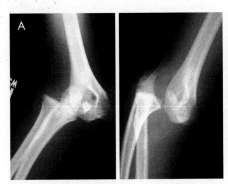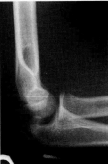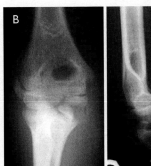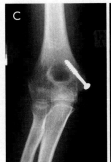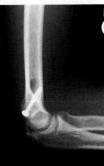

Figure 8-39. A) An elbow dislocation with medial epicondyle fracture. B) Trapped medial epicondyle following reduction. C) Emergent reduction and fixation.

Pitfalls—Medial Epicondyle Fractures

Missing a medial epicondyle that is entrapped in the joint can lead to significant loss of motion and disability (Fig. 8-39).

The ulnar nerve may be irritated or stretched at the time of injury, reduction, or surgery; this ulnar neuropathy is usually transient. Some patients develop a late ulnar neuritis, likely secondary to irritation by callus or a chronic valgus instability.

Nonunion is common in displaced fractures treated non-operatively; however, this rarely leads to clinical problems (with the possible exception of late ulnar neuritis).

Even with anatomic healing, the elbow may become stiff following healing of a medial epicondyle fracture, so early motion is recommended by most surgeons.

LATERAL EPICONDYLE FRACTURES

The center for the lateral epicondyle ossifies late (age 8-13) and is often irregular, causing beginners to confuse it with a fracture (Fig. 8-40). The extensor muscles originate on the lateral epicondyle and may be responsible for avulsion injuries. Very few true fractures of lateral epicondyle are seen; therefore there is no consensus on the need for or type of treatment. Minimally displaced fractures can be casted for 4-6 weeks.

SUMMARY

Distal humerus fractures come in many varieties that change as the child grows and growth centers appear. Treatment options vary based on the type of fracture and age of the patient. It is important not only to understand each fracture and its associated complications, but to have a thorough knowledge of normal elbow development and anatomy to be able to return each child to the best function possible.

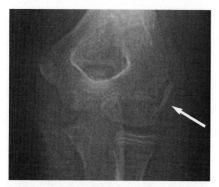

Figure 8-40. As the lateral epicondyle begins to ossify (arrow), it is frequently mistaken for a fracture. This picture represents a normal elbow in an 11-year-old girl.

Suggested Readings

Benesahel, H. et. al. Fractures of the Medial Condyle of the Humerus in Children. J of Pediatric Orthopedics, 6:430-433, 1986.

Blount WP. Fractures in children. Williams and Wilkins 1955.

Campbell CC, Waters PM, Emans JB, Kasser JR, Millis MB. Neurovascular injury and displacement in type III supracondylar humerus fractures. J Pediatr Orthop. 1995 Jan-Feb;15(1):47-52.

Cramer KE, Green NE, Devito DP. Incidence of anterior interosseous nerve palsy in supracondylar humerus fractures in children. J Pediatr Orthop. 1993 Jul-Aug;13(4):502-5.

Culp RW, Osterman AL, Davidson RS, Skirven T, Bora FW Jr. Neural injuries associated with supracondylar fractures of the humerus in children. J Bone Joint Surg Am. 1990 Sep;72(8):1211-5.

Davids JR, Maguire MF, Mubarak SJ, Wenger DR. Lateral condylar fracture of the humerus following posttraumatic cubitus varus. J Pediatr Orthop. 1994 Jul-Aug;14(4):466-70.

Delee, JC, et al. Fracture-separation of the distal humerus epiphysis. JBJS 1980; 62:4-51.

Flynn JC, Richards JF Jr. Non-union of minimally displaced fractures of the lateral condyle of the humerus in children. J Bone Joint Surg Am. 1971 Sep;53(6):1096-101.

Gillingham BL, Rang M. Advances in children's elbow fractures. J Pediatr Orthop. 1995 Jul-Aug;15(4):419-21.

Haraldson S. Osteochondrosis deformans juvenelis capituli humeri including investigation of the intra-osseous vasculare in the distal humerus. Acta Orthop Scand. [suppl], 38. 1959.

Kilfoyle RM. Fractures of the medial condyle and epicondyle of the elbow in children. Clin. Orthop. 1965 July-Aug;41:43-50.

Kim HT, Song MB, Conjares JN, Yoo CI. Trochlear deformity occurring after distal humeral fractures: magnetic resonance imaging and its natural progression. J Pediatr Orthop. 2002 Mar-Apr;22(2):188-93.

Lee SS, Mahar AT, Miesen D, Newton PO. Displaced pediatric supracondylar humerus fractures: biomechanical analysis of percutaneous pinning techniques. J Pediatr Orthop. 2002 Jul-Aug;22(4):440-3.

Mohammad S, Rymaszewski LA, Runciman J. The Baumann angle in supracondylar

fractures of the distal humerus in children. J Pediatr Orthop. 1999 Jan-Feb;19(1):65-9.

Mubarak SJ, Carroll NC. Volkman's contracture in children: Aetiology and prevention. J Bone Joint Surg Br. 1979 Aug;61-B(3):285-93.

Reitman RD, Waters P, Millis M. Open reduction and internal fixation for supracondylar humerus fractures in children. J Pediatr Orthop. 2001 Mar-Apr;21(2):157-61.

Sabharwal S, Tredwell SJ, Beauchamp RD, Mackenzie WG, Jakubec DM, Cairns R, LeBlanc JG. Management of pulseless pink hand in pediatric supracondylar fractures of humerus. J Pediatr Orthop. 1997 May-Jun;17(3):303-10.

Skaggs DL, Mirzayan R. The posterior fat pad sign in association with occult fracture of the elbow in children. J Bone Joint Surg Am. 1999 Oct;81(10):1429-33.

Skaggs DL, Cluck MW, Mostofi A, Flynn JM, Kay RM. Lateral entry pin fixation in the management of supracondylar fractures in children. JBJS Am. 2004 Apr;86-A(4):702-7.

9

Elbow—Proximal Radius and Ulna

Maya Pring ❧ Dennis Wenger ❧ Mercer Rang

INTRODUCTION

In the last edition, all fractures about the elbow were presented in a single dose. Advancement in orthopedic knowledge and further understanding of the remarkable variety of children's elbow injuries makes this a less viable option now. With the increased participation in "extreme sports" we have noted a marked increase in previously less common elbow injuries in children including radial head fractures and injuries to the coronoid process. Placing the entire spectrum of elbow fractures in a single chapter would make it very long and we hope that our arbitrary separation into distal humerus and proximal forearm segments will not confuse the reader.

Anatomy

The elbow joint does not have inherent bony stability; the collateral ligaments and capsule serve as the major joint stabilizers (Fig. 9-1). The collateral ligaments connect the distal humerus to the ulna, the annular ligament

> *"What does not destroy me, makes me stronger"*
> —*NEITZSCHE*

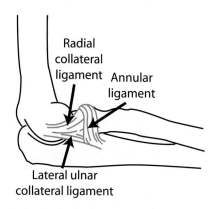

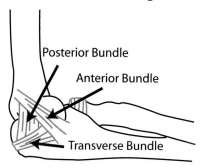

Lateral view of elbow ligaments

Medial view of elbow ligaments

Figure 9-1. The capsule and ligaments give stability to the elbow.

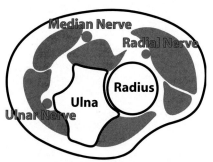

Figure 9-2. Cross section at the level of the elbow.

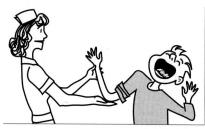

Figure 9-3. Examining an injured child can be very difficult.

maintains the radioulnar joint, and the interosseuos membrane helps to maintain the spatial relationship between the radius and ulna.

The brachial artery, median nerve, and radial nerve all coursing anterior to the elbow joint are at risk for stretch injury with a proximal forearm fracture or elbow dislocation. The ulnar nerve, running medially just behind the medial epicondyle, may be stretched, torn, or entrapped in the joint at the time of injury or during reduction. The posterior interosseous nerve, coursing anterior to the radial head and anterolateral to the radial neck, can easily be injured when the proximal radius is fractured or dislocated (Fig. 9-2).

Initial Exam

As discussed in the prior chapter, it can sometimes be difficult to distinguish between an injured and an infected elbow in a young child. Be wary in puzzling cases and order a complete blood count (CBC), sedimentation rate, and C-reactive protein when the etiology of joint swelling is unclear.

Once the area of concern is identified, a skin exam will rule out an open fracture, with the standard neurovascular exam then performed (see Chapter 8 for details). The fracture type can sometimes be estimated by gentle palpation; however, this may be difficult or impossible in an uncomfortable young child with a swollen elbow (Fig. 9-3).

Because additional fractures in the same limb are common, always check the joint above and below the area of concern. The contralateral elbow should be examined to determine the normal anatomy and motion for each individual.

Radiographic Issues

Radiographs of the flexed elbow often represent compromise views of the upper forearm and the distal humerus but are the usual starting point. Well-centered AP and lateral views of the proximal forearm and distal humerus may be required to better identify a puzzling fracture. Also, an accurate assessment of angulation and shift can only be measured on films taken at right angles to the plane of fracture angulation.

As previously discussed, a fat pad or "sail" sign may be the only x-ray indication of a pediatric elbow fracture. The actual location of these occult fractures is often not determined until follow-up x-rays show callus formation. Olecranon and radial neck fractures are the most common occult fractures of the proximal forearm (supracondylar fracture most common in the distal humerus).

Plastic deformation or greenstick fractures of the ulna (and occasionally the radius) may cause a radial head dislocation, so it is important to obtain x-rays of the entire forearm including the wrist and elbow when there is a forearm fracture. A line drawn down the center of the proximal radial shaft should pass

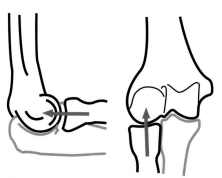

Figure 9-4. The radial head should point directly at the capitellum on both the AP and lateral views.

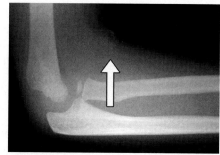

Figure 9-5. Note subtle anterior subluxation of the radial head.

through the center of the ossification center of the capitellum on both AP and lateral views (Fig. 9-4); if not, the radial head is subluxed or dislocated and must be reduced (Fig. 9-5).

PULLED ELBOW SYNDROME (NURSEMAID'S ELBOW)

A pulled elbow is a common early childhood injury. The clinical picture is characteristic; a child between 1 and 4 years suddenly refuses to move an arm and holds the elbow slightly flexed with the forearm pronated. Often, parents think the arm is paralyzed or broken and they rarely mention that the problem began as the child was pulled along or lifted by the wrist—the usual cause in our fast-paced culture (Fig. 9-6). It is remarkable that not all children experience a pulled elbow!

Although a pulled elbow can be readily diagnosed and treated once you have learned to recognize it, do not get lulled into a false sense of security, forgetting to consider other problems. The diagnosis of nursemaid's elbow is now well recognized by most primary care providers and is sometimes overdiagnosed. Unfortunately, some children with other diagnoses end up having painful "pulled elbow" reduction attempts. Conditions that we have had referred to our clinic that were initially treated as a pulled elbow include:

- Septic elbow
- Olecranon fracture
- Radial head or neck fractures (Fig. 9-7)
- Supracondylar fracture
- Septic wrist

Pulled elbow should be a diagnosis of exclusion. In each of the above cases, one or even several reduction attempts had been carried out (unsuccessfully of course). When you encounter the child in this circumstance, the ability to clarify the diagnosis without further terrifying the child defines the art of children's orthopedics. As a "true expert," you may have to once again attempt a reduction, even though less specialized experts have already tried. This is a very tricky environment.

For a true pulled elbow, the x-rays are usually normal. Occasionally, a very slight lateral or distal shift of the radial head can be seen. Ultrasound has been reported to be useful in confirming the diagnosis; however, we have no experience with this technique (Kosuwon).

Salter and Zaltz found that when longitudinal traction is applied to the arm (with the forearm in pronation) the annular ligament partially tears at its attachment to the radius, allowing the radius to move distally, slipping under the annular ligament. When traction is released, the ligament is carried up and becomes impacted between the radius and capitellum (Fig. 9-8). After the age of 5 years, the attachment of the annular ligament to the neck of the radius strengthens and prevents displacement and radial head subluxation. Enlargement of the proximal radial epiphysis with growth may also improve stability.

Treatment—Pulled Elbow

Fortuitous reduction can occur when the x-ray technician supinates the arm to obtain an AP x-ray. Because the x-rays are usually normal, you must rely on the history and your exam to reach the diagnosis. In simple cases, reduction is easy: supinate the flexed elbow and you will feel a click as the subluxed radial head reduces. Often, the elbow must be flexed above 90° with firm supination to achieve reduction. Producing and feeling the click that accompanies successful

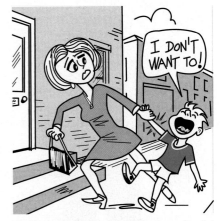

Figure 9-6. The usual mechanism of radial head subluxation in a fast-paced culture.

"Unfortunately, some children with other diagnoses end up having painful 'pulled elbow' reduction attempts"

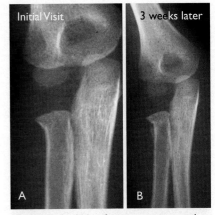

Figure 9-7. We often see masqueraders of a pulled elbow. A) This patient had a radial neck fracture, which was thought to be a pulled elbow. B) Callus was noted on follow-up x-ray.

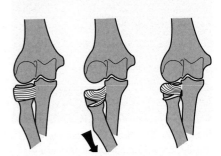

Figure 9-8. With longitudinal traction the annular ligament can partially tear allowing the radial head to move distally.

reduction of the annular ligament can be compared to feeling an Ortolani positive hip reduce for the first time; several successful reductions are required to feel confident of your technique.

After the typical reduction, the child often stops crying, seems more comfortable, and starts to move the arm within a minute or two. No immobilization is required, but the parents should avoid pulling the child or lifting by the arm for the next several years.

Recurrence is relatively common and a child may have repeated subluxations in the first 3-4 years of life. Repeat injuries are treated in the same fashion as first-time subluxations, with the problem gradually disappearing by age 5 years; the younger the child, the greater the risk for recurrent subluxation. Recurrences do not produce long-term problems. In a child with multiple recurrences, we sometimes cast for 3 weeks in the reduced position (elbow flexed to 100° with the forearm supinated), allowing the enforced rest and temporary joint stiffness to add stability (Fig. 9-9).

Pitfalls—Pulled Elbow

A few times a year one is faced with a case that does not seem to reduce despite a correct reduction maneuver by an experienced treater. Clearly, the differential diagnosis noted previously is considered. When convinced that we have a true unreducible nursemaid's elbow (not an occult septic elbow or fracture), our approach includes casting the child in a position that technically will reduce the subluxation (elbow flexed to 100°, full supination) for 3 weeks. This usually solves the problem.

There have been a few case reports in the literature of pulled elbows that were completely irreducible with closed means. In these cases, surgical exploration demonstrated that the annular ligament had slipped past the equator of the radial head and become trapped in the radiocapitellar joint.

DISLOCATIONS—ELBOW JOINT

In children, elbow dislocations without a fracture are uncommon. Whenever you encounter an elbow dislocation, assume an associated occult fracture (which may prevent reduction). The most common example is a medial epicondyle fracture, which frequently becomes entrapped in the joint. A non-concentric reduction should alert the examiner to a trapped fragment, which may be cartilage in younger children (the medial epicondyle ossifies around age 7) or bone in the adolescent (Fig. 9-10). Contralateral films for comparison are critical.

The articular surface of the ulna and of the capitellum may also fracture and prevent concentric reduction. A flap of articular cartilage and subchondral bone lifted off the articular surface may be barely perceptible on the x-ray. Crepitus and a restricted range of motion following reduction should alert you to possible osteochondral fragments in the joint.

More obvious fractures associated with elbow dislocation include lateral condyle, olecranon, and radial neck injuries; these are easily identified on x-ray and are more straightforward in terms of management.

Also, dislocation gives risk to the neurovascular structures, muscles, collateral ligaments, and capsule.

Classification—Elbow Dislocations

Elbow dislocations are described by the position of the radius and ulna in relation to the distal humerus (anterior, posterior, medial, or lateral). They are further

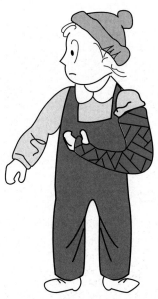

Figure 9-9. For recurrent nursemaid's elbows, we sometimes use a cast in supination and flexion for 3 weeks. This type of cast can also be used in a case where you do not feel the reduction click and the x-rays are normal.

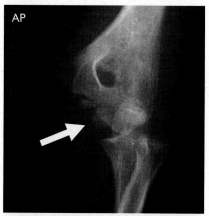

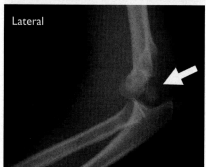

Figure 9-10. Elbow dislocations are usually accompanied by a fracture—Note the medial epicondyle trapped in the joint (arrow).

classified based on whether or not the proximal radioulnar joint remains intact (Table 9-1). Posterolateral dislocations, by far the most common in reported series, are thought to be caused by a fall on the outstretched hand with the elbow extended and abducted. Typically, the radioulnar articulation remains intact with only rare instances of divergent dislocation (radius and ulna separated).

Treatment—Elbow Dislocations

The dislocation should be reduced as soon as possible to relieve pain and improve circulation. Conscious sedation helps to relax the muscles adequately for an atraumatic reduction. An easy method for reduction includes placing the child prone with the elbow flexed over the edge of the bed so that the forearm hangs vertically downward. When the child relaxes, a little pressure over the olecranon with correction of any sideways displacement usually reduces the elbow.

This is a gentle maneuver that does not require the force required for some orthopedic reductions. Avoid hyperextending the elbow prior to reduction because this may further injure the brachialis and neurovascular structures anteriorly. Immediate pain relief can be expected. The child is typically casted for 2-3 weeks to allow soft tissue healing and to avoid the slight risk of recurrent dislocation. Casting longer than 3 weeks should be avoided because the risk of stiffness increases with time in the cast.

Immediate postreduction x-rays should be performed to assess reduction and look for the medial epicondyle. If the medial epicondyle is separated and outside the joint, it can be treated by casting alone if minimally displaced. If markedly displaced, it should be surgically reduced within a few days. If trapped in the joint, prompt open reduction is required.

Pitfalls—Elbow Dislocation

Failure to recognize an entrapped fragment in the joint can lead to destruction of the articular cartilage, non-concentric wear, and early osteoarthritis. In the rare cases of dislocation without fracture, the collateral ligaments of the elbow may be disrupted and even in children this can occasionally lead to instability and require reconstruction.

Nerves and vessels may be stretched and develop a temporary palsy or spasm but most resolve with time. However, neurovascular entrapment following re-

"Failure to recognize an entrapped fragment in the joint can lead to destruction of the articular cartilage, non-concentric wear and early osteoarthritis"

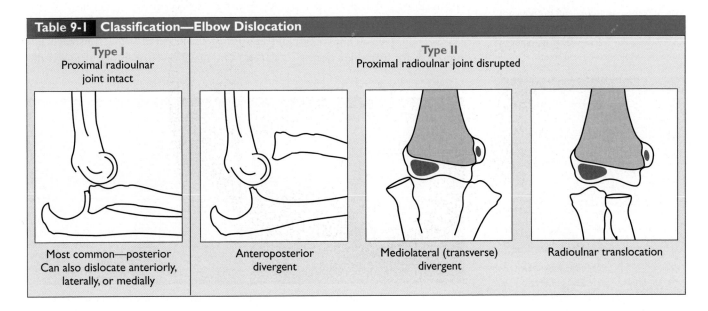

Table 9-1	Classification—Elbow Dislocation		
Type I Proximal radioulnar joint intact	**Type II** Proximal radioulnar joint disrupted		
Most common—posterior Can also dislocate anteriorly, laterally, or medially	Anteroposterior divergent	Mediolateral (transverse) divergent	Radioulnar translocation

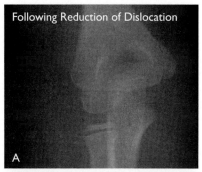

Following Reduction of Dislocation

A

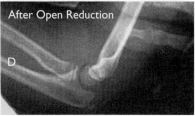

Non-concentric Reduction

B

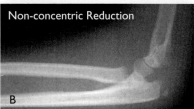

After Open Reduction

C

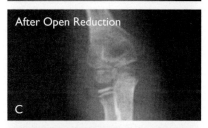

After Open Reduction

D

Figure 9-11. A, B) Child with elbow dislocation reduced elsewhere and referred to us for ulnar nerve palsy. The lateral view suggests non-concentric reduction. C, D) After open reduction, which revealed the unlar nerve was trapped in the joint and was blocking reduction.

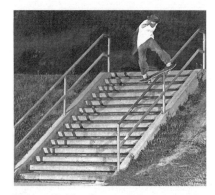

Figure 9-12. Skateboarding down the rails of steps. The new generation ensures that orthopedists will keep busy. (Photo courtesy of T. Hooker.)

duction can lead to disability if not noted and treated promptly. Entrapment of the ulnar nerve is most common with radial and median nerve entrapment occuring occasionally. It may be very difficult to determine if the nerve was only stretched or if it is truly trapped in the joint. A slightly non-concentric reduction on x-ray should alert one to the possibility of soft tissue entrapment that requires surgical intervention (Fig. 9-11).

Heterotopic ossification can develop in the ligaments and capsule following injury, but usually does not cause disability. In rare cases, myositis ossificans develops in the muscles surrounding the elbow, leading to significant loss of joint motion.

PROXIMAL RADIUS: RADIAL HEAD AND NECK FRACTURES

In the previous edition of this book, we noted that children get radial neck fractures and adults get radial head fractures. This circumstance has changed with the adolescent and teenage trends toward participation in extreme sports. We now frequently see radial head as well as radial neck fractures in skateboarders, ATV riders, and other children that participate in high-speed, high-risk sports (Fig. 9-12).

The majority of these fractures are due to a valgus force; some associated with a posterior dislocation; and the remainder accompanied by fractures of the ulnar shaft, reminiscent of a Monteggia fracture. Other fractures around the elbow are present in nearly half of the children with displaced radial neck fractures; look carefully for associated olecranon, coronoid, or distal humerus fractures.

Because the annular ligament holds the radial metaphysis to the shaft of the ulna, when the neck is fractured, the displaced radial head is not only angulated but also shifted laterally as the shaft shifts medially. Pronation and supination depend on the relationship of the radial head to the capitellum and ulna. Significant translation of the radial head separates the center of rotation of the head from that of the shaft, creating a cam-type deformity that inhibits pronation and supination (Fig. 9-13). No available study clarifies how much pure translation is acceptable for later elbow function; therefore we try to minimize translation and do not accept more than 2-3 mm in any direction.

The cartilaginous head of the radius fits the metaphysis like a bottlecap. For this reason, the majority of fractures are metaphyseal, only a few are epiphyseal separations. Epiphyseal separations, when they occur, put the radial head at risk for osteonecrosis because the blood supply is disrupted [the blood supply ascends from a distal source, similar to that of the femoral head, thus each has high risk for avascular necrosis (AVN)]. The usual level of injury through the

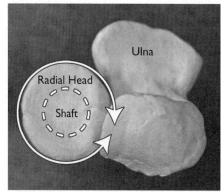
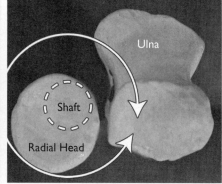

Figure 9-13. If the radial head is not centered on the shaft, pronation and supination will be affected.

metaphysis is just distal to the entry of the vessels, but the blood supply may still be disrupted with significant displacement.

Classification—Radial Head and Neck Fractures

Radial neck fractures can be angulated, translocated, or completely dislocated (Table 9-2). With high-level sports and repetitive motions such as pitching or gymnastics, stress injuries are becoming more common. Rarely, repetitive compressive forces to the radial head and neck may cause osteochondritis dissecans at the joint surface or may injure the physis, creating an angular deformity of the radial neck.

Treatment—Radial Head and Neck Fractures

Tilt of the radial head is better tolerated than translation. Therefore minimally angulated fractures (up to 30°) do not need to be reduced as they will remodel with growth (Fig. 9-14). We usually protect the elbow in a long arm cast for three weeks followed by encouragement of early motion.

For moderately angulated fractures (30°-60°), we try manipulation in the emergency room under conscious sedation. More severely angulated fractures (>60°) are ideally reduced in the operating room with facilities available for open reduction if this is found to be necessary (Fig. 9-15).

Several published methods for closed radial head reduction are reviewed in the following technique tips. Knowledge of each method may save you from opening a radial neck fracture, which increases the risk for elbow stiffness or, at worst, AVN of the radial head. Because of these risks, several of these methods should be attempted before proceeding to open reduction.

If the radial head cannot be reduced to less than 30° of the normal position, a percutaneous pin (under image intensifier guidance) can often be used to lever the head back on to the shaft (Fig. 9-16). Gentle pronation and supination with direct thumb pressure on the radial head may then improve translation.

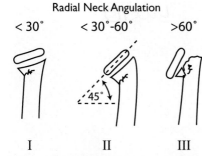

Radial Neck Angulation

< 30°   < 30°-60°   >60°

45°

I   II   III

Figure 9-14. Radial neck fractures with less than 30° of angulation can be casted. With angulation >60°, reduction must be performed. Between 30° and 60° there is some debate as to when reduction is necessary.

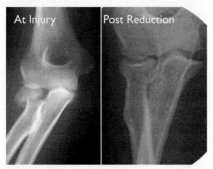

At Injury   Post Reduction

Figure 9-15. Child with radial neck fracture treated by Esmarch bandage method of closed reduction.

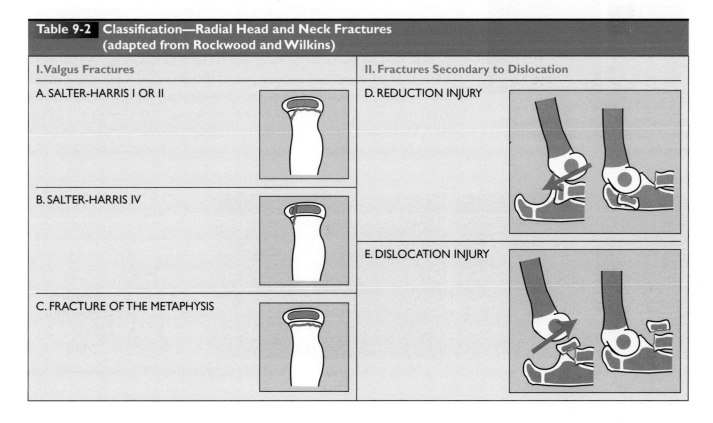

Table 9-2	Classification—Radial Head and Neck Fractures (adapted from Rockwood and Wilkins)		
I. Valgus Fractures		**II. Fractures Secondary to Dislocation**	
A. SALTER-HARRIS I OR II		D. REDUCTION INJURY	
B. SALTER-HARRIS IV			
		E. DISLOCATION INJURY	
C. FRACTURE OF THE METAPHYSIS			

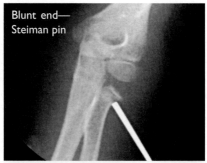

Blunt end—
Steiman pin

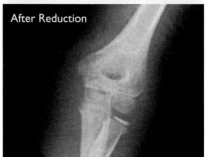

After Reduction

Figure 9-16. A K-wire or Steinmann pin can be used as a joystick for percutaneous/closed reduction.

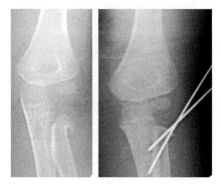

Figure 9-17. If the reduction is found to be unstable, it can be secured with percutaneus K-wires, taking care to avoid the articular surface.

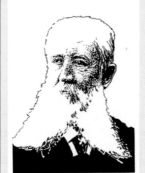

Johann Friedrich August von Esmarch
1823-1908

A German military surgeon who was concerned with blood loss and first aid. During the insurrection against Denmark in 1848-1850, he organized the resistance movement. In 1857 he became Professor of Surgery at Kiel, succeeding Stromeyer, the tenotomist, and marrying his daughter. In 1871 he became Surgeon General of the army and published his description of the bandage that bears his name. He used this to produce a clear, bloodless field for surgery and to diminish the blood loss during amputations in particular.

Occasionally, the radial head can be reduced to the capitellum, but the radial shaft still sits medially preventing normal pronation and supination. Wallace described a novel percutaneous technique for reducing the ulnar translation of the radial shaft to the radial head. A small incision is made on the posterior surface of the proximal forearm at the head of the bicipital tuberosity and a blunt-tipped elevator ("Joker") is passed between the radius and ulna. The radius can then be gently levered laterally while maintaining the position of the radial head with the thumb. The reduction may be stable or can be fixed with a percutaneous K-wire. There have been no reports of AVN or synostosis with this technique.

If attempts at closed reduction and percutaneous reduction fail to give adequate alignment, open reduction should be carried out because late corrective surgery for malunion of the radial neck is very difficult. Vostal showed that the annular ligament or capsule occasionally gets trapped in the fracture, which prevents closed reduction. For open reduction, the Kocher approach is used: The elbow joint is entered laterally between the extensor carpi ulnaris and anconeus. The dissection is kept above the annular ligament and the arm pronated throughout the procedure to protect the posterior interosseous nerve.

The joint is inspected and if any soft tissue remains attached to the radial head, extreme caution should be used to maintain them to protect the blood supply. The radial head can then be manually placed on the shaft. Occasionally, the annular ligament may need to be repaired. Stability should be checked with pronation and supination while directly visualizing the reduction.

Once reduced, these fractures are often stable and do not require internal fixation. If instability is noted intraoperatively, one or two smooth K-wires can be inserted from the lateral proximal radius, just lateral to the articular cartilage, crossing the fracture and engaging the medial metaphyseal or diaphy-seal cortex (Fig. 9-17). The pin should not enter the humerus or cross the radiocapitellar

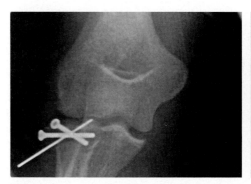

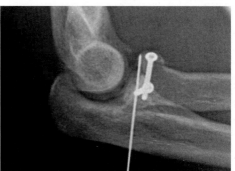

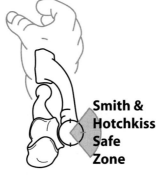

Smith & Hotchkiss Safe Zone

Figure 9-18. Screws and K-wires may be neccesary to fix an intra-articular radial head fracture. These should be inserted through "safe zone" described by Smith and Hotchkiss. (Illustration based on Smith and Hotchkiss.)

TECHNIQUE TIPS:
Radial Neck Fracture Reduction

The Columbus (Ohio) technique. Neher and Torch have described a technique of closed reduction that requires two people to manipulate the head back onto the shaft. A varus force is maintained and the radial shaft is pushed laterally while the radial head is pushed back onto the shaft. (Drawing based on Neher and Torch, see Suggested Readings.)

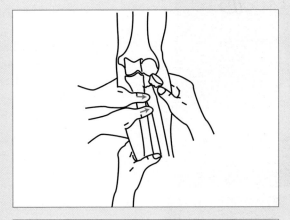

An Esmarch bandage can be wrapped tightly from distal to proximal. The soft tissues help push the radial head back into place (Fig. 9-15).

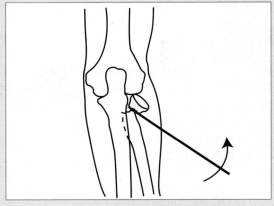

A K-wire or Steinmann pin can be used as a joystick to aid in closed reduction (also see Fig. 9-16).

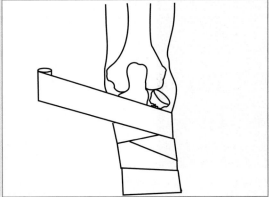

The modified percutaneous technique described by Wallace utilizes a joker between the radius and ulna to lateralize the radial shaft while the radial head is reduced by thumb pressure or K-wire.

(Method or Wallace et al. Children's Hospital—San Diego Treatment outcome of radial neck fractures in children and introduction of a new reduction technique. POSNA—Jacksonville, May 2003.)

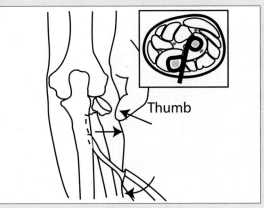

Thumb

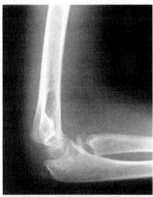

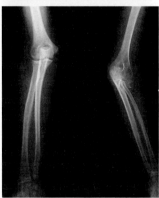

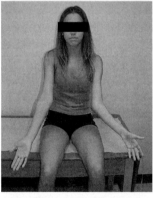

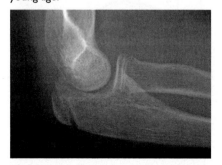

Figure 9-19. Cubitus valgus following a left radial neck fracture with physeal closure (proximal radius), which occured at a young age.

Figure 9-20. This is a normal elbow, the irregular apophysis is often mistaken for a fracture.

joint. Motion should be avoided while the pin is in place with the pin removed early (3 weeks is the maximum).

Intra-articular radial head fractures may require open reduction and internal fixation to maintain joint congruity (gap or intra-articular step off of more than 2 mm) CT scans may be needed to accurately assess displacement. The postero-lateral or Kocher approach is used to expose the radial head. Fragments need to be fixed anatomically. Screws and/or K-wires can safely be inserted through the safe zone described by Smith and Hotchkiss (Fig. 9-18).

In the past, some authors advocated excision of the radial head for comminuted fractures. In growing children, this should be avoided to prevent migration of the radius proximally, which destabilizes the distal radioulnar joint and can cause wrist and elbow pain.

Pitfalls—Radial Head and Neck Fractures

Eventual full flexion and extension of the elbow can be expected in most cases, but some loss of rotation is common. Imperfect results are more common in patients following surgery than in conservatively treated cases; Rang noted a higher correlation with the method of treatment than with the severity of injury. The lesson to be learned is that you should not give up on closed reduction until you have tried every trick you know.

Although rare, synostosis is a hazard on occasion even with closed reduction. The clearance between the proximal radius and ulna is small, and the torn periosteum may create a bridge that allows cross union between the two bones. Not only does synostosis block rotation but it may result in cubitus valgus. Heterotopic ossification may develop following open reduction of radial neck fractures (often seen in the vicinity of the biceps tendon) and correlates with loss of rotation.

Part or all of the radial head may develop AVN. Irregularity of the head and premature closure of the growth plate are common. The carrying angle is often increased in children due to premature physis closure (Fig. 9-19).

Nonunion is rare but disastrous. This may be due to closed reduction where the head is relocated upside down so that the articular cartilage prevents healing. Even if the head is correctly positioned, periosteal interposition may prevent adequate healing.

PROXIMAL ULNA: OLECRANON FRACTURES

The child's olecranon structure differs from an adult with more spongy bone, making the fracture line more difficult to identify. The layer of articular cartilage is thick, allowing occasional osteochondral fractures. The proximal epiphysis (appears at age 8 in girls, 10 in boys) is often irregular and although rarely separated, often is interpreted by primary care givers as a fracture (as in many other instances, a contralateral lateral x-ray may help clarify this, Fig. 9-20).

Although solitary fractures of the olecranon are seen, the majority are associated with fractures or dislocations of the radial neck.

Classification—Olecranon Fractures

Pediatric olecranon fractures are classified as noted in Table 9-3. Adolescent and adult fractures have been classified by Morrey as comminuted or non-comminuted. Oblique fractures and longitudinal split fractures are as common as transverse fractures.

Treatment—Olecranon Fractures

The majority of pediatric olecranon fractures are undisplaced and require only a cast. A cast in extension will reduce the pull of the triceps. When the periosteum is torn, the fragments may separate; therefore if the fracture does not reduce by extending the elbow, there may be interposed periosteum or bone fragments that require open reduction to realign the joint surface.

Displaced fractures are treated with open reduction and internal fixation. The incision should be made just lateral to the subcutaneous border of the proximal ulna and should stay lateral to the tip of the olecranon (avoid putting incisions directly over any subcutaneous bone or in an area that will frequently experience pressure). Keeping the incision a little lateral allows a soft tissue layer between the incision and the bony prominence of the olecranon.

Once the fracture is irrigated with any interposed bone fragments removed, most fractures easily reduce with elbow extension and can be held with a towel clip while fixation is placed. The joint should be checked through a small lateral arthrotomy to ensure a smooth joint surface with no step offs or gaps; this also allows the joint to be irrigated to avoid leaving loose bodies that could further damage the articular surface. Two smooth K-wires and a tension band wire technique provide excellent fixation of the fracture fragments (Fig. 9-21).

The pins should be buried under the skin and left in place until the fracture is completely healed. Percutaneous pins do not supply adequate fixation against the pull of the triceps muscle. Sutures have been suggested (rather than wires) for the tension band, but they are more likely to allow loss of reduction (Fig. 9-22).

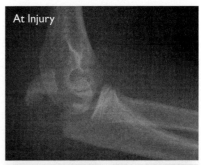
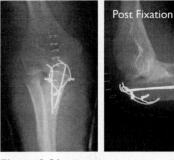

Figure 9-21. Displaced olecranon fractures are best treated with ORIF. This shows the classic fixation with two K-wires and a tension band.

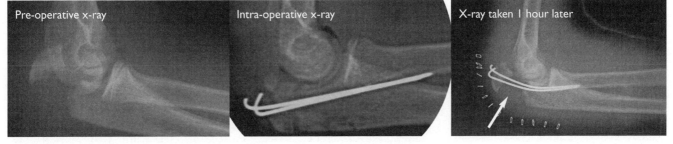

Figure 9-22. Some young children can be treated with K-wires and a suture tension band. However, this x-ray is a good example of what can occur if the child is stronger than the suture. The x-ray taken 1 hour later shows a 2-cm separation due to pull of the triceps. Wire should be used in bigger elbows. See Figure 9-21 for final fixation.

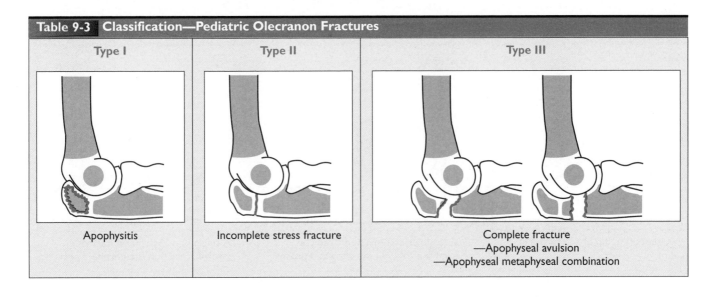

Table 9-3	Classification—Pediatric Olecranon Fractures	
Type I	**Type II**	**Type III**
Apophysitis	Incomplete stress fracture	Complete fracture —Apophyseal avulsion —Apophyseal metaphyseal combination

For more comminuted fractures, a contoured plate and screws often gives better fixation. A 1/3 tubular plate can easily be contoured to the olecranon, and pre-contoured plates are also available for near adult size patients.

Pitfalls—Olecranon Fractures

Comminution at the joint surface, or joint malreduction may lead to early arthritis. The pull of the triceps tends to pull olecranon fractures apart, especially if casted in flexion; this can lead to poor motion and function because of malreduction. There are reports of nonunion, but this is rare in children. Transient neuropraxia of the ulnar nerve may occur secondary to irritation or stretch of the nerve. If the fracture is treated with a cast alone, x-rays should be checked weekly for the first 2-3 weeks to ensure proper healing without late fracture line widening.

PROXIMAL ULNA: CORONOID FRACTURES

The coronoid process remains cartilagenous until the age of 6 years. Most fractures of the coronoid occur in association with elbow dislocation or are associated with other fractures about the elbow.

Classification—Coronoid Fractures

Regan and Morrey classified coronoid process fractures based on the size of the fragment (Table 9-4).

Treatment—Coronoid Fractures

Treatment of coronoid fractures is based on the degree of displacement and the instability of the elbow. In more severe cases, a CT scan will likely be needed to accurately study the injury. Type I and II fractures without associated injuries can be treated with casting for 3 weeks followed by early motion. Casting should be done with the forearm supinated and the elbow flexed to 90°.

Type III fractures typically cause instability of the elbow and require fixation for stabilization. In children, suture fixation through drill holes is typically adequate fixation if the fragment is anatomically reduced (Fig. 9-23). Again, a short time in a cast should be followed with early motion.

At Injury

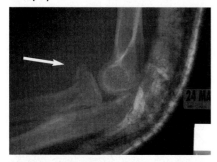

After Open Reduction

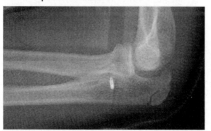

Figure 9-23. Type III coronoid fracture partially hidden by the radial head in this x-ray (indicated by the arrow) resulted in instability of the elbow and was treated with open reduction and suture anchor fixation.

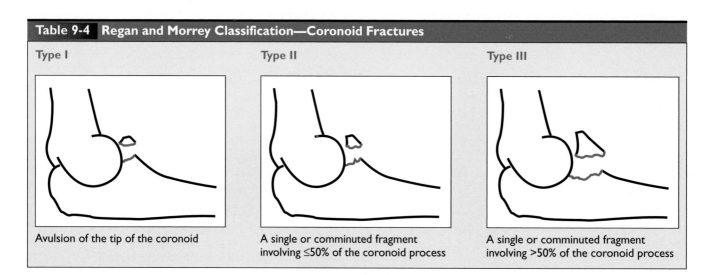

Table 9-4	Regan and Morrey Classification—Coronoid Fractures	
Type I	**Type II**	**Type III**
Avulsion of the tip of the coronoid	A single or comminuted fragment involving ≤50% of the coronoid process	A single or comminuted fragment involving >50% of the coronoid process

Nonunion of type III fractures can lead to chronic elbow instability and recurrent episodes of dislocation. This is rare in children.

MONTEGGIA FRACTURE/DISLOCATION

Radial head dislocation is almost universally accompanied by an ulna fracture or bow in children (Table 9-5). Giovanni Monteggia gave his name to the injury pattern after missing the diagnosis in a young girl in 1814. Lincoln and Mubarak reviewed so-called isolated anterior radial head dislocations and found that each case included a subtle greenstick fracture or plastic deformation of the ulna, suggesting that the term isolated radial head dislocation is a misnomer in children. Most are actually subtle variations of a Monteggia fracture. Straightening the ulna is important to stability of the radioulnar joint because even a slight ulnar bow can push the radial head out over time (if not immediately) (Fig. 9-24).

Confusion may arise when a child with a preexisting congenital or pathologic dislocation falls on the elbow with the ensuing radiographs read as an acute injury. In puzzling cases, examine and radiograph both elbows. The diagnosis of long-standing dislocation can be made (a) if the condition is bilateral or (b) if unilateral, when the affected radius is longer, the radial head misshapen, the capitellum hypoplastic, the distal humerus grooved, and/or ossification more advanced than on the opposite side (Fig. 9-25).

Treatment—Monteggia Fracture/Dislocation

The three critical elements required to treat radial head dislocations include:

1. Straightening the ulna
2. Reducing the radial head
3. Minimizing forces that will redislocate the radial head

Even a slight ulnar bow can keep the radial head dislocated, and therefore the ulna needs to be corrected to its anatomic position. Greenstick ulna fractures or ulnae with plastic deformation can often be straightened in a closed fashion and maintained with a cast alone; however, this reduction may require general anesthesia as it takes a significant amount of force to reshape a bent ulna. We have often used the readily available small oxygen tank (ever-present in ERs and

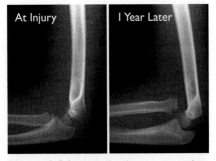

Figure 9-24. Initially this x-ray read as normal following trauma. One year later the radial head was found to be dislocated and the slight residual bow of the ulna was noted.

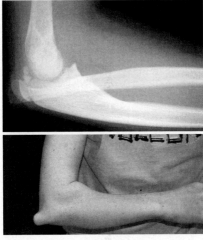

Figure 9-25. Congenital dislocations of the radial head have a different appearance than acute dislocation. This is a severe example; rarely will it be so obvious.

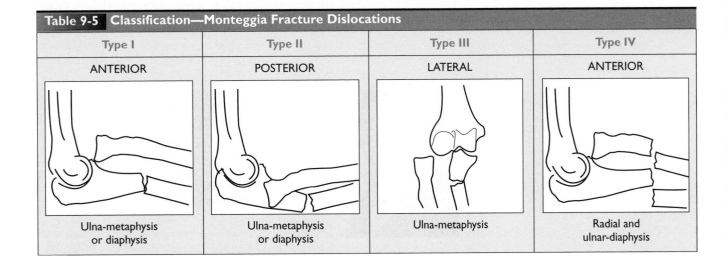

Table 9-5 Classification—Monteggia Fracture Dislocations			
Type I	**Type II**	**Type III**	**Type IV**
ANTERIOR	POSTERIOR	LATERAL	ANTERIOR
Ulna-metaphysis or diaphysis	Ulna-metaphysis or diaphysis	Ulna-metaphysis	Radial and ulnar-diaphysis

At Injury

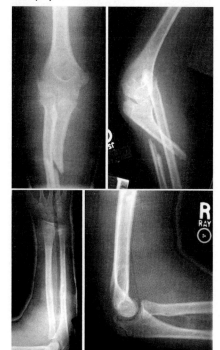

After Closed Reduction

Figure 9-26. This less subtle Monteggia fracture was treated with closed reduction and casting. The patient went on to have complete healing and normal motion.

At Injury   After Closed Reduction

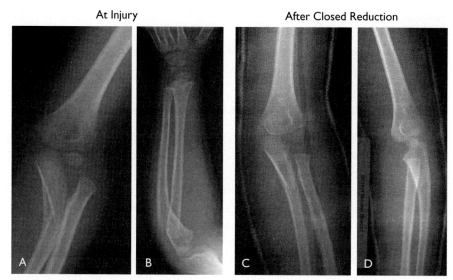

Figure 9-27. A,B) Type III Monteggia fracture/dislocation. C,D) This lateral dislocation was reduced and casted in relative extension.

ORs) as a fulcrum to bend the arm back to its normal position. Perfect alignment may require completing a greenstick ulna fracture.

Experienced surgeons can often reduce and maintain Monteggia fractures using closed methods (Fig. 9-26). Maintaining anatomic alignment of the ulnar fracture sometimes requires open reduction and fixation with a plate and screws or an intramedullary pin. An ulna fracture extending through the olecranon, disrupting the joint surface, usually requires open reduction to restore the joint surface plus either K-wires and a tension band or a contoured plate and screws.

The radial head is usually easily reduced once the ulna is straight. For type I and type III anterior dislocations, your thumb can be positioned directly over the radial head to guide it into place as the elbow is supinated and flexed. Lateral and posterior dislocations tend to require a cast in extension to maintain the reduction (Figs. 9-27, 9-28). Neviaser reported a child whose radial head buttonholed through the capsule and required open reduction. However, the majority of radial head dislocations associated with the Monteggia pattern can be treated with closed methods (although the ulna fracture may have to be opened and fixed—Fig. 9-29).

The Kocher posterolateral approach is recommended for the rare occasions in which open reduction of the radioulnar joint is needed. The forearm should be kept in pronation during the exposure to prevent injury to the posterior interosseous nerve. The annular ligament may need to be repaired or reconstructed to maintain the reduction.

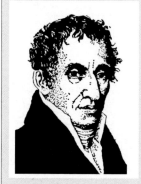

Giovanni Monteggia
1762–1815

Monteggia was born at Lake Maggiore, Italy. He studied in Milan where he became professor of surgery. He is particularly remembered for his description of a fracture dislocation of the forearm that he described in the same year that Colles described his fracture.

At Injury

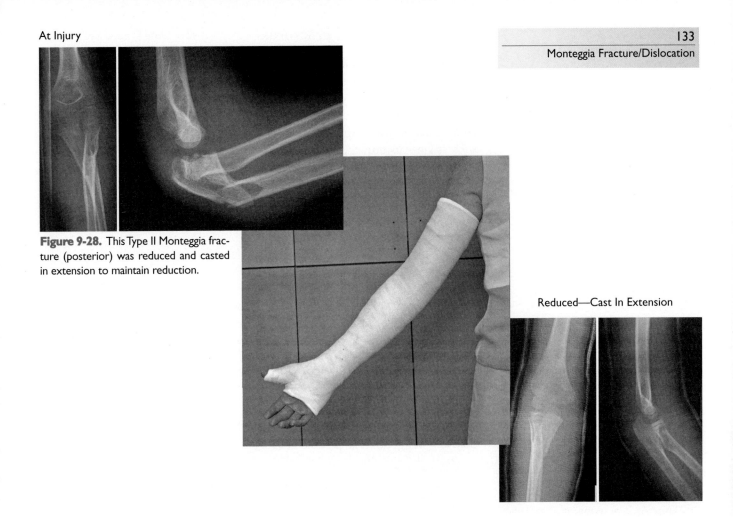

Figure 9-28. This Type II Monteggia fracture (posterior) was reduced and casted in extension to maintain reduction.

Reduced—Cast In Extension

Following reduction of anterior dislocations, the forearm should be immobilized in 90°-100° of flexion with near full supination to keep the radial head reduced while the ulna fracture heals. Flexion minimizes the pull of the biceps, which is the major deforming force in anterior dislocations. Supination gives maximum stability to the joint, reducing the force of the supinator muscle, which may deform the proximal ulna. Check films are taken in 7-10 days to confirm maintained alignment.

"Failing to recognize a subtle radial head dislocation can lead to catastrophe"

At Injury   After Reduction

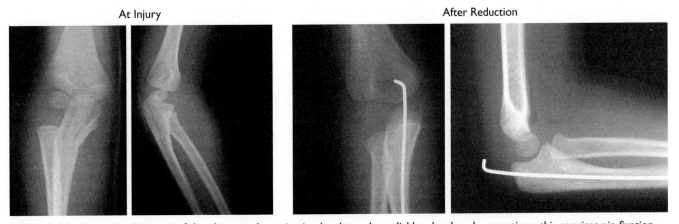

Figure 9-29. Anatomic alignment of the ulna must be maintained to keep the radial head reduced—sometimes this requires pin fixation.

Pitfalls—Monteggia Fractures

Failing to recognize a subtle radial head dislocation can lead to catastrophe. Late reconstruction is often difficult with less than perfect results. For persistent subluxation/dislocation or delayed diagnosis cases, several operative methods have been proposed to reduce the radial head. Bell-Tawse proposed annular ligament reconstruction with a strip of triceps tendon. Other surgeons have used material such as lacertus fibrosis, forearm fascia, palmaris longis, or fascia lata to reconstruct the annular ligament. An ulnar osteotomy with or without annular ligament reconstruction may be necessary to keep the radial head reduced. Motion following surgery may be limited by stiffness. Every effort should be made to make the correct diagnosis early. Always look at the radial-capitellar joint first when assessing an arm or elbow x-ray!

SUMMARY

Proximal forearm fractures can be very complex in terms of both diagnosis and treatment. Subtle fractures are easily missed and can lead to long-term disability. Even in the best surgeons hands, many proximal forearm fractures lead to stiffness and pain.

Suggested Readings

Bado, JL. The Monteggia Lesion. Clinical Orthopedics 50:71-86, 1967.

Beaty JH. Rockwood and Wilkins fractures in children. 5th ed. Philadelphia, Lippincott, Williams, and Wilkins 2001.

Bell Tawse AJ. The treatment of malunited anterior Monteggia fractures in children. J Bone Joint Surg Br. 1965 Nov; 47(4):718-23.

Gicquel P, Maximin MC, Boutemy P, Karger C, Kempf JF, Clavert JM. Biomechanical analysis of olecranon fracture fixation in children. J Pediatr Orthop. 2002 Jan-Feb;22(1):17-21.

Gillingham BL, Rang M. Advances in children's elbow fractures. J Pediatr Orthop 1995 15(4)419-28.

Gonzalez-Herranz P, Alvarez-Romera A, Burgos J, Rapariz JM, Hevia E. Displaced radial neck fractures in children treated by closed intramedullary pinning (Metaizeau technique). J Pediatr Orthop. 1997 May-Jun;17(3):325-31.

Kay RM, Skaggs DL. The pediatric Monteggia fracture. Am J Orthop. 1998 Sep;27(9):606-9.

Kosuwon, W. et al. Ultrasonography of pulled elbow. JBJS 75B:421-22, 1993.

Letts M, Locht R, Wiens J. Monteggia fracture-dislocations in children. J Bone Joint Surg Br. 1985 Nov;67(5):724-7.

Lincoln TL, Mubarak SJ. "Isolated" traumatic radial head dislocation. Journal of Pediatric Orthopedics 14:454-457, 1994.

Neher CG, Torch MA. New reduction technique for severely displaced pediatric radial neck fractures. J Pediatr Orthop. 2003 Sep-Oct;23(5):626-8.

Regan W., Morrey, BF. Classification and treatment of coronoid process fractures. Orthopedics 15:845-848, 1992.

Salter, RB, Zaltz, C: Anatomic investigations of the Mechanism of Injury and Pathologic Anatomy of Pulled Elbow in Young Children. Clin Orthop, 77:134-143, 1971.

Skaggs DL. Elbow Fractures in Children: Diagnosis and Management. J Am Acad Orthop Surg. 1997 Nov;5(6):303-312.

Smith GR, Hotchkiss RN. Radial head and neck fractures: Anatomic guidelines for proper placement of internal fixation. J Shoulder Elbow Surg. 1996 Mar-Apr;5(2 pt 1):113-7.

Triantafyllou, SJ et al, Irreducible pulled elbow in a child. A case report. Clin Orthop 284:153-155, 1992.

Vocke AK, Von Laer L. Displaced fractures of the radial neck in children: long-term results and prognosis of conservative treatment. J Pediatr Orthop B. 1998 Jul;7(3):217-22.

Weisman DS, Rang M, Cole WG. Tardy displacement of traumatic radial head dislocation in childhood. J Pediatr Orthop. 1999 Jul-Aug;19(4):523-6.

10

Radius and Ulna

Mercer Rang ❧ *Philip Stearns* ❧ *Henry Chambers*

INTRODUCTION

The influx of extreme sports and activities has increased a child's risk for fracture. Even children at a young age participate in these more risky activities. When a child falls off a bike, scooter, or skateboard, the upper extremity bears most of the force, particularly the forearm and wrist because the arms are often used to brace one's fall: This is a variation of the parachute reflex (Fig. 10-1). The parachute reflex protects the vital organs often at the expense of the forearm.

Fractures of the radius and ulna, especially about the wrist, are the most common children's fractures. In many ways, these fractures are different from those of adults:

■ Shattering injuries of the articular surfaces of each end of the radius are less common.
■ The bones may bend or plastically deform without a complete fracture.

> *"Convictions are more dangerous enemies of truth than lies"*
> —NIETZSCHE

135

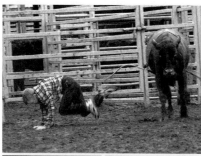

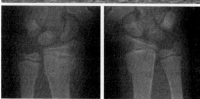

Figure 10-1. Children of every age enjoy a variety of sports. This junior bull rider suffered bilateral distal radius fractures from this fall. (Photo courtesy of R. Knudson.)

- Nonunion is rare.
- Fractures of the shafts of both bones of the forearm can usually be managed closed, therefore requiring reduction and casting skills that adult forearm fractures do not.
- Forearm fractures in children have remodeling potential, which does not exist in adult forearm fractures.

ANATOMY AND PATHOLOGY

The forearm bones are subcutaneous in the lower half of the forearm. The quality of reduction can be appreciated, not only by the surgeon but also by the patient when the cast comes off.

Forearm rotation has a range of 180°, perhaps the greatest range of rotation of any joint in the body. Although a decrease of rotation by 50% may go unnoticed for most activities, fractures should be reduced well so that patients will regain full rotation.

Loss of rotation is a common problem after forearm fractures. Knight and Purvis found residual rotational deformity of between 20° and 60° in 60% of cases. Evans found malrotation deformity of more than 30° in 56% of cases with the distal fragment pronated so that supination was lost.

Fractures have been produced in cadavers and plated with various types of malunion to determine the effects of each.

- Ten degrees of malrotation limits rotation by 10° (Fig. 10-2).
- Ten degrees of angulation limits rotation by 20° (Fig. 10-3).
- Bayonet apposition does not limit rotation.
- Pure narrowing of the interosseous distance is important in proximal fractures. (Narrowing impedes rotation by causing the bicipital tuberosity to impinge on the ulna.)
- Malalignment of fractures of the ulnar metaphysis increases the tension on the articular disc so that the head of the ulna is not free to rotate (Fig. 10-4).

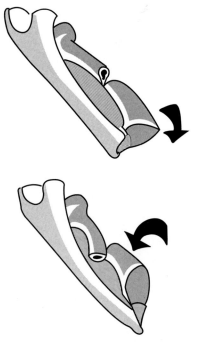

Figure 10-2. Malrotation limits movement. Ninety degrees of pronation deformity, as shown here, limits pronation to the midposition, because the proximal radioulnar joint has reached the limit.

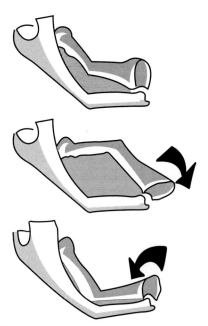

Figure 10-3. Angulation malunion limits rotation, because the interosseous membrane cannot widen and narrow.

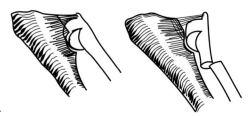

Figure 10-4. Angulation of the distal ulna prevents rotation of the ulna.

ASSESSING THE PATIENT

Some injuries to the forearm are more obvious than others. First, observe the extremity to see how the child holds it and if there is deformity. With severe deformity, the child will be difficult to examine due to pain, fear, and other concerns. The joints above and below the suspected site of injury are examined to rule out other injuries. The Monteggia injury is the classic (Chapter 9); however, supracondylar fractures are commonly seen along with a distal radius fracture.

Assessment is important but may be difficult in a very unhappy child. Pulses, nerve function, and forearm compartment status are noted. Document only what you can confirm (Chapter 8). Look at the forearm in its position of displacement. You should be able to tell from the shape of the arm how the distal fragment lies in relation to the proximal part.

It sometimes helps if first the part of the arm below the fracture is blocked off from vision with a hand and then the part above. If the upper part of the arm lies in supination, and the distal part looks as if it is pronated, a simple supination force on the hand will reduce the fracture. The first person that sees the child has a great advantage, because he/she is the only one who can see the limb as it lies (Fig. 10-5). Prior vigorous splinting may make this analysis problematic.

The skin exam is critical. Often, there is a small puncture wound where a bone end stuck through the skin and then retracted back. The spike of bone may have pulled debris and bacteria back inside with it. If you can express hematoma out through a puncture hole, it should be considered an open fracture and treated appropriately.

Despite the presence of closed fascial spaces in the forearm, the risk of ischemic contracture is low if a well-padded splint or split cast is used. Nerve injuries are also rare but can occur from stretch or laceration.

RADIOGRAPHIC ISSUES

Standard AP and lateral views of the forearm are the usual films performed when a child has a forearm injury. A separate elbow film may be needed to evaluate the relationship between the radial head and the capitellum (Monteggia injury). Beware the forearm film that does not clearly show the radial head–capitellar relationship or because the x-ray technician has placed the name plate over this vital area.

Radius

The radius is a curved bone that is pear-shaped in cross section. Malrotation of the radius is recognized by a break in the smooth curve of the bone and by a sudden change in the width of the cortex (Fig. 10-6).

Angulation

Angulation that produces a volar apex or prominence is conventionally described as volar angulation or bowing. Some describe the distal fragment as being dorsally displaced or tilted. If the distal fragment is tipped in the palmar direction, a dorsal angulation is created. This is worth stating clearly because telephone conversations about fractures are frequently plagued by semantic ambiguities (Chapter 3).

Rotation

X-rays are two-dimensional so it is difficult to recognize and understand rotational deformity. A supination or pronation force causes most fractures. For

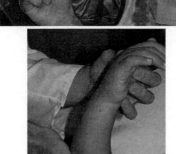

Figure 10-5. Typical deformity in a forearm fracture. A fracture with this deformity (apex dorsal angulation) often is most easily reduced by supination.

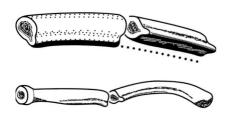

RADIAL MALROTATION

Figure 10-6. A change in the diameter of the radius, the width of the cortex, and the smooth curve of the radius indicate malrotation.

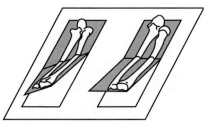

Figure 10-7. Angulation is usually associated with rotation. Use a strip of paper to prove this yourself.

"Prior to the discovery of x-ray films, surgeons had to guess the position of the proximal fragment, and some surgeons still do"

example, when a child extends the hand to break a fall, the pronated thenar eminence hits the ground first and an immediate supination force is applied. The radiographic appearance of this fracture seems to be apex volar angulation, but the displacement is usually rotational. Test this for yourself with a strip of paper, as shown in Figure 10-7. If the surgeon considers only the angulation and corrects it, the rotational deformity will remain uncorrected. An apex volar fracture is often more accurately reduced by applying a pronation force to the hand, whereas an apex dorsal fracture is usually better reduced with a supination force to the hand.

Prior to the discovery of x-ray films, surgeons had to guess the position of the proximal fragment, and some surgeons still do, using the traditional argument that muscle pull determines the position of the proximal fragments. Classic dogma included that "in the case of fractures above the insertion of pronator teres, the proximal fragment is invariably pulled into supination by supinator muscles. The fracture should be immobilized in supination. Fractures below the insertion of pronator teres are invariably pulled into pronation by this muscle and should therefore be immobilized in this position." Although this theory is often repeated and has certain logic, it is often not true.

Position of Bicipital Tuberosity

The bicipital tuberosity is a good landmark for understanding rotation. It normally lies medially when the arm is fully supinated, posteriorly in mid-position, and laterally in full pronation (Fig. 10-8). This method is better applied in older children who have a more prominent tuberosity.

In complete fractures, the rotational position of the proximal fragment can be identified by this method, and reduction becomes more scientific. The distal fragment is lined up in the same degree of rotation as the proximal fragment, which usually maintains its normal position.

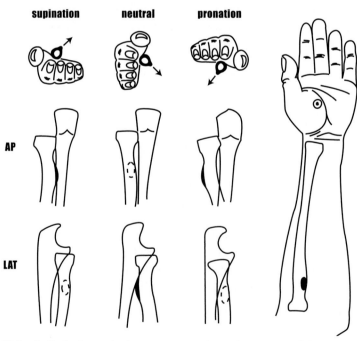

Figure 10-8. (Left) the bicipital tuberosity as a guide to the rotation of the proximal radius. (Right) If you cannot remember where the bicipital tuberosity should be, put an ink mark on your palm at the site indicated. The prominance of the tuberosity always points in this direction.

Application

The previous theories must be learned and applied when reducing forearm fractures. Although useful in achieving reduction, casting in distorted positions of rotation makes x-ray analysis difficult. Except for extreme cases, we apply a long arm (above elbow) cast in neutral rotation (after using rotational theory to achieve reduction). Follow-up x-rays are much easier to analyze (clear AP and lateral views). A compromise seems best. Rotational and angular concepts are used to achieve reduction; then when possible, the cast is applied in neutral or near neutral rotation to allow production of more easily interpretable x-rays.

DISTAL FRACTURES—PHYSEAL

Salter-Harris Type I Injuries

Type I injuries are seen in younger children, are seldom much displaced, and are diagnosed on clinical suspicion more than by radiographic findings (Fig. 10-9). Swelling and tenderness at the growth plate, despite normal radiographs, are our grounds for making this diagnosis. The radiograph may demonstrate a slight widening of the physis. Protection for 3 weeks in a cast or removable splint provides adequate treatment. You may think this is over-treatment, but the entity is common, real, and painful. A cast relieves the symptoms and stops the parents worrying and telephoning. On follow-up exam callus formation may be seen on the radiograph confirming the diagnosis. In general, only cases with more severe trauma would have follow-up to rule out occult physeal injury.

Salter-Harris Type II Injuries

Type II injuries are the most common, usually associated with posterior displacement (volar angulation) and are frequently accompanied by a chip off the ulnar styloid (Fig. 10-10).

This angulation pattern is often referred to as a Colles fracture (although Colles described it in adults). For typical volarly angulated Type II fractures, wrist flexion alone may not maintain the reduction, because the wrist joint

"Although useful in achieving reduction, casting in distorted positions of rotation makes x-ray analysis difficult"

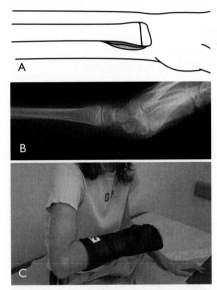

Figure 10-9. Typical SH I fracture. A) Diagram illustrating bleeding and swelling but without displacement. B) X-ray at injury (normal). C) Treatment—either cast or splint (if patient is cooperative) can be used.

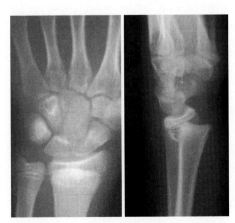

Figure 10-10. The typical SH II fracture of the distal radius (with volar angulation) can be reduced with a hematoma block or conscious sedation.

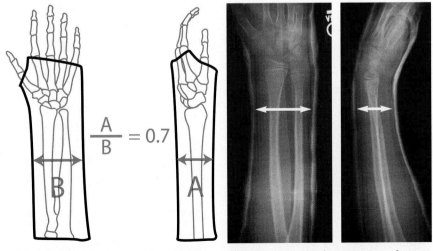

$$\frac{A}{B} = 0.7$$

Figure 10-11. Hyndman et al. studied the ratio of the cast width for maintaining fracture reduction. The lateral diameter (A) must be significantly less than the AP diameter (B) to maximize molding and stability.

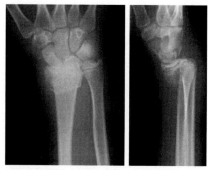

Figure 10-12. Smith variant or fracture with anterior displacement of the distal fragment are common following falls from scooters. This is also a Salter-Harris II injury.

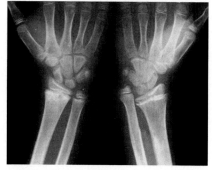

Figure 10-13. Following a severe Type II injury of the right distal radius, this patient had a physeal closure and a resultant wrist deformity. Earlier recognition could have allowed better treatment.

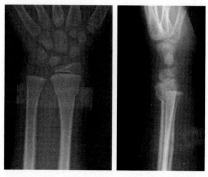

Figure 10-14. Classic buckle fracture of distal radius, best noted on lateral view.

flexes easily to 80° before the capsule tightens enough to exert any influence on the distal fragment. Thus in addition to moderate wrist flexion, three-point molding must be optimized (Chapter 5).

We often use a long arm (above elbow) cast, although Hyndman and then Galpin (POSNA—2004) have demonstrated that a short arm (below elbow) cast can maintain many reductions if the AP and lateral cast diameter ratios are correct (excellent molding required—Fig. 10-11).

Distal physeal fractures can also be seen with anterior displacement (dorsal angulation—Smith variant) due to a fall from a bike, scooter, etc. These Smith-variant fractures are easily reduced by direct pressure (with appropriate anesthesia). The reduction maneuver and molding are reversed (from Colles pattern) when the cast is applied (Fig. 10-12).

In 4-6 weeks, the fracture will be united and the cast can be removed. If a reduction was performed, the child should return to clinic in 1 week for an x-ray check to ensure maintenance of reduction. Severe loss of reduction, up to 10 days after the original injury, is usually re-reduced under general anesthesia. If more than 10-14 days past injury, this re-reduction may damage the physis, thus the fracture is left in its malreduced position with hope for remodeling. In rare cases, a late osteotomy will be required.

It is important to discuss the risks of physeal closure with the family. We follow these children at 6 months and even 1 year after the fracture has healed to assess for premature closure. X-rays of both wrists are taken at follow-up visits and, if there is suspicion of early closure, a CT or MRI can help to further evaluate possible closure.

Salter-Harris Type III and IV Injuries

Injuries that involve the joint surface are less common in children and can be difficult to see on the radiograph. For these injuries the step offs, depressions, or gaps at the joint surface as well as physeal congruity are best evaluated with a CT scan.

If significant displacement is seen (>2 mm in any direction), reduction is required. This can be performed arthroscopically or more typically with a dorsal or volar incision, depending on where the joint damage is located. Plan your incision to get maximum exposure of the joint injury. When possible, we try to minimize internal fixation and use percutaneous pins that are removed after 3-4 weeks, prior to starting motion. If more permanent fixation is required to maintain the reduction, all fixation must be countersunk or very low profile; the tendons and nerves will either be gliding over your metal or catching and tearing on your screw heads and plate edges with attempts at wrist motion. There are very low profile and contoured periarticular plates that can be used as a buttress if needed.

Growth

The distal end of the radius is a classic site for growth disturbance owing to bridging of the physes. Thus all physeal fractures must be followed closely. With radial physeal closure and ulnar overgrowth, a wrist deformity may begin to appear (Fig. 10-13). These children should be radiographed every 3-6 months for signs of a bony bridge so that prompt resection can be carried out.

DISTAL FRACTURES—ABOVE PHYSIS

Buckle or torus fractures are common and usually thought by the family to be a sprain. When the pain persists for several days and an x-ray is ordered, the diagnosis is usually accompanied by guilty feelings on the part of the parent for not bringing the child in right away. The radiograph demonstrates a "buckle" or wrinkle in the cortex of the radius (Fig. 10-14). Buckle fractures can be treated either with a below-elbow cast or Velcro splint, depending on the child's activity level.

Minimally angulated fractures require good casting, often a hematoma block or no anesthesia. Fractures that are apex volar in angulation require a three-point flexion type mold as shown in Figure 10-15. These should be followed in 7-10 days to ensure alignment.

Fractures with apex dorsal angulation require an extension type mold. These also should be followed within 7-10 days (Fig. 10-16).

Also, be wary of nondisplaced fractures that are complete through the volar cortex. These fractures may tip into apex volar angulation; therefore a cast should be applied with a flexion type mold. A follow-up x-ray should also be obtained in 7-10 days. We have seen these fractures angulate in the cast.

Complete Fracture—Both Bones

Complete fractures of the radius and ulna can be very challenging to manage (Fig. 10-17). Reduction may be difficult and unstable, particularly in children less than 2 years, in older children, in proximal fractures, and in those that are comminuted or oblique. If both bones are overlapping, reduce them by increasing the deformity as described on the following page. Charnley's analogy to re-engaging a gear is important in understanding why the deformity must be made worse before it can be reduced. Simple distal pull or simple angular forces will not do.

There are several general rules to guide you:

1. Good reductions last better than poor reductions, particularly in a well-molded cast.
2. In young children (<10) bayonet apposition is adequate if rotation is correct, if the interosseous space is preserved, and if there is no angulation.
3. Immobilize the fracture in the position in which the alignment is correct and the reduction feels stable. Immobilization with the elbow in extension may be the best position for fractures in the proximal one third of the forearm.
4. Minor reduction improvements can be made at 1-2 weeks when the fracture is sticky (wedging—Fig. 10-18—or change cast and re-manipulate).
5. Be prepared to carry out open reduction and internal fixation, particularly in children older than the age of 10 rather than accept a poor reduction.
6. Always warn the parents before you reduce the fracture that re-manipulation is often necessary later and that there will be a bump when the cast comes off.

At Injury   After Reduction

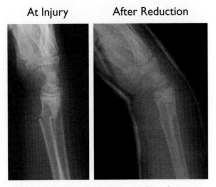

Figure 10-15. Fractures with volar angulation (Colles pattern) can be reduced and maintained with a three-point mold.

At Injury   After Reduction

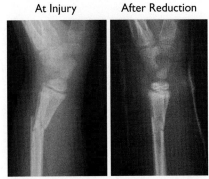

Figure 10-16. For a fracture with dorsal angulation (Smith pattern), an extension mold maintains the reduction. (This patient was very obese thus the cast diameter on the lateral view appears to be too great but in fact could not be improved due to patient size.)

Loss of Reduction   After Wedging

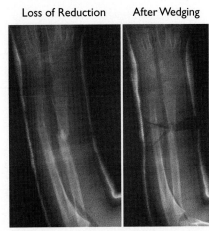

Figure 10-18. Loss of reduction in a both bone forearm fracture can be corrected with a wedge or recasting. This case was corrected by wedging, which must be done very carefully to avoid skin necrosis.

Initial Deformity   After Reduction

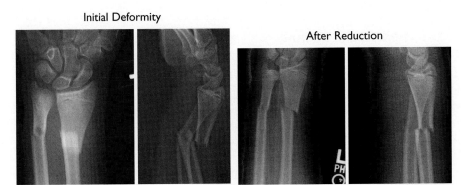

Figure 10-17. Distal both bone forearm fractures can be reduced by using the method of Charnley, described on the next page.

Closed Treatment of Forearm Fractures

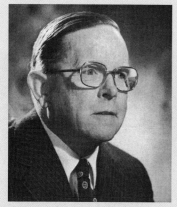

John Charnley
1911–1982

John Charnley, one of the most remarkable surgical innovators of the 20th century, is best known for his work in developing a total hip replacement for the treatment of degenerative arthritis in adults.

Many young orthopedists do not realize the importance of Charnley's work in fracture treatment. After serving in World War II, Charnley returned to the Manchester Royal Infirmary where, working with the famed Sir Harry Platt, he developed an extensive experience in the closed treatment of fractures, leading to his classic text *The Closed Treatment of Common Fractures* (See Suggested Readings).

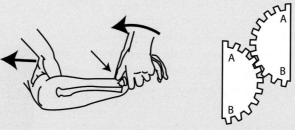

Fracture fragments locked

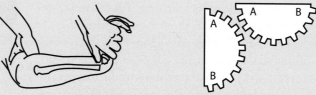

Disengage fragments by increasing the deformity

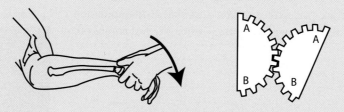

Reduce the fracture

To reduce a fracture the fragments must be disengaged by recreating the injury. This can then be re-engaged in proper alignment to assist with reduction.

(Source: Charnley J. *The closed treatment of common fractures.* Edinburgh: Livingstone, 1980. [Figures reproduced with permission])

Solitary Distal Radial Fractures

The ulnar styloid is usually avulsed. It may be more difficult to reduce a fracture of only one bone as the intact bone will not allow the typical reduction maneuvers. Armed with strong thumbs and awareness of the periosteal hinge, you can usually reduce these fractures closed. If the fragments are still in cortex-to-cortex apposition, repeat the maneuver with more thumb pressure. Be careful not to dislocate your own thumb in the process, as a surgeon in our group did. An OR reduction with K-wire fixation is sometimes required.

Galeazzi's Fracture

The classic Galeazzi fracture (Table 10-1) is a fracture of the radius (usually at the junction of the middle and distal thirds) with dislocation of the distal radioulnar joint; it is less common than Monteggia's injury. These fracture-dislocations are often missed because one focuses in on the distal radial fracture and ignores the subluxation or dislocation of the distal radioulnar joint. When looking too hard for these injuries, it is easy to become confused, as a slightly oblique x-ray of a normal wrist will make the ulna look subluxed. A trick is to look at the the ulnar styloid, it should be pointing at the triquetrum on all radiographic views including obliques.

MIDSHAFT

Midshaft Greenstick Fractures

Minimally displaced fractures are very common. The deformity may be corrected with corrective pressure while the cast is setting. No reduction effort is made as the cast is applied. Then, as it is setting, a smooth corrective three-point mold is applied. Without a good mold, the bone may slowly bend as it heals (Fig. 10-19).

Angulated greenstick fractures of the midshaft require slight overcorrection to take the spring out of the fracture. You will often hear a crack as the bony hinge yields. If this is not done, the deformity may reappear in the succeeding weeks. On the other hand, a too vigorous maneuver (big doctor, small patient)

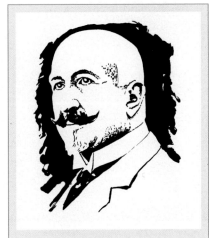

**Riccardo Galeazzi
1866–1952**
Galeazzi directed the orthopedic clinic in Milan for 35 years. He was a contemporary of Monteggia. Galeazzi described a fracture of the distal radius with subluxation of the distal radioulnar joint.
Italian eponynms remain among the most popular and most frequently quoted in contemporary orthopedic discussion. Why? First, Italy has been (and remains) a center for orthopedic ideas. In addition, Italian names have a pleasant way of rolling off the tongue, making those who quote them seem a bit wiser.

Table 10-1 Classification—Galeazzi Fractures	
Type I (Most Common)	**Type II**
Dorsal Subluxation of the Ulna	Volar Subluxation of the Ulna
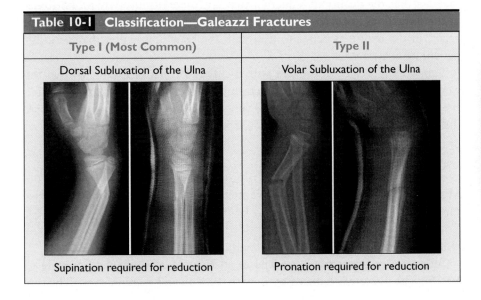	
Supination required for reduction	Pronation required for reduction

Initial Fracture   4 Weeks Later

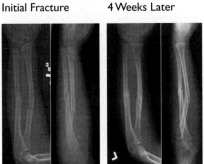

Figure 10-19. This both bone forearm fracture originally appeared to have acceptable alignment, but the radius slowly bowed while in the cast, resulting in malunion with loss of motion.

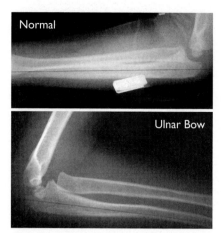

Figure 10-20. Plastic deformation is much harder to correct and often requires fracturing the bone to straighten it.

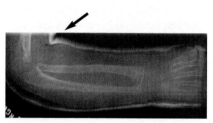

Figure 10-21. Be very careful not to bend the elbow while applying the cast—the fiberglass will dig in and produce a sore (note arrow—cast material kinked at elbow crease, resulted in skin ulceration in the cubital fossa).

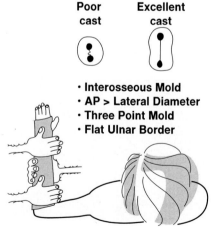

Figure 10-22. The ability to provide a careful three point mold with the cast relatively narrow in its dorsal to volar dimension is critical to maintenance of forearm fracture reduction.

may create more severe displacement. The periosteal tube is intact and will help maintain reduction. Supination injuries are pronated and then given a push to get rid of the anterior angulation, at which time a crack is often heard. The cast should be well molded to prevent further angulation.

Plastic Deformation

Some fractures do not appear to break any cortex yet the arm has a terrible bend to it (Fig. 10-20). The radiograph shows a bent appearance of either or both of the radius and ulna. These are difficult injuries to treat and should be taken to the OR to obtain reduction under general anesthesia. These fractures do not re-model and the child is left with an angulated and rotated forearm. A large amount of force is necessary to reduce these fractures, usually over a rigid object such as an oxygen canister.

Maintaining Reduction

Examine the radiograph to determine the position of the proximal fragment (use the bicipital tuberosity as a guide). Try to line the distal fragment up with the proximal fragment. It is always difficult to hold the limb while the cast is being applied and two people are required, one to maintain the reduction and the other to apply a well-molded cast—holding the thumb and index finger, with slight flexion and ulnar deviation, often helps. Be very careful not to bend the elbow during or after applying the cast—the fiberglass will dig in and produce a sore (Fig. 10-21).

Mold the cast well. The cast should have a straight ulnar border, it should be compressed so the side-to-side dimension is wider than the dorsal to volar dimension, there should be a good interosseous mold and three-point molding at the fracture (Fig. 10-22), and the elbow must be at a perfect right angle. Supracondylar molding just above the elbow should prevent the cast from telescoping up and down the arm. It is difficult to manage all of these factors at one time, so at least while learning, we recommend applying the cast in two stages, a well-molded short arm cast can be extended to an above elbow cast. Some argue that a well-molded short arm cast is more effective than the typical poorly applied long arm cast.

Reduction is confirmed by fluoroscan views with formal x-rays made for the record and for subsequent comparison. Carefully analyze the final films. Remember that the quality of reduction that is accepted is inversely proportional to the difficulties involved in changing it. If the position is not satisfactory, try again. In the end, it is better to deal with the issue now rather than in a 50-patient clinic next week.

Support the weight of the cast with a cuff and collar or a sling, so that the weight of the cast will not act as a deforming force at the fracture site. Include the thumb in the cast if the fracture is very unstable or if the cast is applied with the elbow in extension.

Other Methods

Many authors advocate an alternative method of reduction for midshaft fractures: Traction is used to reduce and hold the limb while the cast is applied. Counter traction is provided by a padded sling around the arm. An assistant pulls on the hand while the surgeon manipulates the bone ends.

Alternatively, finger traps attached to an IV pole can hold the fingers (Fig. 10-23). The fracture is reduced again with traction and manipulation. The cast is then applied, and the sling is pulled out. Some object to this method because the intact periosteum must be stretched to allow the overlapping ends to jump into end-to-end contact. It is like trying to force a door shut when something is in the way of the hinge.

A combination of the two concepts provides a nice compromise. Finger traps optimize longitudinal traction while deft thumbs apply an angular and rotational correction. Clearly, time and experience will be needed for you to develop your best method. The reduction should be checked radiographically weekly for 3 weeks to see if there is any loss of reduction.

When is a Closed Reduction Acceptable?

Price tells us that if the child is younger than 9, then 15° of angulation can be accepted. Those children older than 9 should not have more than 10° of angulation. Malrotation of up to 45° can be accepted in children younger than the age of 9 years, while only 30° should be accepted for those older than 9 years. Shortening is not usually a problem. It is important to remember that the more proximal the fracture is, the less likely it is to remodel with time. Fractures near the physis will remodel in the plane of motion, but rotational deformities do not remodel efficiently.

Open Reduction

Traditional plate fixation, commonly advised for adults, is not needed for most children. Semitubular or compression plates require a large exposure in small arms. They then require removal, which predisposes the child to refracture.

Most centers now use intramedullary (IM) nailing techniques using a flexible titanium nail system (Metazeau) or IM K-wires or Steinman pins for internal fixation in children with open, unstable, or otherwise uncastable forearm fractures (Fig. 10-24, Fig. 10-25).

The term "Nancy nail" is commonly used to describe flexible nailing because the concept was studied and then widely used and publicized by Metazeau in Nancy, France. After widespread use in Europe, the method is now widely accepted worldwide.

It is controversial as to whether it is necessary to fix both the radius and ulna in a both bone forearm fracture. Stability of the forearm is the key to success. If fixation of one bone gives adequate stability for casting, you may get away with only fixing one of the fractures.

"Traditional plate fixation, commonly advised for adults, is not needed for most children"

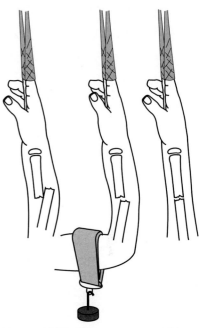

Figure 10-23. Finger traps can aid in reduction of forearm fractures.

"The term 'Nancy nail' is commonly used to describe flexible nailing because the concept was studied and then widely used and publicized by Metazeau in Nancy, France"

At Injury   After Surgery

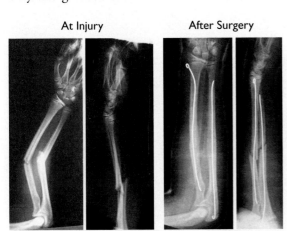

Figure 10-24. K-wires can be used for intramedulary fixation in younger children with severely angulated fractures that fail closed reduction.

At Injury

After Surgery

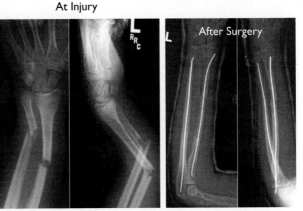

Figure 10-25. In older children, flexible titanium intramedulary nails give better fixation.

"Fractures at or distal to the metadiaphyseal junction can be treated with percutaneous fixation because intramedullary fixation may cause an ulnar angulation at the fracture site"

Under general anesthesia, the fracture is evaluated under fluoroscopic control. If there is an open fracture, the bone ends are débrided in the standard fashion. The fractures may be reduced if possible. Sometimes the fracture will need to be opened to remove entrapped muscle or periosteum through a small incision. Do not try to manipulate the fractures over and over again as we have had a few cases of compartment syndrome after multiple attempted closed reductions and IM fixation. Occasionally, it will be difficult to reduce both of the bones at the same time and one is faced with the decision of which bone to place the pin in first. We usually choose the one that was most difficult to reduce (usually the radius).

Fractures at or distal to the metadiaphyseal junction can be treated with percutaneous fixation (Fig. 10-26) because IM fixation may cause a significant ulnar angulation at the fracture site. These fractures are metaphyseal and heal quickly, so percutaneous pins can be removed after 3-4 weeks. In more distal fractures, it may be necessary to place the K-wire across the physis (we haven't had a physeal closure yet).

Diaphyseal fractures do not do well with percutaneous K-wire fixation; we have had complications of loss of reduction after pin removal at 4 weeks and osteomyelitis from leaving the pins out of the skin. IM fixation is preferred for shaft fractures. K-wires can be used for small children, Steinmann pins can be used, or flexible titanium nails can be used as described by Metazeau.

The starting point for a radius fracture is distal. If possible, one should place the pin (or rod) proximal to the distal radial physis starting on the radial side. Some physicians use Lister's tubercle on the dorsal aspect of the distal radius as a starting point. A small incision is made carefully looking for and protecting the superficial branch of the radial nerve. A drill just slightly larger than the pin or rod should be used. The pin or rod should be prebent to make passage down the bone easier. The tip is curved to bounce off the far cortex after insertion. A gentle long C shape improves three-point contact and reduction stability.

After the pin is across the radial fracture, the ulna pin can be placed. It can be placed through the proximal apophysis or just distal to the apophysis on the lateral aspect of the ulna. We recommend reversing the prebent titanium nails and passing the straight end in the ulna.

Some authors prefer to place the ulnar pin from distally because it is easier to view under fluoroscopy. One must put a smaller bend on the tip, as the ulnar diaphysis intramedullary space is often fairly narrow. It is important to bury the

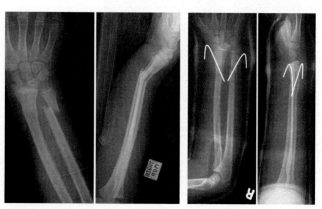

Figure 10-26. Fractures at or distal to the metadiaphyseal junction can be treated with percutaneous fixation if unstable.

For the radius, make a small incision on the dorsal-radial aspect of the wrist, just proximal to the physis. Care must be taken to protect the superficial branch of the radial nerve.

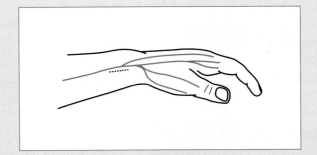

An oblique hole is made in the dorsal-radial metaphysis with a drill (only drill one cortex). Gently widen the hole by spinning the drill and lowering it so that it is near parallel to the shaft.

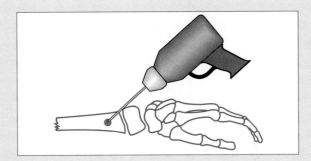

A prebent K-wire or flexible titanium nail is passed to the fracture site. This must be bent so that on entry, when the far cortex is encountered, the pin bounces off the cortex and can be directed down the shaft. We recommend a 20°-30° bend at the tip and an additional gentle bend 1-2 cm from the tip.

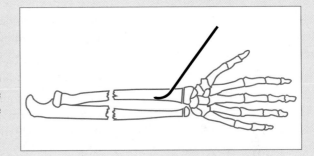

Fluoroscopy or direct visualization (if open fracture) is used during fracture reduction. The bent tip of the pin can be used to aid the reduction and the pin is passed into the proximal radius—stopping short of the physis (usually at the level of the bicipital tuberosity). The pin is cut close to the bone, leaving enough length to allow for later removal but not so prominent that the skin will be tented. The skin is closed over the tip.

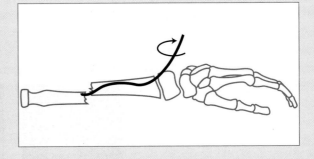

For the ulna, if the pin is inserted through the tip of the olecranon, one has a straight shot down the shaft. The prominent pin with little soft tissue coverage is often bothersome to the patient; lateral starting point on the olecranon allows the pin to be buried but requires a slight curve at the tip and may be trickier to pass.

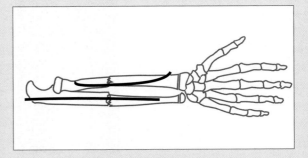

(Variation of technique described by Lascombes, Prevot, Ligier et al.—see Suggested Readings.)

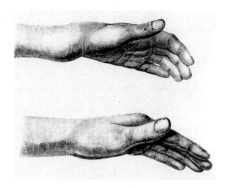

Figure 10-27. John Poland's classic 1896 text included this illustration of a boy whose fracture remodeled (pre x-ray era).

pin below the skin, as these fractures often take longer to heal because of an open fracture, the need for open reduction, and/or the fact that it is diaphyseal. We still use an above elbow cast for these fractures for 6 weeks. The pins can be removed at 6 months or whenever there is complete healing of the fractures.

REMODELING

Children's forearm fractures have an amazing capacity to improve their radiographic appearance with the passing of the months (Figs. 10-27, 10-28). Friberg has shown that fractures at the distal end of the radius will correct at the rate of about 1° a month or 10° a year as a result of epiphyseal realignment. However, diaphyseal malunion is unforgiving. The bone may round off on radiographs so that the site of the fracture disappears, but the arm looks just as crooked and lacks just as much rotation as when the cast was removed. This should be described as "rounding off" rather than "remodeling."

A few rules may help:

1. Only crude predictions can be made about remodeling.
2. Perfect function can only be promised when the fracture remains perfectly aligned.
3. Bayonet alignment or overlapping may be unstable but can be compatible with acceptable alignment.
4. Realignment of a malunited fracture occurs as a result of epiphyseal growth. The malunion does not straighten. For every 10° of metaphyseal malunion, a year's growth should lie ahead for correction.
5. Diaphyseal malunion that blocks more than 50% of rotation and looks ugly should be treated by osteoclasis not benign neglect.

Gandhi noted that angulation at the distal end corrects well if the growth plate has five or more years of activity. Some degree of angulation can be accepted in children younger than the age of 10.

In the midforearm, angulation corrects poorly and limits rotation. Every effort should be made to maintain a reduction free of angulation or rotation.

| Day of Injury | 6 Weeks Post Injury | 6 Months Post Injury | 1 Year Post Injury |

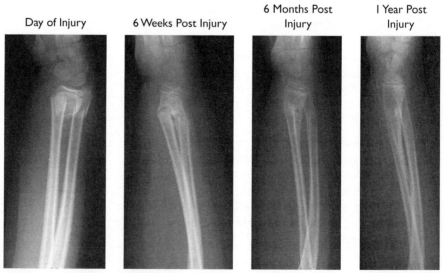

Figure 10-28. Distal fractures with residual angulation have good potential for remodeling if the patient has remaining growth.

REFRACTURE

A small proportion refracture within a few months. These are more difficult to manipulate and may require general anesthesia to achieve reduction. Late refracture (up to 1 year post injury) may be seen (Fig. 10-29). One can try a protective splint post-casting, but it is rarely used for more than a few weeks. The risk for refracture must be explained to the family so that the responsibility for guarded activity is theirs.

Price has noted that late re-fractures are more common when the initial reduction is less adequate with residual angulation. The physically dynamic patient requires the most perfect reduction

MALUNIONS

Fractures of the forearm and wrist are the most common injuries in childhood. Although the majority are easily treated, the occasional case will be underestimated or the patient will miss follow-up appointments and return with poor result.

So what should you do with the child who presents with malunion a few weeks after the cast has been removed at Elsewhere General Hospital? Angular deformity at the distal end in a young child always improves. Rotational deformity at the distal end, midshaft deformity, and deformities in teenagers do not remodel well. It does not help to send these individuals away with reassuring words. They must either accept what they have or accept correction. The parents have already been disappointed once. The choice of correction lies among:

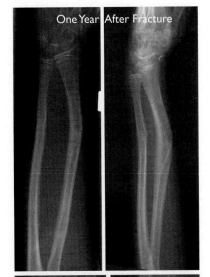

1. Manual osteoclasis. Don't try this. The bone will break at a distance from the malunion and leave you with a dog-legged arm.
2. Drill osteoclasis. This is the method of choice. Make a 5-mm incision over the malunion. Use a drill guide or a trocar to protect the soft tissues as you make several holes in the bone with a powered drill. Drill both the radius and ulna, keeping away from the nerves. Crack the bone and immobilize it in a cast, sometimes with the elbow in extension. Take x-ray films frequently.
3. Osteotomy and plating (Fig. 10-30). Trading a scar for a deformity is a basic tenet of orthopedics. The cosmetic disadvantage has lead us to avoid plating in primary fracture treatment, but it is the most exact method.

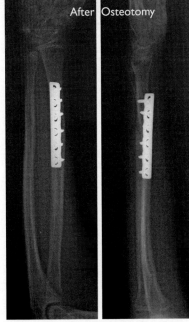

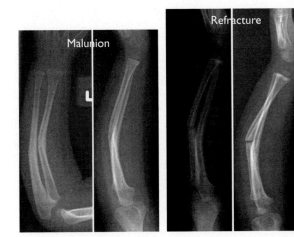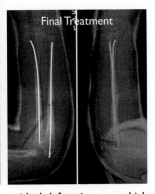

Figure 10-29. Both bone forearm fractures that heal with residual deformity are at high risk of refracture.

Figure 10-30. Malunions with resultant loss of function are best treated with osteoclasis or osteotomy and internal fixation.

SUMMARY

A knowledgeable pediatric care provider can treat the majority of these injuries in a closed fashion. Forearm fractures in children require reduction and casting skills as nowhere else in the body. It is important to study and understand the mechanics of fractures and their reduction. These fractures also need to be followed closely as they may drift in the cast and cause significant deformity and loss of function.

Suggested Readings

Blackburn N, Ziv I, Rang M: Correction of the malunited forearm fracture. Clin Orthop 1984;188:54-57.

Chess DG, Hyndman JC, Leahey JL, Brown DCS, Sinclair AM: Short arm plaster cast for distal pediatric forearm fractures. J Ped Orthop 1994;14:211-213.

Flynn, J.M. Pediatric forearm fractures: decision making, surgical techniques and complications. AAOS Instructional Course Lectures, 51:355-360, 2002.

Galpin, RD et al, A Comparison of Short and Long-Arm Plaster Casts for Displaced Distal-Third Pediatric Forearm Fractures: A Prospective Randomized Trial. POSNA Instructional Course Lectures. 2004.

Jones, K., Weiner, D. The management of forearm fractures in children: a plea for conservatism. J Ped Orthop., 19:811-815, 1999.

Lascombes P, Prevot J, Ligier J, et. al. Elastic stable intramedullary nailing in forearm fractures in children: 85 cases. J Pediatr Orthop 10:167-171, 1990.

Lee, S., Nicol, R.O., Stott, N.S. Intramedullary fixation for pediatric unstable forearm fractures. Clin. Orthop., 402:245-250, 2002.

Price CT, Scott DS, Kurzner ME, Flynn JC. Malunited forearm fractures in children. J Ped Orthop 1990;10:705-712.

Shoemaker SD, Comstock CP, Mubarak SJ, Wenger DR, Chambers HG: Intramedullary Kirschner wire fixation of open or unstable forearm fractures in children. J Ped Orthop 19:329-337, 1999.

Trousdale RT, Linscheid RL: Operative Treatment of malunited fractures of the forearm. J Bone Joint Surg Am 1995;77:894-902.

Verstreken L, Delronge G, Lamoureux J: Shaft forearm fractures in children: Intramedullary nailing with immediate motion: A preliminary report. J Ped Orthop 1988;8:450-453.

Walsh, H.P.J.; McLaren, C.A.N.; and Owen, R.: Galeazzi fractures in children. J Bone and Joint Surg., 69-B:730-733, 1987.

11

Hand

C. Douglas Wallace ❧ *Dennis Wenger*

INTRODUCTION

Hand injuries in the pediatric population frequently lead to an emergency room visit for evaluation and management. The mechanisms vary from the proverbial fall on an outstretched hand to torsional injuries of the digits in sports, crush injuries from children dropping heavy objects on their own or others' hands, plus a myriad of other causes from the vigorous lifestyle of a normal, active child.

Due to the intricate nature of hand function, attention to detail is required in managing these injuries. Children are well known for their ability to remodel fractures that have healed with some angulation. Pediatric hand fractures are no exception to this; however, certain limitations exist in the remodeling capacity of a pediatric hand injury. Similar to forearm fractures, hand fractures that occur close to a physis have substantially greater ability to remodel than those that occur distant to the physis.

Angular malalignment directly adjacent to a phalangeal physis may be well tolerated and remodel in time, whereas malalignment distally in the same phalanx may lead to permanent deformity and dysfunction. Malrotation has not been demonstrated to remodel in hand injuries.

> *"Most people would succeed in small things, if they were not troubled with great ambitions"*
>
> —*HENRY WADSWORTH LONGFELLOW*

151

"Due to the intricate nature of hand function, attention to detail is required in managing these injuries"

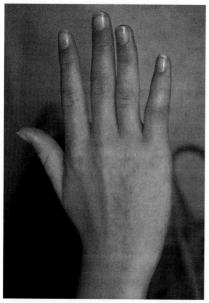

Figure 11-1. Angular malalignment is usually easy to detect with the digits extended. This patient has a fracture of the little finger proximal phalanx.

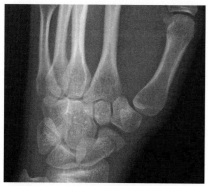

Figure 11-2. This subtle distal pole scaphoid fracture was apparent only on the scaphoid (oblique) view of the wrist.

This short chapter will present only the most common children's hand fractures. Many specialized texts are available for more complex injuries.

PHYSICAL EVALUATION

Evaluation of a child's hand injury can be challenging because children in general fear strangers, particularly those in white coats. A child with a painful hand injury can be extraordinarily uncooperative and difficult to evaluate.

Nonetheless, the responsibility falls on the treating physician to evaluate the child's hand for important characteristics that can be gleaned from careful observation of the child's hand with minimal contact.

One should look closely at the child's hand for evidence of rotatory or angular malalignment (Fig. 11-1). This can occasionally be seen with observation alone. More accurate assessments can be made by combining observation with gentle manipulation of the hand to study the functional alignment of each joint within the hand. Specific observation of the rotation of the nail beds with the digits both extended and flexed aid in determining rotatory problems.

Angular malalignment is usually easy to detect with the digits in an extended position; however, on occasion the swelling in juxtaarticular fractures can mask angulation.

When palpating the digits for tenderness, the examiner should consider the structures that pass beneath and the potential for underlying damage. Vascular assessments, specifically the digital Allen's test, are more practical for the older, more cooperative child. Certainly, capillary refill and digital color can be readily evaluated even in a very young, screaming child.

Neurologic function of an acutely injured digit is difficult to assess, particularly in the uncooperative child. Sharp/dull discrimination and two-point discrimination becomes a reasonable measurement of nerve function beginning at approximately age 5 years.

RADIOGRAPHS

Standard AP and lateral plain films (plus obliques as needed) are generally adequate to assess hand injuries (Fig. 11-2). Oblique views are very helpful to assess metacarpal fractures. In the presence of tenderness in the anatomic snuffbox, a more detailed evaluation of the scaphoid is warranted and a scaphoid oblique should be obtained. In cases of ulnar-sided wrist pain, one can consider an intra-articular contrast MRI in an attempt to elucidate injury to the triangular fibrocartilage complex (TFCC) and interosseous ligaments.

INITIAL MANAGEMENT

Following examination and initial imaging studies, definitive versus temporizing treatment should ensue. When immobilizing interphalangeal joints, extension is the preferred position unless there are reasons in regards to correcting an angular rotatory deformity to position the digits otherwise. The metacarpopha-

---

Common Abbreviations Used by Hand Surgeon

MP = metacarpal-phalangeal	IP = interphalangeal (finger)
PIP = proximal interphalangeal (finger)	CMC = carpal-metacarpal joint
DIP = distal interphalangeal (finger)	TFCC = triangular fibrocartilage complex (at distal radioulnar joint)

langeal joints should be immobilized in flexion to put the collateral ligaments on stretch and speed recovery of flexion/extension (Fig. 11-3). If the nature of the injury precludes this position, then the injury should be managed primarily with the attention to soft tissue tensions as a secondary consideration. Despite poor attention to proper mobilization techniques, children often will regain motion rapidly with minimal deficits nonetheless.

When immobilizing a child with a suspected scaphoid injury, a thumb spica component should be added to the immobilization device.

INDIVIDUAL INJURIES

The vast majority of pediatric hand fractures can be treated non-operatively. Injuries frequently requiring surgical intervention include mallet finger deformities with loss of articular congruity, phalangeal neck fractures with extension or malrotation, intra-articular fractures of the interphalangeal joints, and a more generic set of fractures that occur secondary to a crush injury.

PHALANGEAL FRACTURES

Distal Phalangeal Fractures

Tuft fractures are frequent and the vast majority requires solely symptomatic treatment with protection and splinting for several weeks to allow early healing of the soft tissue and osseous damage. The patient may return to activities when comfortable.

Mallet Finger

The pediatric mallet finger (named mallet because of its appearance if not treated) is important to recognize due to potential long-term disability from missed injuries (Fig. 11-4). The mallet finger generally occurs from a jamming type injury, loading the DIP joint.

There may or may not be a fracture involved. Classically, in the pediatric population this involves the Salter-Harris III injury in which the extensor mechanism is attached to the epiphyseal fragment that displaces dorsally. Although this is the most frequent etiology of the juvenile mallet finger deformity, these can also be due to a tendinous disruption with a negative radiograph.

Management of the mallet finger involves extension splinting across the DIP joint. It is important to ensure maintenance of congruity of the distal interphalangeal joint on the lateral view. In cases where the distal phalanx migrates volarly with loss of the articular congruity on the distal aspect of the middle phalanx, operative intervention is warranted (Fig. 11-5). The degree of displace-

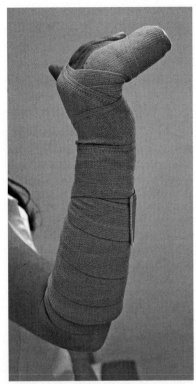

Figure 11-3. Properly positioned ulnar gutter splint. When immobilizing the hand, ideally the MP joints should be flexed and the IP joints extended to avoid contracture of the intrinsic muscles. This is less important in children as they rarely get stiff following injury.

At Injury   After Surgery

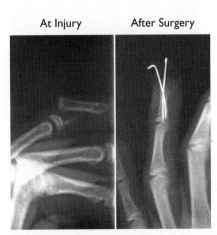

Figure 11-5. Open physeal fracture with nail bed disruption requiring débridement, repair, and K-wire fixation.

At Injury   In Splint   8 Weeks Later

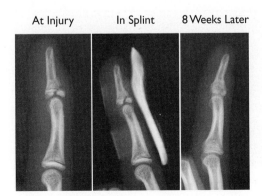

Figure 11-4. Classic Salter-Harris III fracture that leads to a mallet finger if left untreated. This child was treated with the dorsal "suspension" splint method of Lester et al. (see next page).

ment of the dorsal fragment in general is not the indication for surgical intervention, rather, the articular congruity is.

It is also important to stress that splinting should be in extension but not hyperextension. Generally, a dorsally placed splint that in length proceeds from the PIP joint to a point distal to the tip of the finger held on with tape produces adequate immobilization. Minimal extension may be added to the splint. A lateral radiograph centered on the DIP joint should be obtained to evaluate articular congruity. The splint can be adjusted as necessary to provide the best closed alignment. With preserved articular congruity, 6 weeks of uninterrupted splinting should be adequate to treat this injury.

At the termination of immobilization at 6 weeks, the splint can be worn while the child is active for an additional 1 to 2 weeks but taken off for bathing and sleeping purposes to allow gentle reintroduction of motion to the DIP joint.

Indications for surgical intervention in a mallet finger include volar subluxation of the distal phalangeal fragment. With loss of articular congruity, long-term function of the joint cannot be ensured. Therefore closed versus open reduction and pin fixation is warranted in this instance.

In addition to this, a Salter-Harris I versus II fracture of the base of the distal phalanx with significant angulation will have the appearance of a typical mallet finger deformity but be associated with a nailbed disruption and open injury. In

Suspension Taping Method for Mallet Finger Treatment

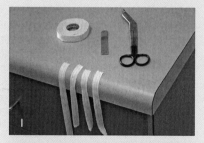

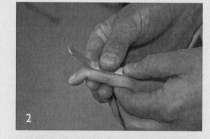

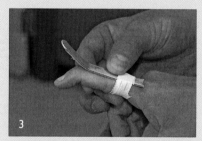

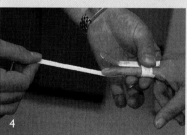

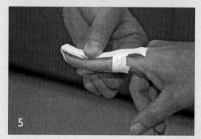

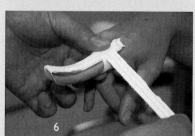

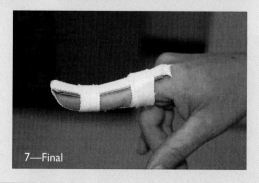

The longitudinal taping "suspension taping" method of dorsal splinting to treat a mallet finger.

Modified from Lester B et al. (see Suggested Readings). Note that Lester advised leaving the PIP joint free—in children (hand is smaller) we usually incorporate the PIP joint as well to be sure the splint doesn't slide off.

these instances, the fingertip droops with bleeding from the eponychial fold. Radiographs generally reflected an intact epiphysis; however, the metaphyseal component is angulated. Treatment includes recreating the deformity for exposure, irrigation, and débridement of any foreign material from the fracture site; careful reduction of the nail back into the eponychial fold; and fracture reduction, often with K-wire fixation.

A congenital deformity that can mimic a mallet deformity and present as such is called a Kirner deformity. A Kirner deformity of the distal phalanx is formed in a hooked configuration, which gives the finger the appearance of a drooping tip (Fig. 11-6). This has been known to be overlooked until the child has an injury to the digit, the parents' attention focuses on this, and the child is brought in for evaluation of the finger injury. A lateral radiograph generally will establish the diagnosis due to the characteristic curved growth pattern of the distal phalanx.

PHALANGEAL NECK FRACTURES

The pediatric phalangeal neck fracture can be a diagnostic dilemma in a very young child. In general, these injuries tend to have the distal fragment pushed into an extended position (with apex volar angulation). In the older child, this is obvious on x-ray because the volar subcondylar fossa has been obliterated by the extension of the condyles. In the young child with nonossified condyles, it can be extremely difficult to detect. The only indication may be a swollen interphalangeal joint with some malalignment of the shafts. Even then, it may not be apparent on plain radiographs.

Management of these injuries often entails reduction and pin fixation with cross K-wires (Fig. 11-7). The key is to restore adequate flexion to the digit. As the distal condylar fragment extends, the fossa into which the articulating phalanx should enter disappears. A resultant loss of flexion with abutment of the base of the next phalanx on the neck of the more proximal phalanx can result in a permanent loss of flexion. Although children can remodel this deformity over time, it may be necessary in cases of delayed diagnosis to perform an osteoplasty to recreate a phalangeal neck fossa to allow flexion of the interphalangeal joint. The key is to catch this when the fracture is fresh, reduce the extension with direct pressure and/or flexion, and cross pin the condyles into position.

In addition to extension deformities, translation and angular deformities can also be seen with phalangeal neck fractures (Fig. 11-7). A phalangeal neck fracture with mild angulation can often be reduced under digital block anesthesia. With careful taping to the adjacent digit, this can hold the fracture in a corrected position that is reasonably stable, allowing closed treatment. If this proves inadequate, pin fixation can be added to manage the injury.

PHALANGEAL SHAFT FRACTURES

Phalangeal shaft fractures are common in adolescents who are involved in more vigorous sporting activities. These patients must be evaluated for rotatory and angular malalignment. Again, special attention paid to alignment of the fingernails with fingers extended is helpful in determining rotatory alignment (Fig.11-8).

In addition to this, careful closing of each individual digit should show a consistent pattern of the finger aiming toward the scaphoid tubercle volarly. One can place a dot in the palm at the center of the nail on the uninjured hand to show the normal alignment and then flex the fingers of the injured hand individually placing a dot at the center of the nail on the palm to indicate the ro-

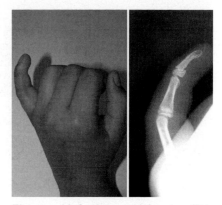

Figure 11-6. Kirner deformity—This congenital deformity of the distal phalanx of the fifth finger can be confused with a fracture.

"Phalangeal shaft fractures are common in adolescents who are involved in more vigorous sporting activities"

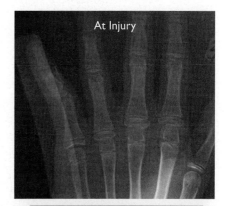

At Injury

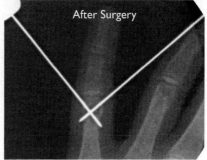

After Surgery

Figure 11-7. Angulated and unstable phalangeal neck fracture requiring reduction plus percutaneous K-wire fixation.

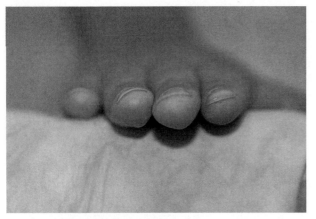

Figure 11-8. Assessment of fingernails with digits extended suggests malrotation of the ring finger.

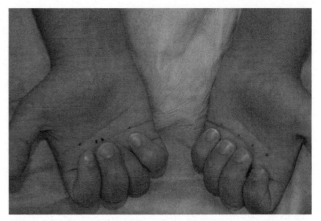

Figure 11-9. Drawing dots on the palm at the point where the flexed fingertips reach the palm helps to detect malrotation. The left hand is normal. The ring finger is malrotated in the right hand.

tatory alignment of the digits (Fig. 11-9). Rotatory malalignment must be treated to prevent permanent deformity.

PROXIMAL PHALANGEAL FRACTURES

The fracture at the base of the small finger proximal phalanx that results in abduction of the digit is known as an "extra-octave" fracture (Fig. 11-10). These are usually Salter-Harris II fractures, which can be managed simply with digital anesthesia block and gentle reduction consisting of flexion at the metacarpophalangeal joint with concomitant adduction of the small finger toward and under the ring finger. Placing a pencil between the ring and small fingers provides an efficient fulcrum (Fig. 11-11). Placing the MP joint in flexion tensions the collateral ligaments, which allows reduction of the shaft to near anatomic reduction. This can be immobilized in intrinsic plus position with the involved digit and the adjacent digit carefully protected in a cast.

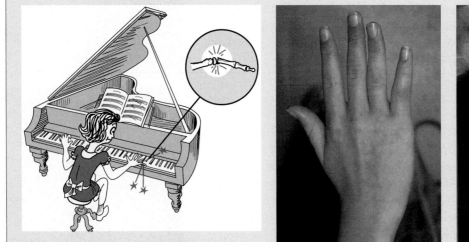
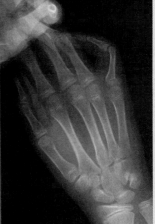

Figure 11-10. The so-called extra-octave fracture of the fifth finger. Left untreated, the child could have a greater hand span at the piano.

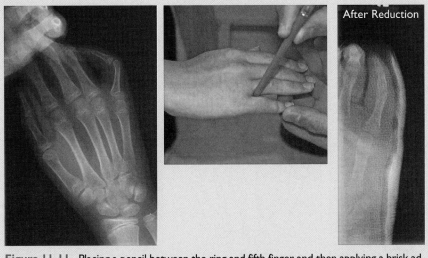

Figure 11-11. Placing a pencil between the ring and fifth finger and then applying a brisk adduction force to the small finger provides efficient reduction of an "extra-octave" fracture.

At Injury

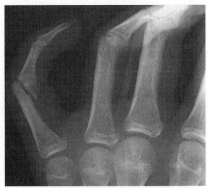

After Reduction

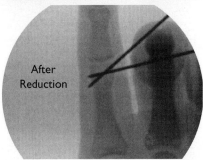

Figure 11-12. Intra-articular phalangeal condyle fracture. Treatment by closed reduction and percutaneous K-wire fixation.

INTRA-ARTICULAR FRACTURES

Another fracture requiring special attention is the phalangeal intra-condylar intra-articular fracture. Minimal depression of the phalangeal condyle will result in obvious angular deformity as well as possible premature joint degeneration due to incongruity of the joint surfaces. Anatomic reduction of the joint surface is critical for proper management of these injuries. Even a half millimeter of displacement can lead to angulation and some degree of loss of ultimate function. In fresh injuries, reduction can be accomplished with a digital block, use of ligamentotaxis for reduction of the fracture, and pin fixation utilizing smooth K-wires (Fig. 11-12). In a cooperative adolescent patient, this can be done with local anesthesia in the clinic/small procedure room setting, using a portable fluoroscopy imaging device. A battery-operated pin driver is an excellent tool for simple management of these fractures.

If anatomic reduction is not attainable in a closed setting, then open reduction with as anatomic as possible restoration of the joint surface is indicated. The K-wire fixation in the vast majority of phalangeal fractures should be left in place 3 to 4 weeks, followed by a gentle motion program.

METACARPAL FRACTURES

Metacarpal fractures can occur at the head and neck region, shaft, or base, similar to phalangeal fractures. The most common metacarpal neck fracture involves the distal end of the small finger metacarpal (Fig. 11-13). This is commonly called a boxer's fracture that in the modern world seems more commonly due to "boxing" (hitting) a wall rather then hitting a human.

Although significant angulation can be tolerated in this region due to the mobility at the base of the small finger metacarpal, reduction is often indicated to improve alignment and minimize the need for remodeling. The general guidelines for management of adult metacarpal neck fracture, as a rough rule, can also be applied to children (Table 11-1).

Metacarpal shaft fractures occur more commonly with torsional injuries and are often seen in contact sports when players collide with an oblique blow that is transmitted to the metacarpal shaft. These tend to be spiral fractures.

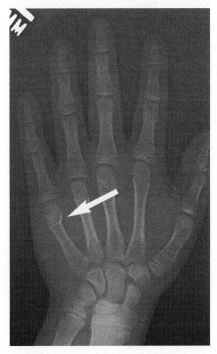

Figure 11-13. Typical fifth metacarpal (boxer's) fracture in an adolescent.

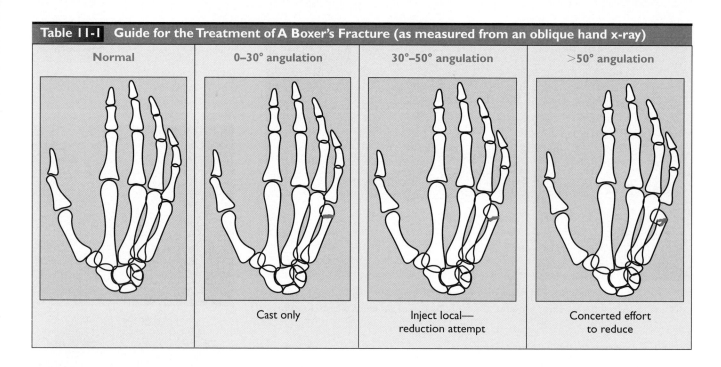

Normal	0–30° angulation	30°–50° angulation	>50° angulation
	Cast only	Inject local—reduction attempt	Concerted effort to reduce

Table 11-1 Guide for the Treatment of A Boxer's Fracture (as measured from an oblique hand x-ray)

Alignment is key and assessment of alignment should be performed with the digits both extended and flexed at the metacarpophalangeal joint. In theory, metacarpophalangeal joint flexion in the intrinsic plus position should maintain rotational alignment of the fracture (Fig. 11-14). In those instances, controlling anterior/posterior angulation is all that should be necessary with reduction and casting.

Open reduction and internal fixation are rarely indicated with the exception of poor rotatory control, entrapment of the extensor mechanism of the fracture spike, and inability to control alignment, particularly in a transverse fracture (Fig. 11-15).

Several metacarpal base fractures are of note in the hand. The small finger metacarpal may sustain a fracture dislocation at the carpometacarpal level.

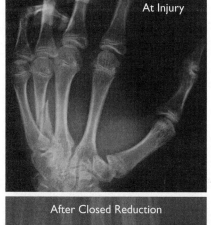

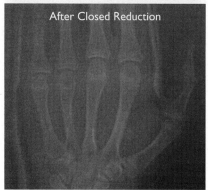

Figure 11-14. This fourth metacarpal fracture was treated with closed reduction and casting with the MP joints in a position of function.

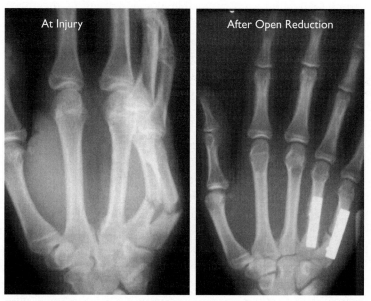

Figure 11-15. Fracture of both the fourth and fifth metacarpals in a teenage boy. Fracture reduction could not be maintained; therefore open reduction plus internal fixation were performed.

These may be treated with reduction and immobilization if the reduction is stable. If not, they require closed versus open reduction with pin fixation across the CMC level and potentially between the metacarpals as well to maintain length.

In some instances, comminution is present at the base of the small finger metacarpal, which is intra-articular. The degree of comminution may be difficult to assess without the assistance of a CT scan for both severity assessment as well as preoperative planning (if necessary).

THUMB INJURIES

Several injuries are unique to the thumb metacarpal and/or have enough attention paid to them to warrant separate discussion.

Base of Metacarpal

Injuries to the thumb carpometacarpal region occur in children as well as in adults. Bennett fractures (intra-articular fracture of the CMC) can occur and tend to be in the adolescent to young adult population. These require treatment similar to adults to stabilize the CMC level with accurate reduction and pin fixation.

Extra-articular fractures are more common. These tend to occur in younger children as a Salter-Harris II versus metaphyseal injury. Although some remodeling is possible, an accurate reduction is optimal. Often, this can be obtained with a local anesthesia block and gentle manipulation consisting of traction with direct pressure volarly over the apex of the deformity with support under the metacarpophalangeal joint (Fig. 11-16). Care must be taken not to hyperextend the metacarpophalangeal joint in the process.

A thumb spica cast with careful molding to hold the position of the fragments is applied. In cases of severe deformity, loss of reduction, or inability to attain adequate reduction, pin fixation should be performed. Generally, this can be performed percutaneously.

Gamekeeper's Thumb

Metacarpophalangeal joint injuries, relatively common in the teenage population, are often associated with contact sports. A bony or soft tissue gamekeeper lesion can occur in this group. The diagnostic dilemmas in the adult population are also seen in the young adult/adolescent population. When tenderness is identified at the metacarpophalangeal joint level of the thumb, radiographs should be obtained prior to stressing the ligaments because a bony gamekeeper lesion may be present and further displacement of the fragment should be avoided. Surgical criteria are similar to those in the adult population. Accurate reduction of the volar/ulnar portion of the proximal phalanx of the thumb is important for ligamentous stability (Fig. 11-17).

Dislocations

Metacarpophalangeal joint dislocations are reported in the pediatric population. The proximal phalanx usually displaces dorsally on the metacarpal head and neck region. There are both reducible and irreducible forms.

In general, the more easily reducible form has hyperextension at the metacarpophalangeal joint with mild proximal migration of the base of the proximal phalanx of the thumb. Dislocations less amenable to closed management tend

In Cast After
At Injury | Attempted Reduction | 4 Weeks Later

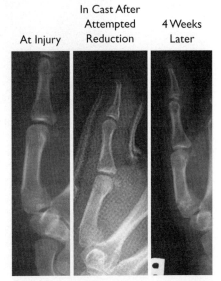

Figure 11-16. Base of metacarpal thumb fracture with moderate angulation, the joint is not involved. Slight reduction was gained and the final result was satisfactory.

At Injury | After Surgery

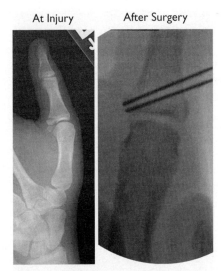

Figure 11-17. This teenage lacrosse player presented with thumb MP joint pain after an injury. After diagnosis as a gamekeeper's thumb (with bony avulsion), surgical reduction was performed.

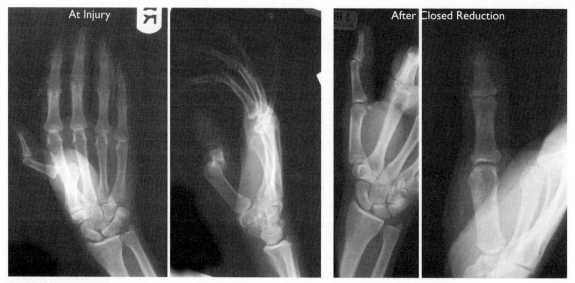

Figure 11-18. Typical thumb MP joint dislocation in a teenager. A translational force (not distraction) allowed closed reduction).

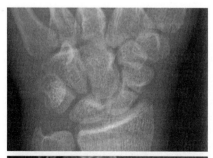
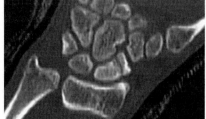

Figure 11-19. The so-called anatomic snuffbox is formed by the extensor and abductor tendons of the thumb. The scaphoid bone lies just under the center of the triangle. A patient with a scaphoid fracture will likely be very tender in this area.

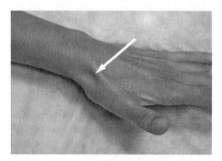

Figure 11-20. Delayed union—scaphoid waste fracture in a 15-year-old boy who fell at football practice. Note lack of callus despite 10 weeks of immobilization.

to be dislocated dorsally, with the phalanx and metacarpal shaft colinear. When reducing a metacarpophalangeal joint dislocation after obtaining radiographs to rule out fracture component, one must be careful to not distract the metacarpophalangeal joint. Rather than distraction, the reduction maneuver entails gentle translation of the base of the proximal phalanx along the dorsum of the metacarpal head and neck region to bring it back onto the distal aspect of the metacarpal (Fig. 11-18). By preventing distraction, one may avoid entrapping the volar plate between the metacarpal and proximal phalanx. Immobilization should be with the metacarpophalangeal joint in a gently flexed position for approximately 4 weeks. Occupational therapy is often necessary to regain motion in this joint.

CARPAL INJURIES

Scaphoid (carpal navicular) fractures are often seen in vigorous, athletic, adolescent boys and occasionally in girls. This is generally from sport or fall on an outstretched hand. Not uncommonly, there is a delay in presentation, particularly if the child is hesitant to report the injury to the family.

At presentation, the classic tenderness in the anatomic snuffbox region (Fig. 11-19) should be evaluated. AP, lateral, and scaphoid oblique view are helpful to clarify the diagnosis. Scaphoid waist fractures certainly occur in the older child and adolescent population. In addition, distal pole fractures are more common than in adults.

Distal pole fractures can be treated in a below elbow thumb spica cast for approximately 6 weeks and then gentle return to activities.

Waist fractures are a bit more precarious (Fig. 11-20). If there is no displacement, the injury appears stable, and swelling is mild to moderate, a below elbow thumb spica cast can be applied for 4 weeks followed by radiographs, then recasting for an additional 4 weeks. If there is minimal displacement or a question of stability, a long arm thumb spica cast should be applied for the first 6 weeks followed by a short arm thumb spica cast for an additional 4 weeks.

In cases of delayed presentation, the scaphoid fracture anatomy is critical in determining treatment. Despite having mild to moderate cystic changes in a scaphoid fracture in a teenager, closed management can be successful with a nondisplaced injury.

The Boat-Shaped Bone

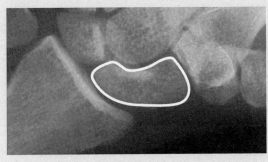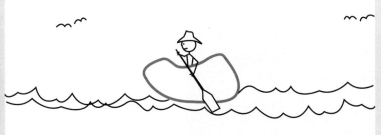

A navicular bone (shaped like a boat—from Latin navis = ship, navicula = small boat, skiff) is found in both the hand and the foot. Rather than requiring one to clarify the hand navicular as a "carpal" navicular, most use the term scaphoid (from Greek—scapho = something dug or scooped out).

A CT scan is helpful in determining the anatomy of the scaphoid to look for a humpback or flexion deformity. If the osseous alignment appears appropriate, a course of closed management can be attempted prior to considering open management.

Surgical treatment is indicated for a delayed union that shows no evidence of healing, a displaced scaphoid fracture, and a scaphoid fracture that is associated with carpal instability/ligament injuries (Fig. 11-21). The current method of choice for fixation of scaphoid fractures appears to be a variable pitch screw that provides compression as the screw is placed. This can be a cylindrical or tapered design. In cases where there is delay in presentation and collapse of the scaphoid, bone grafting may be necessary to restore scaphoid anatomy. This can be obtained from the iliac crest or the distal radius with care to avoid injury to the distal radial physis.

"The current method of choice for fixation of scaphoid fractures appear to be a variable pitch screw that provides compression as the screw is placed"

Ligament Injuries

Although scapho-lunate injuries are not impossible, they are rare in children. On the other hand, injuries such as the transscaphoid perilunate dislocation have been reported in this age range.

At Injury   After Open Reduction

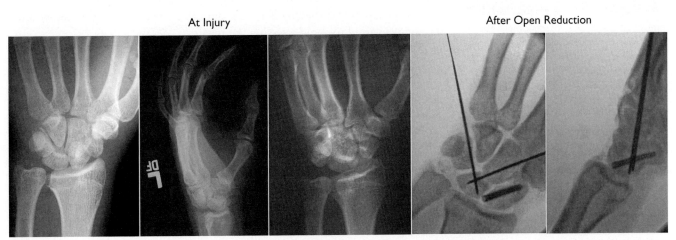

Figure 11-21. This teenager had a serious fall in sports with a scaphoid fracture plus carpal dislocation. Treatment included open reduction, stabilization of the dislocation with K-wires, and fixation of the scaphoid fracture with a variable pitch screw.

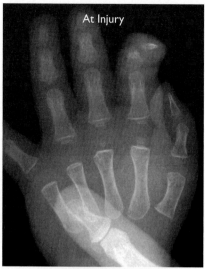

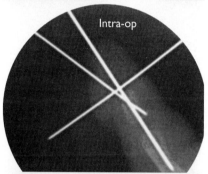

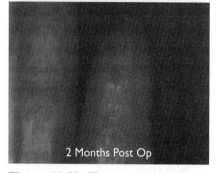

Figure 11-22. This preschooler had a television set dropped on his index finger. His crush injury was treated with débridement and pinning.

On rare occasion, in conjunction with other injuries of the distal radius or wrist region, ulna-sided wrist pain develops. This can be related to an ulnar styloid nonunion, although complaints from this are rare.

Triangular fibrocartilaginous complex (TFCC) injuries occur in older children. In cases of ulna-sided wrist pain with an unclear diagnosis, an arthrogram contrast MRI of the wrist may delineate the pathology. This can be particularly helpful in evaluating the TFCC. TFCC injuries may be amenable to arthroscopic evaluation and débridement versus repair, depending on the nature of the injury.

CRUSH INJURIES—DIGITS

Crush injuries to the hand or digits can be difficult and challenging to treat (Fig. 11-22). The severity of injury can range from the simple soft tissue contusion and/or tuft fracture up through virtual or complete amputation of the digit. The crush-injured digit tends to heal less well and over a longer period of time than the digit that sustains an injury with a less severe mechanism. For comminuted fractures, open reduction and internal fixation may be necessary.

One should anticipate a delay in healing and the need for pin placement for a prolonged period of time, at least 6 weeks. The family should be counseled regarding the long-term prognosis and outcome from crush injuries. These include poor nail development, stiffness, and/or angular deformity. Proper counseling of the family should be undertaken preoperatively. Crush injuries to the entire hand can also occur and management is similar to what is done for adult injuries. Release of compartments may be required in severe cases.

NERVE AND TENDON INJURIES

Both nerve and tendon lacerations can and do occur in children. The mechanism tends to be from grasping and/or playing with sharp objects. Certainly, in the older child, altercations with knives can be implicated. Halloween is a particularly risky time of the year (pumpkin carving is a slowly aquired skill).

Tendon repairs should be performed primarily. When the profundus and superficialis tendon are disrupted, most likely only repair of the profundus is indicated. Early occupational therapy is indicated in the older child, (perhaps age 6-8). In younger patients, we use, a mitten-type cast with the wrist flexed 30°, with the hand carefully positioned as if holding a ball but with nothing actually within the hand. In such a cast, the child can volitionally wiggle the fingers within the cast, although not generating any force of significance. Due to age, detailed occupational therapy is not an option. Hence, the need to allow some motion yet casted to avoid stressing the repair.

Suggested Readings

Barton NJ: Fractures of the phalanges of the hand in children. Hand 1979;2:134-143.

Bogumill GP: A morphologic study of the relationship of collateral ligaments to growth plates in the digits. J Hand Surg 1983;8:74-79.

Campbell RM Jr. Operative treatment of fractures and dislocations of the hand and wrist region in children. Orthop Clin North Am. 1990 Apr;21(2):217-43.

Dixon GL Jr, Moon NF: Rotational supracondylar fractures of the proximal phalanx in children. Clin Orthop 1972;83: 151-156.

Fischer MD, McElfresh EC: Physeal and periphyseal injuries of the hand: Patterns of injury and results of treatment. Hand Clin 1994;10:287-301.

Hankin FM, Janda DH: Tendon and ligament attachments in relationship to growth plates in a child's hand. J Hand Surg 1989;14B:315-318.

Hastings H, Carroll C: Treatment of closed articular fractures of the metacarpophalangeal and proximal interphalangeal joints. Hand Clinics 1988;4(3):503-527

Le TB, Hentz VR. Hand and wrist injuries in young athletes. Hand Clin. 2000 Nov;16(4):597-607.

Leonard MH, Dubravcik P: Management of fractured fingers in the child. Clin Orhtop 1970;73:160-168.

Lester B, Jeong GK, Perry D, Spero L: A simple effective splinting technique for mallet finger. Am J Orthop. 2000 Mar; 29(3):202-6.

Mahabir RC, Kazemi AR, Cannon WG, Courtemanche DJ. Pediatric hand fractures: a review. Pediatr Emerg Care. 2001 Jun;17(3):153-6.

Mintzer CM, Waters PM. Surgical treatment of pediatric scaphoid fracture nonunions. J Pediatr Orthop. 1999 Mar-Apr;19(2): 236-9.

Moore RS Jr, Tan V, Dormans JP, Bozentka DJ. Major pediatric hand trauma associated with fireworks. J Orthop Trauma. 2000 Aug;14(6):426-8.

Nofsinger CC, Wolfe SW. Common pediatric hand fractures. Curr Opin Pediatr. 2002 Feb;14(1):42-5. Review.

12

Pelvis and Hip

Maya Pring ❧ *Mercer Rang* ❧ *Dennis Wenger*

INTRODUCTION

The osteoporotic bone of an elderly lady is very different from the tough, growing bone of a child. Greater violence is required to produce a hip or pelvic fracture in a child. For example, most trochanteric fractures are bumper injuries in children of 6 or 7 years, the age when the greater trochanter is at the level of a car bumper (Fig. 12-1), and most pelvic fractures are the result of high-speed motor vehicle accidents.

It is misleading to apply the mass of information about adult fractures to children, and the small number of papers that relate specifically to children present widely varying statistics that are almost impossible to compare. If this were a more common injury, perhaps we would all know more about the best methods of treatment.

Luckily, unlike adults, children tolerate cast immobilization. The chance of union is excellent in a young child with an undisplaced intertrochanteric hip fracture. In a cast, a child will not develop bed sores or deep vein thrombosis or lose the will to live, but malunion is a real hazard. If a displaced fracture of the neck is reduced closed and held in a cast, coxa vara is almost a certainty.

Initial Exam

Occasionally, a child will fall from a countertop or the back of a couch and strike the floor in just the right way, sustaining an isolated sub- or intertrochanteric femur fracture. However, more commonly, hip and pelvis fractures

"We can be absolutely certain only about things we do not understand"
—*ERIC HOFFER*

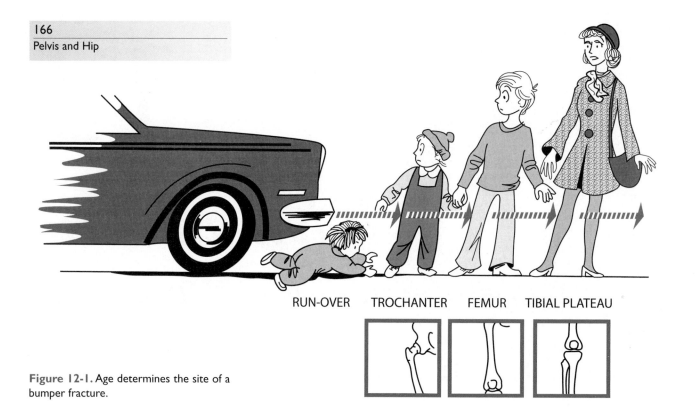

RUN-OVER   TROCHANTER   FEMUR   TIBIAL PLATEAU

Figure 12-1. Age determines the site of a bumper fracture.

"Pelvic fractures may be accompanied by genitourinary and/or gastrointestinal injury"

in children are the result of high-energy violence and are associated with other injuries. In these cases, the initial exam needs to concentrate on identifying any life-threatening injuries including head, spine, thoracic, abdominal, pelvic, neurologic, and vascular trauma. A coordinated plan to care for each injury must be established. The hip exam itself must be gentle to avoid further disruption of blood supply (especially femoral neck).

Associated Injuries

Pelvic fractures may be accompanied by genitourinary (GU) and/or gastrointestinal (GI) injury. It is important to look for blood at the urethral meatus and to check for hematuria; a retrograde urethrogram/cystogram should be obtained if clinically indicated (Fig. 12-2). Abdominal, vaginal, and rectal exams are performed by or together with the general surgery team; blood at the anus suggests injury to the lower GI tract that can contaminate a pelvic fracture; this can be worse than an open pelvic fracture if missed. The rectal exam can also identify a displaced prostate indicating transection of the urethra.

Specific Exam

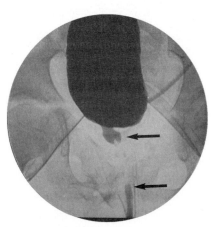

Figure 12-2. This child was run over by a truck. Cystogram and retrograde urethrogram show complete disruption of the urethra (arrow) and elevation of the bladder. Always remember to check for GI and GU injuries when the pelvis is fractured.

Instability of the pelvis can often be felt with a compression test, testing for both lateral and anteroposterior instability. This test should not be repeated by multiple examiners as there is risk for compounding the damage already done by the fracture. Feel the pulses and test active movements in both legs. Subtle neurologic injuries are easily missed—always test sacral sensation. When the sacroiliac (SI) joint is dislocated, the lumbosacral trunk, superior gluteal nerve, and obturator nerve are at risk. However, as will be described later, children rarely have true SI joint disruption, typically they fracture through the physis adjacent to the SI joint. Sacral fractures can rupture the sacral roots, or the foramina can be compressed causing compression of the sacral roots.

Blood Loss

In the field, prior to arrival at the hospital, hemorrhage from a pelvic fracture can often be partially controlled by binding the pelvis with a sheet wrapped tightly around the patient at the level of the AIIS. This will close down fractures and tamponade the bleeding during transport or until further treatment can be rendered.

Extraperitoneal hemorrhage to some degree is common and in most cases is allowed to tamponade with blood transfusion given as needed. In a few instances, bleeding can be massive and well concealed. An arteriogram may be required to identify the site of bleeding, and coils can be placed by the interventional radiologist to stop the bleeding.

Reading Pelvic X-rays

The pelvis is a very complex three-dimensional structure and analyzing films can be difficult. Fractures are difficult to see and can occur through growth areas such as the triradiate cartilage, which makes x-ray interpretation difficult.

The ischio-pelvic syndesmosis is even more puzzling, and may mimic a fracture (Fig. 12-3). This syndesmosis often fuses assymetrically, making interpretation difficult. Further complexity is added by Ogden's noting that in very rare instances this syndesmosis can be the site of a stress fracture in a young jogger.

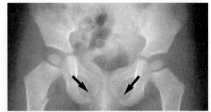
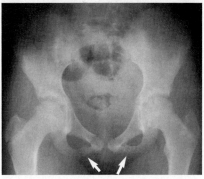

Figure 12-3. A) In this young child, note the ischium and pubis beginning to fuse. B) In this older child, the synchondroses had an almost expansile appearance. This is a normal finding and should not be confused with a fracture. These syncondroses may close asymmetrically, adding further confusion.

HIP DISLOCATION

Dislocation is more common than femoral neck fracture in childhood and fortunately carries far fewer risks for complications than does adult dislocation (Fig. 12-4). This is likely due to hip joint laxity in the child as well as the fact that the acetabular growth cartilage (adjacent to labrum) is not yet ossified, with the true socket not as deep as in the fully ossified adult. The hip of a child younger than the age of 5 is usually dislocated by a fall with minimal trauma. As age increases, the degree of violence required to dislocate the hip escalates (age 6-10—athletic injuries, automobile accidents thereafter). A more violent dislocation is more likely to be associated with fracture of the acetabulum or femur and sciatic nerve damage.

A recent traumatic dislocation can hardly be confused with a long standing paralytic dislocation for which the treatment is entirely different. On the other hand, recurrent dislocation of the hip in a child with Down's syndrome may be confusing. The bone looks normal, and only the classic facial features of Down's syndrome clarify the diagnosis.

Classification

The femoral head can be dislocated either anteriorly or posteriorly or rarely into the obturator foramen (Table 12-1). A hip is most commonly dislocated posteriorly causing the limb to be held in a shortened, flexed, adducted, and internally rotated position. Anterior dislocations cause the limb to extend, abduct, and externally rotate. Traumatic obturator dislocations (or intrapelivc dislocations) are very rare in children but have been reported. The hip tends to be held in flexion, abduction, and external rotation, but this is more variable.

Treatment

It is not merely kind to reduce a dislocated hip as soon as possible; early closed reduction will almost always succeed, whereas each passing hour makes the need for open reduction more likely (Fig. 12-5). Prompt reduction also reduces the incidence for avascular necrosis (AVN) (although the incidence of AVN is much lower in children as compared to adults).

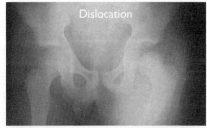
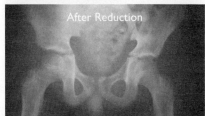

Figure 12-4. This child dislocated his hip during a simple slip and fall. Reduction was easy and protected with a hip spica for 4 weeks.

Table 12-1 | Hip Dislocations

Anterior	Posterior	Obturator
Hip extended abducted and externally rotated	Hip short, flexed, and internally rotated	Hip flexed, abducted, and externally rotated

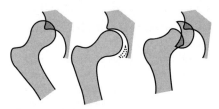

Figure 12-5. Complications recognized after reduction. An acetabular fragment or avulsion from the femoral head may block complete reduction. A type I injury to the physis may become evident.

Reduction of anterior and posterior dislocations are easy if adequate muscle relaxant is used. A posterior dislocation is reduced by flexing the hip and the knee to 90° and applying traction while the leg is externally rotated.

Anterior dislocation is best reduced by pulling the leg in extension, abduction, and internal rotation. After reduction, the hip should move freely without crepitus. A post-reduction pelvis x-ray and CT scan should be obtained to confirm that the hip is concentrically reduced without intra-articular fragments. The x-ray sign of fragment entrapment may be only a subtle joint space widening when comparing the injured to the normal hip.

After reduction, we apply a hip spica for 4 weeks to allow capsular healing. Movement usually returns quickly, and myositis ossificans is rare in children. Radiographic review should continue for a year to detect AVN.

Obturator dislocations should be taken to the operatinge room for open reduction. They are usually irreducible by closed methods.

Pitfalls

Problems are unusual. During a reduction, an unrecognized proximal femoral epiphyseal separation may become apparent. In such a case, the neck, not the head, reduces into the acetabulum. Such a circumstance mandates open reduction and pinning.

A trapped intra-articular fragment is easily overlooked if a post-reduction CT scan is not obtained (Fig. 12-6). A fragment in the joint requires arthro-

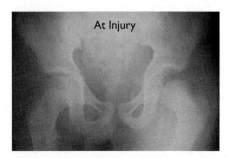

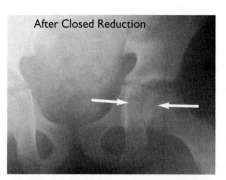

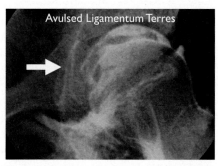

Figure 12-6. Following reduction, a widened joint space is indicative of a fragment in the joint. In this case, the arthrogram and subsequent open reduction revealed an avulsion fragment of the femoral head with the attached ligamentum teres.

tomy for removal of the fragment or fixation of large fragments. This can be a posterior acetabular rim fragment, the ligamentum teres with an avulsed head fragment, or both.

The overall incidence of AVN in the literature is 10% or less. Delayed reduction and severe injury are the most important causes. Recurrent dislocation of the hip is a rare sequel to traumatic dislocation.

Voluntary Dislocation of the Hip

Some teenaged girls complain that they can feel the hip dislocate. The usual cause is a snapping hip, in which the tensor fascia lata jumps across the greater trochanter as the girl rotates her hip. Once learned, some teenagers seem to have a morbid preoccupation with repeating the maneuver. Some very convincingly impress the neophyte examiner as being a dislocation. Treatment is by stretching (physical therapy) and only very, very rarely surgery (incision in tensor fascia). An extremely rare cause is a true voluntary dislocation, a condition that was described by Broudy and Scott.

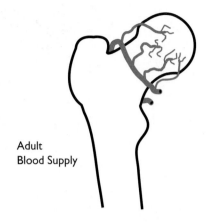

Adult
Blood Supply

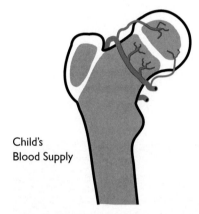

Child's
Blood Supply

Figure 12-7. The adult has intraosseus vessels that supply the femoral head. Children with open physes have a more tenuous blood supply as vessels do not cross the physis.

HIP FRACTURES

Anatomy and Physiology—Hip

The following differentiate hip fractures in children as compared to adults:

1. The periosteal tube in a child is much stronger than in an adult; many fractures are undisplaced in children.
2. The proximal femoral bone (with the exception of the physis) is much stronger in children and requires a large force to break it, whereas the osteoporotic bone in the elderly is easily fractured with a simple fall.
3. The hardness of a child's bone and the small diameter of the femoral neck are often not suited to fixation with standard adult fixation devices.
4. The proximal femoral physis is a point of weakness in the skeletally immature child; fractures that cross this growth plate may lead to physeal arrest that can cause coxa breva or coxa vara. Although a fracture heals, deformity may progress with growth.
5. The blood supply of the head is different (Fig. 12-7). When the physis is still open, blood vessels do not cross the physis so the blood supply to the head is tenuous and easily disrupted. AVN may result from complete division of the vessels, kinking of the vessels that remain intact, or tamponade by hemarthrosis within the hip capsule.

Classification

Pediatric hip fractures (from the femoral head to the lesser trochanter) have been classified by Delbet (Table 12-2). More distal fractures of the femur including subtrochanteric fractures are discussed in Chapter 8.

Treatment

Type I Fractures (Transphyseal)

The femoral head separates from the neck through the physis. In very young children, this injury is most likely to occur when a child has been run over by a car but may also be seen in abused infants. In children, great violence is required, and there are usually associated injuries. In adolescents, an acute Type I

Table 12-2 Delbet Classification of Pediatric Hip Fractures

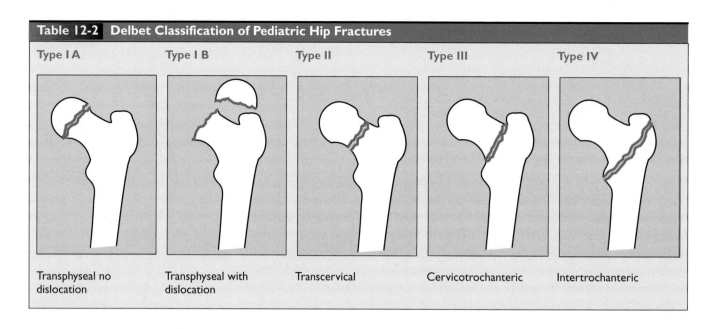

Type I A	Type I B	Type II	Type III	Type IV
Transphyseal no dislocation	Transphyseal with dislocation	Transcervical	Cervicotrochanteric	Intertrochanteric

injury is seen, which is difficult to differentiate from an acute (unstable) slipped capital femoral epiphysis (SCFE) (see next section).

Traction has been advised for type IA fractures with no displacement in very young children, but in most cases, spica cast immobilization is used. In displaced fractures in infants, closed reduction is relatively easy, and the reduction should be held in a one-and-a-half hip spica. Displacement can occur in the cast, and frequent radiographs should be taken to detect this. If pin fixation is required (rare), it should be done with smooth pins because pinning may aggravate the tendency for premature fusion.

If the head is dislocated (type IB), urgent open reduction is mandated (Fig. 12-8). Canale and Bourland described five cases of traumatic separation accompanied by dislocation and all developed AVN with four of the five developing degenerative arthritis. The young patients required leg-length equalization. Traumatic separation of the proximal femoral epiphysis is a severe injury, and the parents should be warned that problems are more likely than not.

Type II and III Fractures—Transcervical and Cervicotrochanteric

The perils of these injuries are great, with AVN reported in up to 50% of cases. Although more common in displaced fractures, AVN can occur in undisplaced fractures. Premature closure of the physis can occur as a sequel to AVN, leading to a short femoral neck and a weak lever arm for the abductor muscles, a short

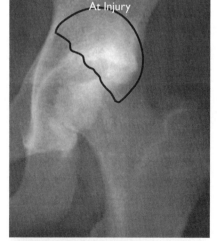

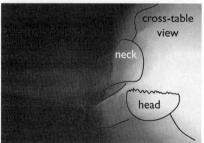

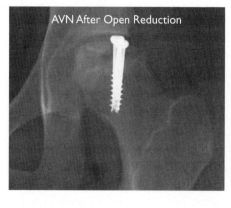

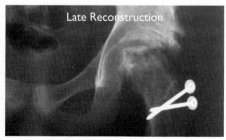

Figure 12-8. This 15-year-old boy suffered a severe type IB injury with marked head displacement. Despite immediate open reduction, he developed AVN. Late construction included femoral head recontouring, bone grafting, and a shelf acetabuloplasty.

leg, and limitation of abduction owing to greater trochanter overgrowth (Fig. 12-8). Delayed union, nonunion, and drifting into coxa vara are also common.

Nondisplaced Fractures

Nondisplaced neck fractures in young children (younger than 4 or 5 years) have some inherent stability, and the safest way to protect them is in a one-and-one-half hip spica with the leg held in internal rotation and abduction for 6-8 weeks. This is only advised for a truly undisplaced injury. The fracture should be checked frequently for change in alignment. In older children, pinning is technically easier and reduces the chances of displacement.

Displaced Fractures

Muscular forces across the hip joint tend to produce coxa vara in displaced fractures (i.e., fractures in which the periosteum has been torn). Cast fixation after reduction does not neutralize these muscular forces, and loss of reduction in a spica cast is almost certain. For displaced fractures, the conservative approach is internal fixation (Fig. 12-9). In the classic text *Treatment of Fractures in Children and Adolescents,* Weber et al. state "We regard every fracture of the femoral neck in a child as an emergency situation which requires operative intervention with a minimum of delay. Rapid action is essential to allow anatomically precise reduction and stabilization as well as evacuation of the intracapsular hematoma." We adhere to this A-O recommendation for all displaced femoral neck fractures. Although some surgeons might try a closed reduction and pinning (as in treating an elderly patient), the open approach seems to provide the most predictable results (Fig. 12-10).

The anterolateral or Watson-Jones approach gives excellent exposure for reduction and fixation of femoral neck fractures. This approach utilizes the interval between the tensor fascia lata and gluteus medius, with the abductors retracted to expose the capsule. The capsule is opened to release the hematoma and to allow exact fracture reduction. The fracture can be anatomically reduced with the aid of a periosteal elevator, traction, and internal rotation. The fracture is fixed with cancellous screws avoiding the physis if possible.

Most authors express a preference for threaded pin or screw fixation. The metaphysis is composed of hard bone (unlike the adult metaphysis), providing a "good bite" for screws or threaded pins. It is usually unnecessary to cross the physis, but in high fractures do not hesitate to place a pin (temporarily) across the

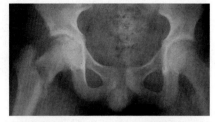

At Injury

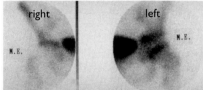

right   left

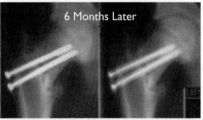

6 Months Later

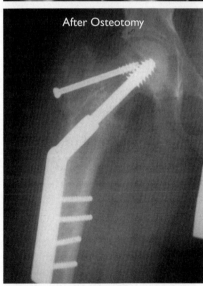

After Osteotomy

Figure 12-9. This 13-year-old boy fell on wet grass and presented with a femoral neck fracture. The bone scan showed decreased blood flow in the right hip. Despite anatomic reduction and pinning, he developed mild AVN and coxa vara. Late treatment included a valgus osteotomy.

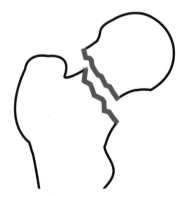

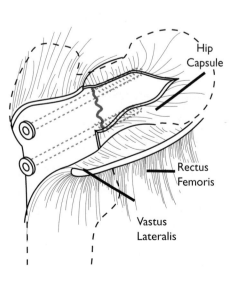

Hip Capsule

Rectus Femoris

Vastus Lateralis

Figure 12-10. Weber et al. emphazised the need for urgent open reduction in this injury (see Suggested Readings). An anterolateral Watson-Jones approach allows a safe, extensive exposure to the capsule.

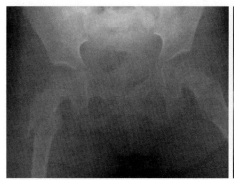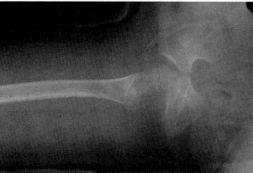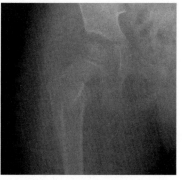

Figure 12-11. This intertrochanteric fracture in a 6-year-old child was treated with casting and went on to heal appropriately without surgical intervention.

physis. If pins are placed across the physis, they should be smooth and be removed as soon as possible to avoid interfering with growth. There are also several lag screw-plate systems available now in children's sizes. The capsule is loosely closed once fixation is secure.

A child does not need rapid rehabilitation. Apply a hip spica for 6-8 weeks to protect the hip (ruptured soft tissues—capsule, vessels) in hopes of decreasing the chance for AVN. Remember the load on the hip imposed by straight leg raising can approach that imposed by walking. A belt-and-suspenders approach is needed to prevent nonunion, coxa vara, and AVN.

Type IV (Intertrochanteric Fractures)

In young children, most intertrochanteric fractures can be reduced and held in skin traction. When callus is present at 3-4 weeks, a one-and-one-half hip spica should be applied (Fig. 12-11). The chief indication for internal fixation is irreducibility or inability to hold the fracture in traction because of other injuries.

Operative treatment used for older children can be difficult, because considerable comminution or separation of the greater trochanter may be present without being obvious on radiographs. Always obtain high-quality films before starting surgery. Older children usually require ORIF with a plate and screws or a lag screw with side plate.

Avulsion Fractures—Lesser Trochanter

Avulsion fractures of the proximal femur are not included in the previous classification system but are worthy of mention in this section. We frequently see avulsion fractures in young aggressive athletes. Avulsion fractures of the lesser trochanter can be caused by the pull of the iliopsoas in sprinters. These typically heal with conservative treatment and do not result in noticeable hip flexor weakness. Crutch use and partial weight bearing for 3-4 weeks typically gets athletes back into competition.

Avulsion Fractures—Greater Trochanter

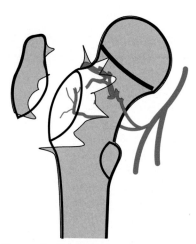

Figure 12-12. Periosteal stripping is the suggested mechanism for femoral head AVN secondary to greater trochanteric avulsion.

The greater trochanter can be avulsed by the abductors, usually associated with a severe twisting fall (Fig. 12-12). Although this injury may appear relatively benign, the posterior circumflex vessels traverse dangerously close to the fracture plane and may be disrupted at the time of fracture (probably in relation to associated periosteal stripping). If the fracture is allowed to heal in a significantly displaced position, the abductors will be weak and Trendelenburg limp will result. ORIF is the preferred method of treatment for displaced fractures; however, the technique should be cautious to avoid increasing the risk for AVN of the femoral head (which is substantial) (Fig. 12-13).

Pitfalls

Ratliff emphasized AVN as the main cause of poor results in proximal femoral fractures (Table 12-3). MacEwen reports that type IB injuries (complete head separation and dislocation) have the highest rate of AVN (80-100%), followed by type IA and type II (50%), and type III (27%). Type IV (intertrochanteric) fractures have the lowest reported rate of AVN (14%).

AVN is best detected early with a bone scan or MRI but is often apparent radiographically after several months and probably always within a year. Radiographs should be obtained regularly (every 2-3 months) during the first year. The first x-ray signs of AVN include the head does not become osteoporotic and does not grow, and the cartilage space becomes wider. These signs appear long before signs of gross density, fragmentation, and deformity of the head. Slight disturbance of circulation produces coxa magna luxans creating a large head that is poorly covered by the acetabulum.

Coxa vara is the most common deformity following cast treatment of proximal femoral fractures; it results in a shortened limb and abductor weakness and may predispose to future fractures of the femoral neck.

Nonunion is rare, but when it occurs, bone grafting is advocated with valgus osteotomy if there is coxa vara.

SCFE (vs. Transphyseal Fracture)

As noted before, an acute SCFE and a type 1A transphyseal fracture are similar images by x-ray but occur in different patient populations. Ratliff noted that acute fractures occur up until age 8-9 years and that acute (unstable) slips occur in teenagers, often with predisposed anatomy (obesity, retroversion of the femoral neck—Table 12-4). SCFE, a pathologic process and not necessarily the result of trauma, will be discussed here because it is within the spectrum of physeal fractures. In the most basic terms, SCFE is the result of a "sick" physis that is unable to support the weight of the child. The femoral neck becomes progressively more retroverted until the femoral head slides off the neck through the physis. The trauma that is associated with an acute SCFE is typically less severe than the trauma required to fracture a healthy proximal femur.

Classification

SCFEs are traditionally classified as acute (pain <2 weeks), chronic (pain >2 weeks) or acute on chronic (sudden worsening of chronic pain).

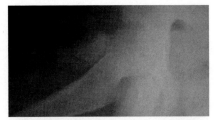
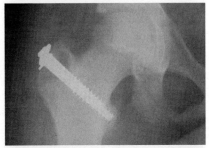
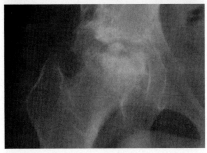

Figure 12-13. An avulsion of the greater trochanter can result in AVN of the femoral head.

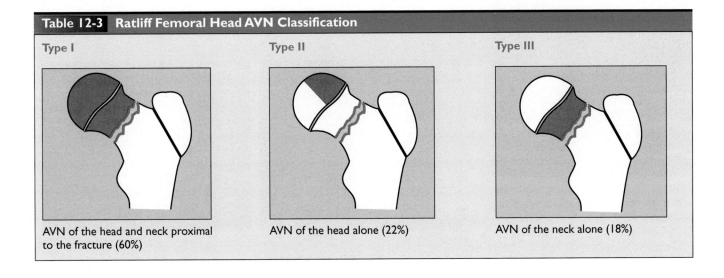

Table 12-3	Ratliff Femoral Head AVN Classification	
Type I	**Type II**	**Type III**
AVN of the head and neck proximal to the fracture (60%)	AVN of the head alone (22%)	AVN of the neck alone (18%)

Table 12-4	Differentiating a Fracture from a Slip (modeled from Ratliff)	
Characteristic	Transphyseal Fracture	Slipped Capital Femoral Epiphysis
Age incidence	Child under 9 y/o	Child 11–16 y/o
Onset	Sudden, following injury	Gradual or sudden
Mechanism of injury	Severe violence, e.g., MVA	No injury or minor violence, e.g., fall
Endocrine defect	Not present	Sometimes present

MVA = motor vehicle accident.

Loder modified this into a patient presentation classification describing SCFE as being either stable or unstable. A patient is able to walk unassisted with a stable slip (this correlates to a chronic slip in the traditional classification). Patients with unstable SCFEs are unable to walk due to acute pain (these correlate to acute and acute on chronic SCFE).

Treatment—SCFE

In situ pinning with screws or threaded Steinmann pins is the standard treatment for stable SCFE (Fig 12-14); treatment of the acute (unstable) injury is more difficult and is heavily debated. The tradition was to try traction followed by pin fixation, but this method still led to a high AVN rate. One should consider an aggressive approach that includes emergent open reduction and fixation with threaded screws. Parsch (Stuttgart) emphasizes that open inspection allows reduction to just the right position (avoiding over-reduction) in cases of acute on chronic slip. We favor this approach, which appears to decrease the risk of AVN (Fig. 12-15). The surgical approach is similar to that discussed for open reduction of childhood femoral neck fractures (discussed earlier in this chapter).

PELVIC AND ACETABULAR FRACTURES

The pelvis is like a suit of armor: when it is damaged there is much more concern about its contents than about the structure itself. The problems for the orthopedic surgeon are different at each age. Osteoporotic old people sustain minor fractures in falls that pose neither visceral nor orthopedic problems. Young adults involved in motor vehicle accidents (MVAs) suffer fractures that

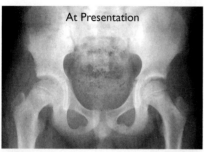

At Presentation

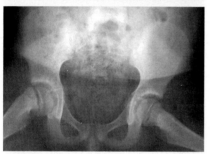

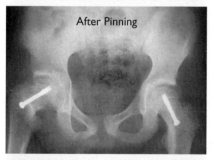

After Pinning

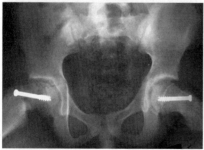

Figure 12-14. This patient presented with a left chronic SCFE and a right acute on chronic SCFE. Both were treated with *in situ* pinning.

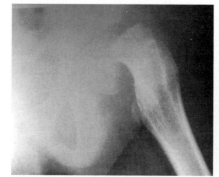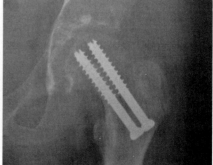

Figure 12-15. This acute SCFE was treated with open reduction and internal fixation. Acute slips are at extremely high risk for AVN.

may be difficult to reduce in addition to life-threatening visceral injuries. Children's fractures are seldom displaced much and can usually be treated with rest and protected weight bearing, but their other injuries may require more attention. On the other hand, teenagers often have severe fractures (Fig. 12-16).

Radiographic Issues

Avoid ordering a frog view of the pelvis if there is any concern for a hip fracture. Although this is the lateral view of the proximal femur that orthopedic surgeons are accustomed to, placing the child in a frog position risks further displacement of a hip fracture. Instead, order a cross-table lateral (along with an AP pelvis view) for safe radiographic evaluation.

Pelvic ring fractures are better evaluated with inlet and outlet x-rays (tube angled 45° caudad or cephalad, respectively) in addition to the AP view (Fig. 12-17).

Acetabular fractures are initially evaluated with oblique (Judet) x-rays. The obturator oblique x-ray allows evaluation of the anterior column and the posterior rim of the acetabulum. The iliac oblique shows the posterior column and the anterior rim. However, a three-dimensional CT scan is much more accurate and is becoming a standard for evaluation and preoperative planning (if surgery is being considered).

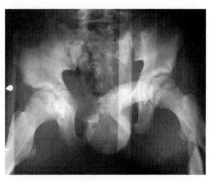

Figure 12-16. This patient was in a severe MVA, he sustained a left femur fracture as well as a vertical shear fracture to his pelvis, fracturing through his SI joint, ischium, and pubis on the left side.

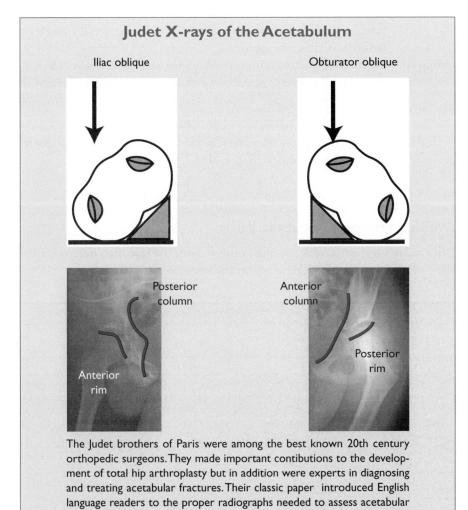

Judet X-rays of the Acetabulum

Iliac oblique

Obturator oblique

Posterior column

Anterior column

Anterior rim

Posterior rim

The Judet brothers of Paris were among the best known 20th century orthopedic surgeons. They made important contibutions to the development of total hip arthroplasty but in addition were experts in diagnosing and treating acetabular fractures. Their classic paper introduced English language readers to the proper radiographs needed to assess acetabular and pelvic fractures. Much can be learned by analyzing these oblique views (although CT scans have diminished their mystique).

Inlet View—Helps in Assessing Posterior Ring Pathology

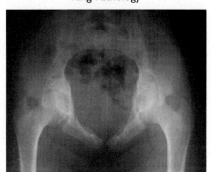

Outlet View—Demonstrates Anterior Ring Pathology

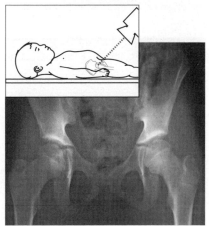

Figure 12-17. Inlet and outlet views show any disruption of the pelvic ring and they are especially good for seeing movement of the SI joint.

A gonadal shield should not be used when obtaining x-rays of possible pelvic fractures—the pathology can easily be concealed by the shield.

MRI studies are rarely needed but when performed have shown interesting differences in adult versus children's SI joint injuries. MRI studies of posterior pelvic injuries have clarified that the vertical displacement in SI joint injuries in children occurs through the non-ossified iliac growth cartilage next to the SI joint and typically does not tear the ligaments, analogous to what one sees at the ankle in a child (physeal separation rather than ligament injury). Thus bony healing is likely in children.

Classification

The most important aspect of understanding pelvic fractures is whether the fracture is stable or unstable. This differentiation provides the basis for whether a pelvic fracture will require operative intervention. A single break in the pelvic ring typically does not render instability to the pelvis; two or more breaks in the ring will destabilize it.

Quinby and Rang classified pelvic ring fractures into three groups:

Group I: Uncomplicated fractures; these are minor and minimally displaced. Signs of abdominal or urologic injury are absent or settle quickly with non-operative treatment.

Group II: Fractures with visceral injuries requiring surgical exploration. These are more severe; the patient may be in shock and require transfusion. The pelvis can conceal a large amount of hemorrhage before it is clinically apparent.

Group III: Fractures associated with immediate massive hemorrhage. Hemorrhage may be from visceral injuries or vascular injury. Even with advanced trauma life support and aggressive management, the mortality of these patients is still high.

Torode and Zieg developed a more detailed classification system for pediatric pelvic fractures, which is summarized in Table 12-5.

Treatment

Avulsion Fractures About the Pelvis

With today's aggressive athletics, the muscles about the hip often overpower the open pelvic apophyses creating avulsion fractures (Fig. 12-18).

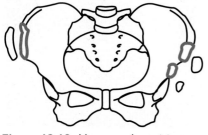

Figure 12-18. Many muscles originate at the pelvis. With strong muscle contraction, the origin of the muscle can be avulsed.

Table 12-5	**Torode and Zieg Classification of Pelvic Fractures**		
Type I	**Type II**	**Type III**	**Type IV**
	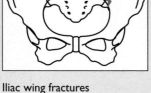	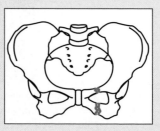	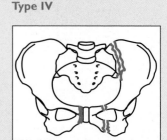
Avulsion fractures	Iliac wing fractures	Simple ring fractures (includes pubic and acetabular fractures)	Fractures producing an unstable segment, (includes straddle, Malgaine, and other unstable fractures)

Type I—Sartorius Avulsion
(Sprinting Injury)

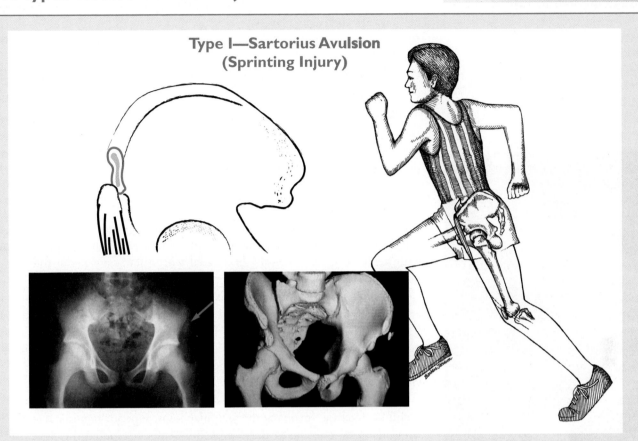

Type II—Tensor Fascia Avulsion
(Rotational Injury)

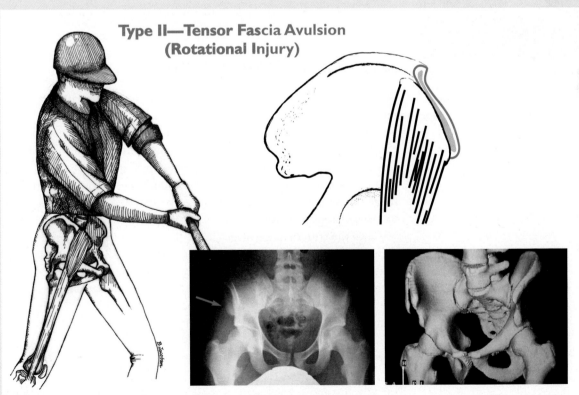

Drawings courtesy of Scott Mubarak.

- The iliac crest apophysis can be avulsed by aggressive twisting as seen in baseball batters.
- The anterior inferior iliac spine is avulsed by the rectus femoris (often seen in soccer and rugby players).
- The anterior superior iliac spine can be avulsed by the sartorius or the tensor fascia lata (seen frequently in sprinters).
- The ischium can be avulsed by the hamstrings (most commonly in hurdlers and gymnasts).

The vast majority of these avulsion fractures heal very well with conservative treatment including protected weight bearing for 3-4 weeks. A very rare patient will develop a painful nonunion that requires operative fixation or excision of the fragment; this is not the first line of treatment.

Fractures of the Pelvic Ring

Stable fractures of the pelvic ring (rami fractures, iliac wing fractures, ishial fractures) that do not involve a joint (acetabulum or SI joint) and are not associated with hemorrhage can typically be treated with a few days of rest followed by protected weight bearing until the fracture heals (usually 4-6 weeks).

Unstable pelvic fractures can be fixed with an external fixator or internal fixation. Pin placement for the external fixator will depend on the location of the fracture and the unstable segment. All orthopedic surgeons should be able to quickly apply a stabilizing pelvic external fixator. These should be positioned to allow access to the abdomen if the general surgeons are planning surgery for a visceral injury.

Many pelvic fractures are now fixed with percutaneous screws. These are very useful for fractures involving the sacroiliac joint, superior ramii, and some iliac wing fractures, but due to the complexity of understanding the three-dimensionality of the pelvis, this percutaneous approach is best left to the experts (Fig. 12-19).

ACETABULAR FRACTURES

Fractures of the acetabulum in the skeletally immature patient are extremely rare. When they occur, they are typically seen as separation through the tri-radiate cartilage. With minimal displacement, fractures of the tri-radiate cartilage can be treated with protected weight bearing; this fracture risks closure of the tri-radiate growth center and subsequent hip dysplasia. Fractures with significant displacement need to be reduced. Smooth pins can cross the tri-radiate cartilage to maintain reduction and should be removed once the fracture is healed to avoid iatrogenic closure.

Once the tri-radiate cartilage closes, fractures of the acetabulum are classified and treated like adult fractures. Three-dimensional CT scan is very useful for understanding the fracture. It is critical to remove any bone or cartilage fragments from the hip joint to avoid further joint destruction. Reconstruction of the acetabulum is best left to the experts; traction is often useful to keep the joint distracted until the time of surgery.

CONCLUSION

Luckily, hip and pelvic fractures are relatively rare in children. It is important to understand and recognize these fractures and their associated injuries. The more severe fractures are produced by high-energy trauma and the associated injuries may be life threatening. Proximal femoral fractures need to be maintained in

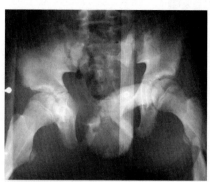

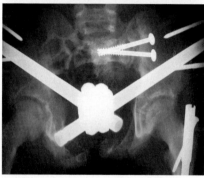

Figure 12-19. This multi-trauma patient was treated with SI joint fixation and an external fixator for his pelvic ring fracture as well as a nail for his subtrochanteric fracture.

anatomic alignment until the fracture has healed. The risk of AVN is significant following both closed and open treatment of proximal femoral fractures. In the rare instance that a pelvic fracture requires operative intervention, this may be best left to the experts as the surgery may be technically difficult and the prognosis is often poor.

Suggested Readings

Bagatur AE, Zorer G. Complications associated with surgically treated hip fractures in children. J Pediatr Orthop B. 2002 Jul;11(3):219-28.

Blasier RD, McAtee J, White R, Mitchell DT. Disruption of the pelvic ring in pediatric patients. Clin Orthop. 2000 Jul; (376):87-95.

Broudy AS, Scott RD: Voluntary posterior hip dislocation in children. J Bone Joint Surg 57A:716, 1975.

Canale ST, Bourland WL: Fracture of the neck and intertrochanteric region of the femur in children. J Bone Joint Surg 59A:431, 1977.

Cheng JC, Tang N. Decompression and stable internal fixation of femoral neck fractures in children can affect the outcome. J Pediatr Orthop. 1999 May-Jun;19(3):338-43.

Davison BL, Weinstein SL. Hip fractures in children: a long-term follow-up study. J Pediatr Orthop. 1992 May-Jun;12(3):355-8.

Demetriades D, Karaiskakis M, Velmahos GC, Alo K, Murray J, Chan L. Pelvic fractures in pediatric and adult trauma patients: are they different injuries? J Trauma. 2003 Jun;54(6):1146-51.

Flynn JM, Wong KL, Yeh GL, Meyer JS, Davidson RS. Displaced fractures of the hip in children. Management by early operation and immobilisation in a hip spica cast. follow-up study. Injury. 2001 Jan;32(1):45-51.

Grisoni N, Connor S, Marsh E, Thompson GH, Cooperman DR, Blakemore LC. Pelvic fractures in a pediatric level I trauma center. J Orthop Trauma. 2002 Aug;16(7):458-63.

Haddad RJ, Drez D: Voluntary recurrent anterior dislocation of the hip. J Bone Joint Surg 56A:419, 1974.

Hughes LO, Beaty JH. Fractures of the head and neck of the femur in children. J Bone Joint Surg Am. 1994 Feb;76(2):283-92.

Judet R, Judet J, Letournel E. Fractures of the acetabulum: Classification and surgical approaches for open reduction. Preliminary report. J Bone Joint Surg Am. 1964 Dec;46:1615-46

Magid D, Fishman EK, Ney DR, Kuhlman JE, Frantz KM, Sponseller PD. Acetabular and pelvic fractures in the pediatric patient: value of two- and three-dimensional imaging. J Pediatr Orthop. 1992 Sep-Oct;12(5):621-5.

Mehlman CT, Hubbard GW, Crawford AH, Roy DR, Wall EJ. Traumatic hip dislocation in children. Long-term followup of 42 patients. Clin Orthop. 2000 Jul; (376):68-79.

Metzmaker JN, Pappas AM. Avulsion fractures of the pelvis. Am J Sports Med. 1985 Sep-Oct;13(5):349-58.

Morsy HA. Complications of fracture of the neck of the femur in children. A long-term follow-up study. Injury. 2001 Jan; 32(1):45-51

Musemeche CA, Fischer RP, Cotler HB, Andrassy RJ. Selective management of pediatric pelvic fractures: a conservative approach. J Pediatr Surg. 1987 Jun;22(6):538-40.

Nikolopoulos KE, Papadakis SA, Kateros KT, Themistocleous GS, Vlamis JA, Papagelopoulos PJ, Nikiforidis PA. Long-term outcome of patients with avascular necrosis, after internal fixation of femoral neck fractures. Injury. 2003 Jul;34(7):525-8.

Ogden JA. Hip development and vascularity: relationship to chondro-osseous trauma in the growing child. Hip. 1981:139-87.

O'Rourke MR, Weinstein SL. Osteonecrosis following isolated avulsion fracture of the

greater trochanter in children. A report of two cases. J Bone Joint Surg Am. 2003 Oct;85-A(10):2000-5

Pape HC, Krettek C, Friedrich A, Pohlemann T, Simon R, Tscherne H. Long-term outcome in children with fractures of the proximal femur after high-energy trauma. J Trauma. 1999 Jan;46(1):58-64.

Ratliff, AHC: Traumatic separations of the upper femoral epiphysis in young children. JBJS 50B:757, 1968.

Scuderi G, Bronson MJ. Triradiate cartilage injury; report of two cases and review of literature. Clin Orthop 217:179-183 1987.

Silber JS, Flynn JM. Changing patterns of pediatric pelvic fractures with skeletal maturation: implications for classification and management. J Pediatr Orthop. 2002 Jan-Feb;22(1):22-6.

Smith WR, Oakley M, Morgan SJ. Pediatric pelvic fractures.J Pediatr Orthop. 2004 Jan-Feb;24(1):130-5.

Song KS, Kim YS, Sohn SW, Ogden JA. Arthrotomy and open reduction of the displaced fracture of the femoral neck in children. J Pediatr Orthop B. 2001 Jul; 10(3):205-10.

Torode I, Zieg D. Pelvic fractures in children. J Pediatr Orthop. 1985 Jan-Feb; 5(1):76-84.

Weber BG, Brunner Ch, Freuler F. Treatment of Fractures in Children and Adolescents. Springer-Verlag, Berlin Heidelberg 1980.

White KK, Williams SK, Mubarak SJ. Definition of two types of anterior superior iliac spine avulsion fractures.J Pediatr Orthop. 2002 Sep-Oct;22(5):578-82.

13

Femoral Shaft

Maya Pring ❧ *Peter Newton* ❧ *Mercer Rang*

INTRODUCTION

Femur fractures in children are common, with causes ranging from abuse in a neonate to a motorcycle accident in a 16-year-old. Optimal treatment varies according to age (Fig. 13-1). Surgeons who treat children's fractures need to understand the nature of a femoral fracture in each age group and master treatment techniques that allow full recovery of structure and function. In this chapter, we will divide femoral fractures into age groups and present a practical treatment path for each group.

ASSESSING THE PATIENT

In most cases, diagnosis of a fractured femur is straight-forward. After the pedal pulses have been palpated, the leg should be splinted before radiographs are

> *"The surest way to corrupt a young man is to teach him to esteem more highly those who think alike then those who think differently"*
>
> —*NIETZSCHE*

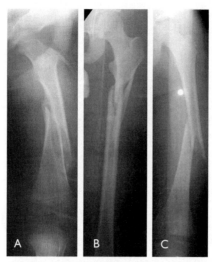

Figure 13-1. Each fracture must be treated differently based on the age of the child and the anatomy of the fracture. A) Spiral fracture in infancy, easy to hold in a cast. B) Proximal fracture in an 8-year-old, hard to hold in cast. C) Shaft fracture in a teenager, will require intermedullary fixation.

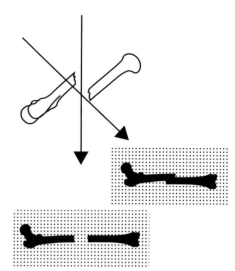

Figure 13-2. A fracture may appear distracted or overlapping depending on the angle at which the radiograph is taken. Judge length with a tape measure.

"Surgeons who treat children's fractures need to understand the nature of a femoral fracture in each age group and master treatment techniques that allow full recovery of structure and function"

taken. A subsequent thorough physical exam and secondary survey are critical because the pain of a femur fracture frequently distracts the patient who may not complain of other possibly life-threatening injuries. Monitor the blood pressure; shock is almost never the result of a femur fracture in childhood and is more likely due to internal hemorrhage (e.g., a ruptured spleen).

Although femur fractures are common and may result from apparently minimal trauma or a twisting injury during ordinary play, if the child is younger than age 5 years, nonaccidental trauma or child abuse should be considered. If there is concern, a skeletal survey and ophthalmologic exam should be obtained with child protection services involved in the evaluation (see Chapter 17). In a study by Nurk et al., 67% of femoral fractures in children younger than the age of 1 year were secondary to child abuse. However, patients between 1-2 years of age were much more likely to sustain their femur fractures through nonabuse mechanisms; only 11% of children age 1-2 sustained fractures from abuse. An orthopedic surgeon's experience in noting that roughhouse play among siblings can lead to an innocent limb fracture in a young child (and that spiral fractures are very common in nonabuse circumstances) can often add clarity to the initial social service inquiry of child abuse.

RADIOGRAPHIC ISSUES

Often, the initial femur film is not of high quality, being one of many x-rays taken quickly in the emergency department as opposed to the more controlled setting of the radiology suite. Polytrauma patients can be difficult to position, and with the many issues that take precedence in their acute medical management true AP and lateral x-rays are unusual.

However, several things can be learned from these early films (location of fracture, angulation, shortening, etc.), and decisions for treatment can usually be made based on these initial films despite their shortcomings. One must be certain that the x-rays include both the hip and knee prior to proceeding with treatment to avoid missing a hip dislocation, femoral neck fracture, or occult knee injury.

The degree of fracture shortening or fragment overlap at the time of initial injury has been used to help determine appropriate management. Staheli has noted that the markedly shortened limb (due to fracture overlap) is not a good candidate for early spica treatment; however, the concept of initial shortening as a determinant of treatment choice cannot be easily applied for several reasons. Figure 13-2 describes the difficulty in assessing fracture distraction or overlap on plain films, both at the time of initial evaluation and later with the patient in traction or a spica cast. The lateral radiograph may be more accurate in assessing true shortening.

Modern emergency medical treatment (EMT) transport includes application of traction in the field (Fig. 13-3), which makes determination of initial shortening (and associated periosteal stripping) difficult. Some have suggested a manual "push test" to determine how much the fracture will shorten. However, this is painful for the awake child and may risk further soft tissue damage; traction should generally not be removed for x-rays or exam until adequate sedation and analgesia have been obtained.

As casting techniques have improved (Chapter 5), we have moved away from the concept of initial shortening as an indicator for traction and cast many femoral shaft fractures that were previously thought not amenable to early spica treatment. Vigilance regarding observation for subsequent in-cast shortening must accompany this approach.

CLASSIFICATION

Several classification methods help determine appropriate treatment for each femur fracture type.

Anatomic Classification

Femoral shaft fractures are typically divided into proximal (subtrochanteric), midshaft, and distal types. (Femoral neck and hip fractures are discussed in Chapter 12; distal physeal and epiphyseal fractures in Chapter 14.)

Deformity Classification

Depending on fracture level, the forces exerted on the fragments by the muscles that remain attached can pull the fracture into varus, valgus, flexion, extension, or rotational malalignment (Fig. 13-4). These forces must be considered and

"Modern EMT transport includes application of traction in the field, which makes determination of initial shortening (and associated periosteal stripping) difficult"

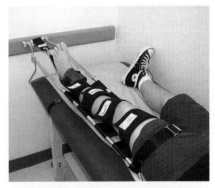

Figure 13-3. For quick transport of a patient with a femur fracture, a Harris traction splint can be used to keep the fracture out to length. These splints cannot be used for more than a few hours as there is a risk of skin necrosis and tourniquet effect at the ankle. The proximal pad pushes against the ischium while traction is pulled through the ankle cuff.

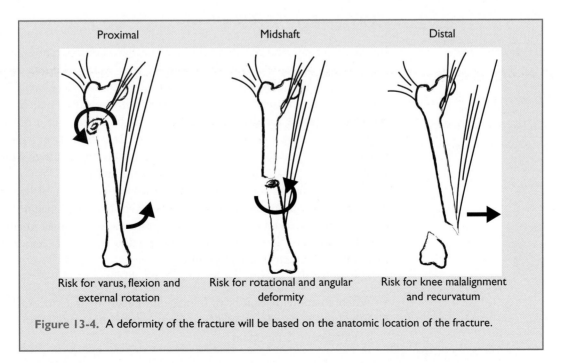

Proximal	Midshaft	Distal
Risk for varus, flexion and external rotation	Risk for rotational and angular deformity	Risk for knee malalignment and recurvatum

Figure 13-4. A deformity of the fracture will be based on the anatomic location of the fracture.

Table 13-1	Simple Treatment Outline—According to Age	
Age of Child	Standard Treatment	Options for More Complex or Open Fractures
<2 years	Single leg spica, or Pavlik harness	Skin traction with delayed casting
2–6 years	Early spica cast	Skin or skeletal traction, plate fixation (submuscular or open), external fixator
6–14 years	Flexible intramedullary nails	Skeletal traction, plate fixation (submuscular or open), external fixator
>14 years	Interlocked intramedullary nails	Skeletal traction, plate fixation (submuscular or open), external fixator

counteracted by the cast, traction, or internal fixation when planning treatment. Poorly applied treatment of any type can worsen the initial deformity and create an unacceptable result.

Age-Based Classification

Contemporary treatment methods have allowed development of an age-related treatment algorithm (Table 13-1) appropriate for institutions where current technology is available and who have an incentive to shorten hospital stays. This algorithm will obviously differ in hospitals where flexible nails and trochanteric entry nails are not available and where lengthy hospital stays (in traction) are more affordable than the latest technology. Traction remains a viable and frequently used treatment method for femoral shaft fractures in any age group.

The reader should recognize that the age cutoffs in this algorithm are not absolute with treatment of each child tailored to the size and activity level of the individual. For example, a 130-pound 6-year-old skateboarder will be treated differently then a 70-pound gymnast of the same age. Larger patients are difficult to manage in a spica and are more likely to be treated surgically.

TREATMENT

Children Age 0-2 Years

"The drama facing the parents of an infant with a fractured femur who requires hip spica immobilization cannot be overestimated"

Because fractures heal readily at this age and have great potential for remodeling, a good outcome is almost certain in very young children regardless of shortening or initial alignment. Surgery is almost never necessary (the rare exceptions being an open fracture or fracture with neurovascular compromise). Treatment choices for the infant include a Pavlik harness or a hip spica cast. (Fig. 13-5). In very young children, often the Pavlik harness provides adequate immobilization and the traditional single leg spica is not required, which greatly simplifies diaper changing and overall care of the child.

The drama facing the parents of an infant with a fractured femur who requires hip spica immobilization cannot be overestimated. Imagine young parents who are panicked about their child's injury and who may in addition feel that they are being accused of child abuse: it takes an experienced, mature team to handle this circumstance gracefully.

The surgeon must consider many issues including:

- Where to apply the spica cast (emergency department, clinic, OR),
- Whether the parents should be present for the spica application (if in clinic or emergency department)

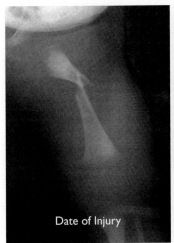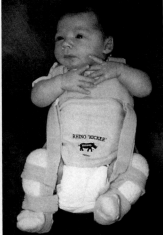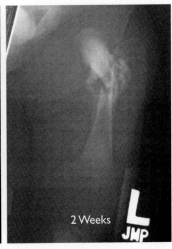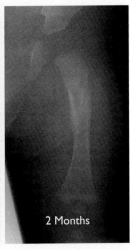

Date of Injury   2 Weeks   2 Months

Figure 13-5. This infant was treated in a Pavlik harness and had quick healing and remodeling of her fracture.

- The need for and advisability of sedation
- Whether the child should be admitted to the hospital for further workup, monitoring, or family teaching about care of the child in a hip spica

Whether this is done awkwardly or well depends on the orchestration of the team leader.

Although an infant with a femoral fracture and newly applied hip spica can be sent home following casting, we have concerns about this concept. Caring for a child of any age in a hip spica is an immense new burden on the parents, and clear instructions are required for the parents to understand cast care, diapering, carrying the child, wheelchair rental and use, etc. We believe that most parents of a child with a new hip spica require careful instruction and teaching, and in our system this is most likely to occur with an overnight hospital admission. Exceptions might include an early morning case where teaching nurses can then provide education during the day.

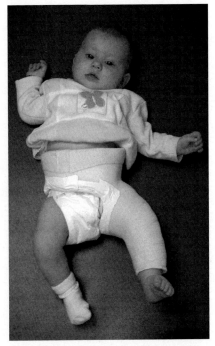

Figure 13-6. Typical spica cast position for a young child.

Application of Hip Spica Cast

Very young children (up to age 2 years) who require little manipulative reduction can have a spica cast applied in the emergency department or clinic, frequently with no sedation or with only minor conscious sedation. Remember that early spica application may prevent overall inspection of the child (abdominal viscera, skin bruising, etc.) and should be avoided if a child abuse workup is ongoing. The spica should be easy to apply with the child awake and in a position that makes care of the child as simple as possible. Usually, the hip is flexed 30° and abducted 30° with the knee in similar flexion (Fig. 13-6).

Children Age 2-6 Years

In this age group, most femoral fractures can be treated with manipulative reduction plus a hip spica cast, commonly referred to as "immediate spica" cast treatment; we avoid this terminology because it implies that both the patient and the doctor are best served by applying the spica cast immediately. We prefer the term "early spica" treatment and often find it better for all involved to admit the child for temporary placement in skin traction (see Techniques Tips—Skin Traction) until the dust has settled. This allows assessment of swelling and possible associated abdominal or other soft tissue trauma, as well as allowing the surgeon to perform the reduction and hip spica application in a comfortable environment at an elective time with an experienced team. This is usually within the first few days after injury.

"We avoid the term 'immediate spica' treatment as it implies a sometimes unnecessary rush to treatment. Often temporary traction with spica application at a scheduled time with 'daytime' personnel is better"

TECHNIQUE TIPS:
Skin Traction

1. For patients >60 pounds
2. Apply adhesive to the skin
3. Pad malleoli and fibular head with cast padding
4. Apply traction tape (fabric-backed foam) down medial and lateral sides of the leg
5. Overwrap the tapes from ankle to knee leaving the foot free
6. Use no more than 5 pounds of weight
7. Use sling or pillow to support the hip and knee in a slightly flexed position (20°-30°)
8. Check skin regularly, as skin blistering and sloughing can occur
9. Regular neurovascular checks—nerves and blood vessels can be compromised
10. Traction used until adequate callus for spica

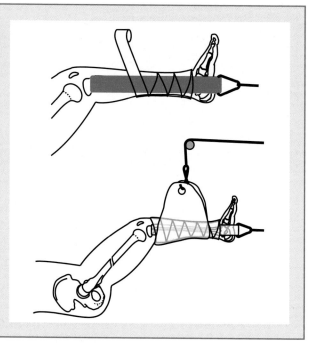

TECHNIQUE TIPS:
Skeletal Traction

1. For patients >60 pounds (can be used on adults as well as children)
2. The distal femur is preferred for insertion of Steinmann pin (tibial pins may sublux the tibia and stretch the knee ligaments or injure the tibial tubercle)
3. Pins may be threaded (better hold) or smooth (easier to insert and remove)
4. Pins inserted from medial to lateral to protect the neurovascular structures, entry point is proximal and parallel to the physis in the metaphyseal flare
5. During pin insertion, hold the leg in the position for traction (usually 90-90) so the skin and fascia are not stretched after pin insertion
6. Apply dressing over pins, followed by a traction bow
7. A short leg cast with anterior loops allows rotation adjustment and prevents equinus contractures
8. Apply enough weight to support the leg, avoid over distraction at the fracture site
9. X-rays in traction should be checked weekly to allow proper adjustment of weight and position to ensure that there is no distraction at the fracture site and that alignment remains acceptable
10. Traction used until adequate callus for spica (good test: no pain with thigh motion—usually 3 weeks)

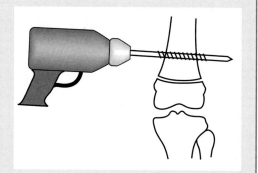

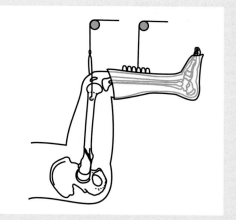

This age group requires greater attention to reduction than does the infant, thus fracture classification becomes more relevant. The goal of manipulative reduction plus spica cast application is to align the distal and proximal fragments in a position most likely to be maintained by the cast (Fig. 13-7). The surgeon must skillfully mold the cast to counteract the forces of the muscles that pull on each fragment.

End-to-end reduction, which is difficult to achieve, is not required because the femur tends to overgrow following fracture. Initial in-cast shortening of 1-1.5 cm is ideal and up to 2-3 cm is often acceptable.

Proximal Fractures

Proximal femoral fractures often prove difficult to align in a spica cast and may require traction or open reduction plus internal fixation. The strong pull of the abductors and external rotators on the greater trochanter pulls the proximal fragment upward and outward. Whether treated in traction or attempted early spica reduction, these patients should be treated with the hip in flexion, abduction, and external rotation to align the shaft with the proximal fragment (90-90 position with the heel over the contralateral tibia). The parents should be warned at the outset that treatment may change. If reduction is lost, the patient may need to be converted to traction or even open reduction and internal fixation to optimize the outcome (Fig. 13-8).

Mid-shaft Fractures

Midshaft fractures tend to drift into varus so the cast should be aggressively molded to create slight valgus initially. It is important to evaluate rotation of the fracture both clinically and radiographically as the proximal fragment will tend to externally rotate.

Cast Position—90°-90° Versus Relative Extension

Twenty years ago, the 90°-90° (hip-knee flexion) cast position became popular (Arkansas Children's Hospital method). The foot/calf segment and abdominal segment were applied first with the two segments then connected (using traction on the distal casted tibia). Although effective in maintaining reduction, Frick as well as Czertak have reported skin problems as well as compartment

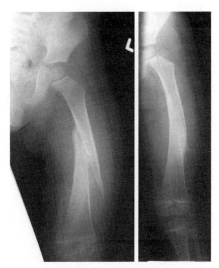

Figure 13-7. Young children have an incredible potential to remodel femur fractures. Fractures need only to be aligned in the cast not necessarily reduced.

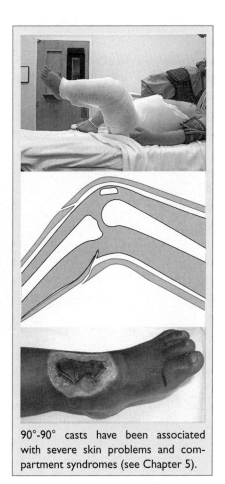

90°-90° casts have been associated with severe skin problems and compartment syndromes (see Chapter 5).

| At Injury | In Traction | In Spica | After ORIF |

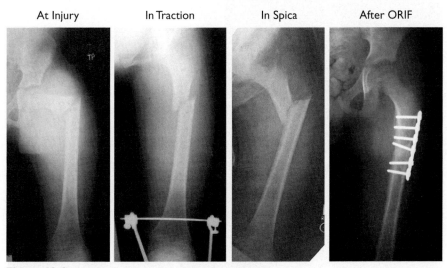

Figure 13-8. Treatment may need to be changed during the course of healing. This patient was initially treated in traction for 3 weeks and then converted to a spica cast. The cast did not maintain the fracture alignment and the family opted for surgery instead of continued traction.

syndromes and skin slough associated with this method. We no longer use the strict 90°-90° position to avoid these risks (also see Chapter 5).

Distal Fractures

For distal fractures, the gastrocnemius tends to flex the distal fragment, causing recurvatum at the fracture site. Flexing the knee will reduce this deforming force. Distal femoral fractures can be aligned with a neutral varus-valgus alignment—with the knee in 10°-20° of flexion. Because of the increased risk for knee malalignment in distal fractures, x-rays should include the proximal tibia to ensure proper positioning in the cast.

Following the Patient—Pitfalls

Early spica treatment is efficient but may blind the surgeon to evolving complications. Changing a selected course goes against the "black and white" nature of many surgeons. Gradual angulation or shortening in the spica must be recognized and dealt with if the reduction becomes unacceptable. The wise surgeon must be flexible and react promptly to changes.

Response to progressive shortening or angulation may include:

- Cast wedging (Fig. 13-9)
- Change to traction
- External fixator application
- Open reduction

Changing to traction or an external fixator is always easier if the parents have been warned of the possible need to return to more traditional methods.

Duration of Treatment

Spica cast immobilization should continue until healing is evident on x-ray; a ball-park rule for weeks of casting is 3 + the child's age in years, up to 12 weeks (e.g., a 4-year-old child is casted for approximately 7 weeks). The fracture should be monitored with weekly x-rays for the first 3 weeks. Because the evolving callus is flexible during this time period, moderate loss of alignment can often be corrected by careful cast wedging.

> *"Proximal femoral fractures often prove difficult to align in a spica cast and may require traction or open reduction plus internal fixation"*

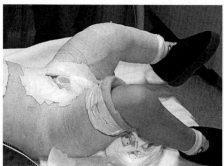
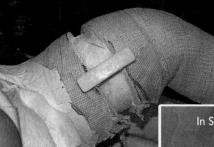
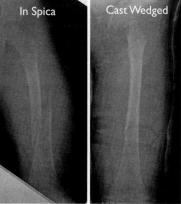
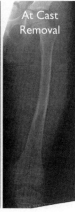
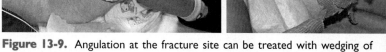

Figure 13-9. Angulation at the fracture site can be treated with wedging of the cast.

TECHNIQUE TIPS:
Application of a Hip Spica for Child with Femur Fracture

(Cast in relative extension minimizes risk to skin and compartments)

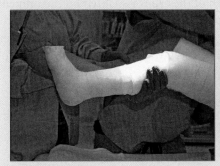

1) Short leg (below knee segment) applied first to help hold the limb. Little traction or pressure can be used and the junction must be well padded (we use felt). Some do not incorporate the foot and add the calf segment last (to avoid skin problems).

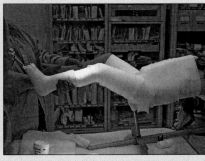

2) Limb positioned in relative extension. Cast padding added. Note temporary spacers under padding over abdomen (use towels or skin tape packs).

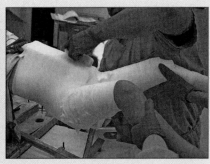

3) Synthetic material rolled on. Again note cast prominence over temporary abdominal protection spacers.

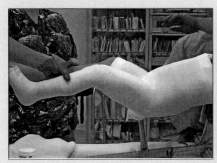

4) Fiberglass completed.

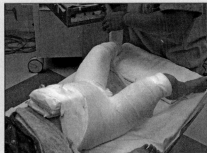

5) View from above—cast complete—note cast has been trimmed down to the umbilicus level to ensure easy abdominal expansion and breathing—The temporary pads will now be removed (once cast hardens).

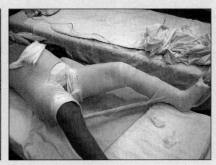

6) Spica cast complete; abdominal pads removed. Wood is attached to opposite thigh for stability.

Pre-Spica film   After Spica

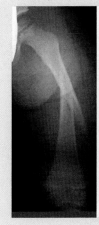
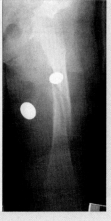

NOTE: We have changed to this more relaxed position, as compared to the 90°-90° position, which has a risk for skin and compartment problems in the calf. Some would not apply the calf segment first nor incorporate the foot to further minimize these risks.

6 Weeks After Injury

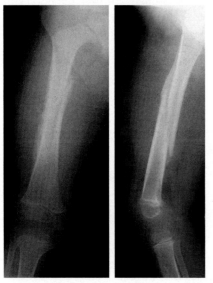

Figure 13-10. Early post-spica x-ray. It is often difficult to determine if the callus is adequate to resume weight bearing.

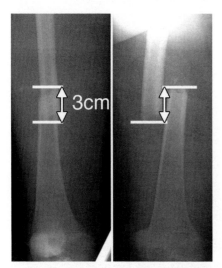

Figure 13-11. In older children and teenagers, shortening needs to be corrected as overgrowth does not occur as frequently.

Activity Level After Spica Removal

Advice for return to activity is perhaps the least standardized part of childhood femoral fracture treatment. Should children use crutches and at what age is crutch training appropriate? Do children fall more and put themselves at higher risk of refracture with crutches? Does physical therapy help? There are no definitive answers, but we will present our observations and recommendations.

One can never be sure of the strength of the callus visualized on the immediate post spica x-ray. (Fig. 13-10) How strong is it? Is there any risk that the femur may bend with weight bearing? When the spica is removed, we describe the fracture as "healing," not healed, accordingly, we advise the parents as follows:

- Each child has an individual healing biology
- We don't know when the child will walk (it could be 2 days or several weeks)
- Take the child home and let him/her sit on the floor and crawl
- Do not help or encourage the child to walk
- Allow to pull to stand when able
- The child will gradually progress to walking and will limp for several months
- Crutches are generally not necessary in this young age group and are poorly tolerated in children younger than 6 to 7 years old
- Physical therapy does not appear to change the outcome

Children Age 6-12 Years

Shortening and malunion are the main risks in this age group because of increasing muscle strength in puberty and decreasing help from overgrowth and remodeling (Fig. 13-11). Classic treatment for an adolescent with a femoral fracture included traction for several weeks (until early callus formation—fracture becomes "sticky") followed by placement in a hip spica for many weeks to allow further healing. This method remains popular in many settings but requires lengthy hospitalizations with intensive maintenance and traction adjustment, which is time consuming for the surgeon, nurses, and orthopedic technician staff.

Our guide to children 0-8 years regarding how to rehabilitate from a fracture and casting is guided by observations in the animal kingdom. The dog on the left required no instruction and rests comfortably after knee surgery.

The dog on the right had a femur fracture and did not have the benefit of casting. She elected 3-legged walking for a month and then resumed her normal quadriped gait.

Cast design crutches and wise surgeon advice will allow most children to heal equally well.

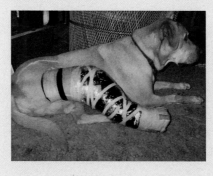

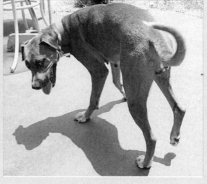

Although traction techniques for femoral fracture treatment are a dying art in many institutions, the method offers many treatment variations and should be understood by all who treat femoral fractures. Although time consuming, traction avoids the risks of anesthesia, surgical fixation, and the almost inevitable later implant removal.

With larger children, care in a spica cast becomes a burden to the family and patient. In much of the developed world where both parents may be full-time employees, keeping a child out of school for an extended period becomes unreasonable (Fig. 13-12). However, in much of the world, families are extended, with multiple family members to care for a child in a spica cast or traction. Also in these circumstances, operating rooms, image intensifiers, fully trained surgeons, and medical equipment are less affordable; treatment choices must fit the culture as well as the injury.

Flexible Nail Methods

The development of flexible intramedullary nail systems in North America (Rush, Ender) and Europe in the last two decades has revolutionized the care of children with fractures in this age group. The elastic titanium Nancy nail method of Metazeau and Lascombes, with further development and popularization by Parsch, Slongo, and others, has become a widely accepted treatment method for adolescents in most centers in the United States and Canada.

The advantages of flexible nails over metal plates or formal intramedullary rods are considerable. Although easy to apply, metal plates on the femur are very difficult to remove without incurring a subsequent femur fracture (too little load sharing). Formal rod systems require a proximal entry site, which may risk damage to the growth center of the greater trochanter or, in a worst case scenario, avascular necrosis (AVN) of the femoral head. The distal entry site for most flexible nail system avoids these risks.

Flexible intramedullary nailing can be accomplished with either stainless steel or titanium implants. Largely, theoretical advantages have led some to advocate one over the other. Stainless steel is stiffer in bending; yet titanium, which is more elastic, may conform and contact a larger area of the medullary canal resulting in improved fixation. One real advantage of the latest titanium implants is the superior tools for insertion (and removal).

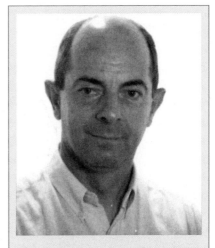

The Flexible Nail Revolution (The Nancy Nail)

Jean Paul Metazeau (Nancy, France) popularized a method called "embrochage centromedullaire elastique stabile" in the early 1980s.

This method, based on principles first developed in Romania, evolved into the current method known in North America as "flexible nailing," which has wide application for treatment of children's fractures.

Lascombe, Parsch, Prevot, Ligier, Slango, Heinrich, Rang, and others helped to make this a widely used method in North America.

(Photo courtesy of Pierre Lascombe.)

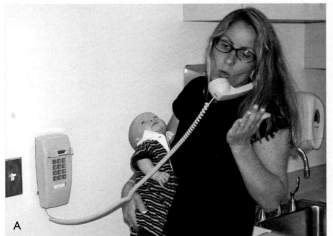
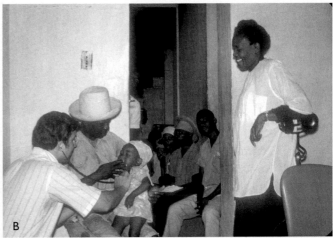

Figure 13-12. A) Modern American mother "always on the go" often with inadequate time or extended family support for time-consuming treatment such as traction. B) Haitian families with a large extended family, all involved in the care of the child, may be more willing to accept treatment methods that require lengthy hospitalization or prolonged attention at home. Photos provided courtesy of Michelle Marks (Left) and Dennis R. Wenger (Right).

TECHNIQUE TIPS:
Flexible Intermedullary Nailing

Distal entry site—2 "C" nails

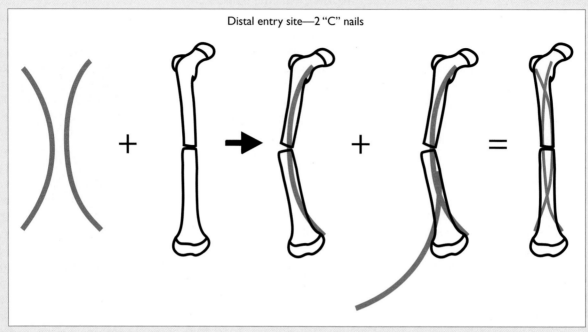

Proximal entry site—"S" and "C" nails

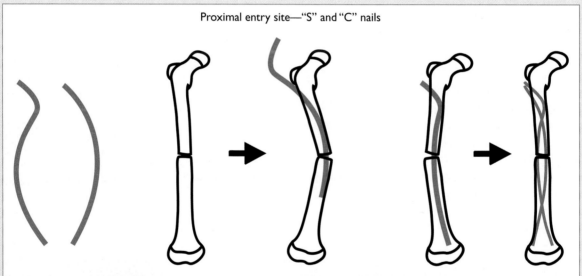

1. Preoperative planning: the narrowest diameter of the diaphyseal canal is measured. The width of each nail should be 35%-40% of this diameter (example, if canal diameter is >1 cm, use two 4 mm nails). Larger diameter nails give better stability and decrease the risk of nonunion, but >80% canal fill risks additional comminution.

2. For most fractures, an entry point 1.5-2 cm above the distal femoral physis in the metaphyseal flare is preferred. One nail should enter from the medial side and one from the lateral side to stabilize varus-valgus angulation. With distal entry sites, the two nails can both be "C" shaped.

3. For distal fractures, consider a proximal entry point on the lateral aspect of the femur and just below the apophysis of the greater trochanter. The nails should be pre-bent: one into a "C" shape and one into an "S" shape so that one ends medially and one laterally in the distal femur.

4. The widest separation of the two nails should be at the level of the fracture. To get the nails into the proximal portion, turn the nail into anteversion as it approaches the femoral neck.

5. Back the nails out 1 cm, cut to leave 1.5-2 cm out of the bone for easy removal, and then tamp back into place.

Variation of technique described by Ligier, Metazeau, Prevot, and Lascombe—see Suggested Readings.

Another controversy regarding flexible nail usage relates to the site of insertion—proximal versus distal. In either case C-shaped segments of the nails should be placed with opposing orientation to provide balanced varus and valgus bending moments at the fracture site. Distal insertion medially and laterally of 2 C-shaped rods makes this a straightforward task. Both nails should be similar diameter and generally pre-bent to a similar degree. Proximal insertion can be accomplished through a single lateral incision (at the level of the greater trochanter). Contouring the nails requires more attention with one C shaped and one S shaped. The two limbs of the S, however, are not of equal length—the proximal limb should be a short sharp curve. The S-shaped rod requires rotation through 180° as it is inserted to turn the lower limb of the S in the opposite orientation of the C. Proximal fixation is most stable if the starting hole is in the lateral femoral cortex just below the flare of the greater trochanter. Fixation of distal femoral fractures is best with the proximal insertion method, whereas in most cases the simpler distal insertion method is used for middle and proximal fracture locations.

Usually inserted from the distal end of the femur, the single most important advantage of the flexible nail system is avoidance of the risk for femoral head AVN. The disadvantages include need for a second surgery to remove the nails, risk of bursitis over the prominent nails, infection, and malunion (especially in larger children with enough weight and muscle force to bend the flexible nails).

Postoperatively, although some surgeons still prefer spica casting, if the fracture is stable, a knee immobilizer and crutches can be used, allowing the patient to ambulate independently and return to school within a week. The learner will likely use a spica more often until the flexible nailing technique has been mastered.

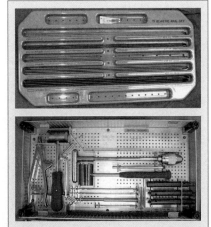

There are now many commercially available titanium elastic nail sets with easy to use insertion instrumentation.

Age 14 Years And Older

Treatment in this age group still provides treatment choices. For extreme traditionalists or those working in an environment where surgical methods are not affordable, traction methods followed by hip spica casting can still be used. Tremendous attention is required to ensure angular control as well as maintenance of equal limb lengths. Smaller children in this age group can still be treated by flexible intramedullary nail systems, which are available in larger diameters (4-4.5 mm).

As patients get larger, the risk for angulation or loss of fracture position increases with flexible nail fixation (Fig. 13-13). For these reasons, older children are commonly treated with formal intramedullary rod fixation. The early generations of intramedullary nails and those typically used in the adult population have a piriformis fossa entry site, which has been shown to put the femoral head at risk for AVN. This risk is greatest when the physes are still open with limited blood flow across the open physis.

Trochanteric Entry Site Intramedullary Rods

Newer intramedullary rods are now available that have a curvature that allows introduction through the greater trochanter. With proper technique, the vascular supply to the femoral head that encircles the base of the femoral neck is completely avoided thus significantly reducing the risk of AVN. This method offers an ideal solution for the older child; fracture stability is maximized allowing early weight bearing with no need for casting or prolonged bed rest. However, expense becomes an issue because the newest and best systems are always more expensive. There is a risk for nonunion if the fracture is fixed with a gap at the fracture site, however, this can be overcome with dynamization of the nail if necessary.

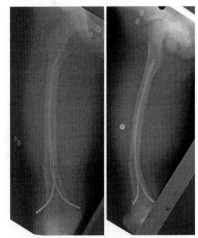

Figure 13-13. As patients get larger, the risk of angulation of loss of alignment with flexible nails increases. Such cases are better treated with a solid nail (trochanteric entry).

TECHNIQUE TIPS:
Interlocking Intramedullary Nails

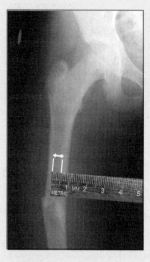

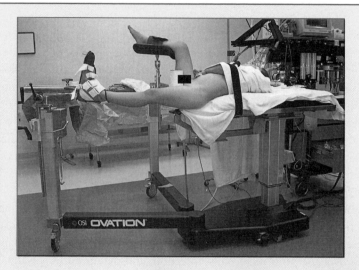

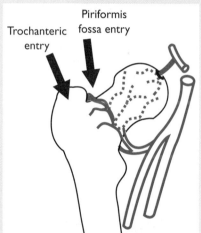

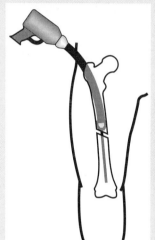

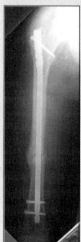

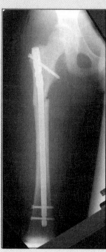

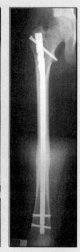

1. Preoperative planning: the narrowest portion of the canal should be measured on the x-ray to determine nail diameter—the canal should be filled with the nail. Use the contralateral leg to determine length—either a plain x-ray or fluoroscopy with a ruler will ensure equal leg lengths. Note the alignment of the uninjured leg to avoid fixing the fractured femur in malrotation.

2. A fracture table with the leg adducted simplifies fracture reduction, fluoroscopy, and nail insertion.

3. The tip of the trochanter is usually palpable even on very large children (if not, c-arm can be used as a guide), a guide pin can be inserted through the skin and into the lateral side of the tip of the trochanter prior to making any incision—this pin should never slip medially into the piriformis fossa as this puts the vascular supply to the femoral head at risk.

4. Using c-arm, the guide pin is inserted through the trochanter and down the proximal shaft, guided by AP and lateral image views.

5. Now a very small (1 cm) incision can be made around the guide pin to allow reaming and nail insertion.

6. Oblique, spiral, and comminuted fractures should have distal interlocking screws placed to maintain length and alignment.

TECHNIQUE TIPS:
Submuscular Plating

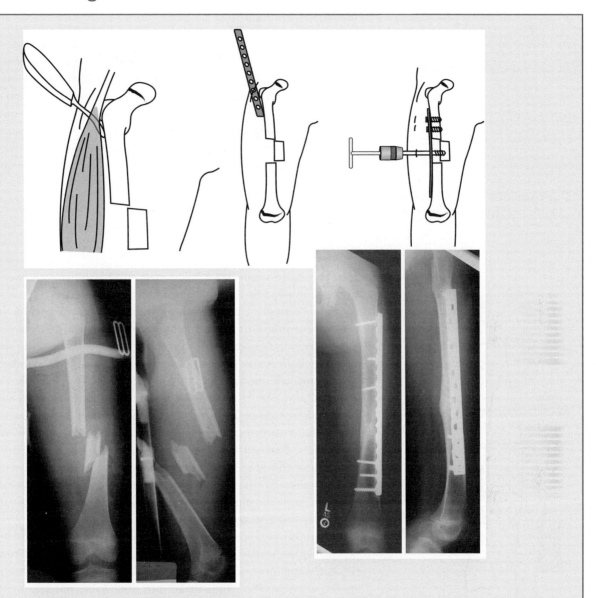

1. Through a small proximal incision, a Cobb elevator can be used to gently separate the periosteum from the overlying muscle.
2. The plate is pre-countoured using the contralateral femur as a template; it is then slid into place extraperiosteally.
3. Proximal screws are inserted percutaneously.

4. Several companies have developed instruments that can be used through a hole in the plate to pull the distal fragment to the plate.
5. Once the fracture is reduced, the remaining screws are inserted.

Published courtesy of Enis M. Kanlic, MD, PhD, Texas Tech University Health Science Center at El Paso.

"The external fixator for treatment of femoral fractures in childhood still has a place on the surgical supply shelf. In our institution it is now just behind the flexible nail set"

Dale Blasier MD—May 2003 POSNA
trauma course, Jacksonville Florida

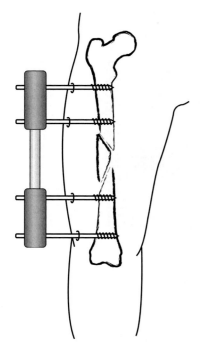

Figure 13-14. External fixation is commonly used for open fractures and unstable patients.

ALTERNATIVE TREATMENT METHODS FOR ANY AGE CHILD WITH FEMUR FRACTURE

Submuscular Plating

Minimally invasive techniques of plating the femur allow little soft tissue disruption, no stripping of the periosteum, and anatomic alignment by an indirect method. This technique has been adapted from adult fracture management and is being used in younger children with excellent results in several centers. A precontoured plate can be inserted through a small incision proximal to the fracture and slid along the lateral femoral cortex to span the fracture. Screws are then inserted percutaneously using fluoroscopic guidance. This technique does necessitate a second surgery to remove the plate, which can be more destructive than its insertion if care is not taken to preserve the soft tissues. There is an increased risk of late fracture through the screw holes following plate removal.

External Fixation

External fixation provides a quick method of stabilizing the fracture if the patient is unstable and is likely to need further procedures such as soft tissue coverage. For example, traction and casting must be avoided when there is concern about spine injury or intraabdominal or intrathoracic injury or if the patient will be making frequent trips to the CT scanner or operating room. These are excellent indications for an external fixator that will stabilize the fracture quickly and not interfere with care of the child's other injuries.

Airplane transportation is also much easier in an external fixator (as compared to a hip spica cast). Thus femur fractures in the children of tourists at ski areas (who must fly home after their holiday) are commonly treated with external fixators. External fixator immobilization can be converted to standard intramedullary fixation or spica casting at a later time. If the fracture is allowed to heal completely with the external fixation in place, there is a continued risk of infection while the pins are in place and significant risk of fracture through the holes following removal of the fixator.

As with external fixators in other locations, half pins should be inserted perpendicular to the shaft and close to the fracture (Fig. 13-14). More pins increase the initial stability but also increase the later fracture risk. The large soft tissue envelope around the femur make infection, pain, and scarring from the pins bigger issues than when used for other bones such as the tibia. For these reasons, many surgeons avoid external fixation if the femur can be stabilized with a different technique.

Open Fractures

Open fractures can be graded according to the Gustillo and Anderson classification (Table 13-2); however, this classification has not been shown to be as valuable in pediatric fractures. Open fractures result from much higher energy mechanisms that should caution the surgeon to look for other injuries. Open fractures should be taken to the operating room within 12 hours for formal débridement and irrigation, or sooner if there is neurovascular compromise. These fractures should be stabilized early with intramedullary nails, plate, or external fixator. Unless there is minimal contamination and soft tissue injury, open fractures should not be placed in a cast.

Table 13-2	Gustilo and Anderson's Open Fracture Classification
Type	**Soft Tissue Injury**
I	Clean wound <1 cm
II	Laceration >1 cm (no extensive soft tissue damage)
III	Massive soft tissue damage, high-energy trauma
IIIA	Adequate soft tissue coverage
IIIB	Contaminated wound, periosteal stripping
IIIC	Arterial injury requiring revascularization

From Gustilo, J Trauma 24:742–6, 1984.

ACCEPTABLE RESULTS

Few issues remain so unsettled as to what angulation or length difference can be accepted following treatment of a femur fracture. The biologic phenomenon of overgrowth due to postfracture growth stimulation has led to a somewhat "laissez faire" approach to maintaining adequate length during treatment in children. In young children, this is often acceptable. In older children, the chance for significant stimulation and correction of limb difference decreases and one may be left with a limb-length difference. Similarly, internal fixation can on occasion stimulate overgrowth to make the limb too long, particularly if plate fixation is used. This may be less common with the use of flexible intramedullary nails but still can occur.

Families seem more concerned about a limb that ends up being short than if it is long. The biologic phenomenon of fracture stimulation and overgrowth seems to carry less "blame," although the effect on gait, spine asymmetry, etc., is equal whether the limb is "too long" or "too short."

Traditionally, orthopedic surgeons have been taught that patients could adapt to a 1-inch limb difference without difficulty. Gross interviewed a group of runners entered in a marathon race regarding whether or not they had lower limb symptoms and then carefully measured them to determine who had a limb-length difference. He found that runners with up to a 2-cm limb length difference did not notice it or did not have symptoms. This is one of the few research papers focusing on this topic; however, the research methodology used does not meet current standards.

We are unwilling to state with certainty the amount of final residual limb, length difference that can be accepted following femoral fracture but believe that 2 cm should be considered as an upper limit. Ideally, one should try to achieve a final difference of 1 cm or less. Anyone who thinks that a 1 1/2 cm limb-length difference is of no consequence should try to wear an insole or shoe lift on one side for a single day. The alterations in stride and knee mechanics are remarkable. Practical knowledge suggests that, as orthopedics becomes more sophisticated and patients become more likely to participate in athletics and vigorous activities throughout a very long life (our life expectancy is extending rapidly), standards of acceptance for limb-length difference will likely diminish.

Monitoring Limb-Length Difference

Finally, a good knowledge of plotting and following length difference and application of contralateral epiphysiodesis to correct any unavoidable difference (prior to growth plate closure) are essential to the orthopedic armamentarium (Fig. 13-15). There are several methods of predicting leg-length discrepancy at skeletal maturity (see Technique Tips—Calculating Leg-Length Discrepancy).

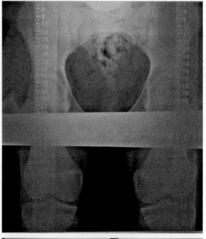
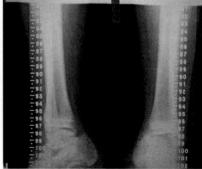

Figure 13-15. A scanogram is commonly used to determine leg-length discrepancy following femoral fractures. Serial studies may be needed to plan epiphysiodesis.

TECHNIQUE TIPS:
Calculating Leg-Length Discrepancy and
Timing Epiphysiodesis

The Green and Anderson growth chart can be used to estimate the growth remaining in a normal distal femur or proximal tibia following consecutive skeletal age levels.
See Anderson, M, Green, WT. JBJS 45A:1-14, 1963.

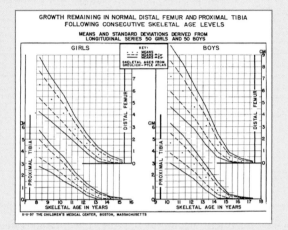

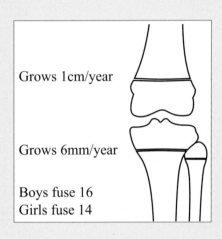

Grows 1cm/year

Grows 6mm/year

Boys fuse 16
Girls fuse 14

The arithmetic method of predicting growth remaining in a normal limb is the least accurate method but can be used for a quick gross estimation of growth remaining in a busy clinic.

Mosley used the Green-Anderson data to develop an elegant graphic method of predicting future growth in children with a leg-length discrepency. This methods requires consecutive evaluations to predict the best time for epiphysiodesis.
See Mosley, CF. JBJS 59A(2):174-9, 1977.

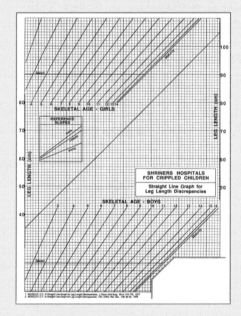

Timing of Epiphysiodesis

$M_\varepsilon = LM/(LM - \varepsilon/\kappa)$

M_ε = multiplier at the age of epiphysiodesis

ε = desired correction by epiphysiodesis

use current **L** and **M**

chose κ =
0.71 for the femur
0.57 for the tibia
0.67 for the femur + tibia

Determine
A_ε = age at epiphysiodesis that corresponds to M_ε from the multiplier table

Herzenberg and Paley's multiplier method offers a more complex calculation that can be used to appropriately time epiphysiodesis for equalization of a leg-length discrepancy on the first visit. For a more detailed description of how to use this method refer to Paley et al. JBJS 82A(10):1432-46, 2000.

Figures reproduced courtesy of the Journal of Bone and Joint Surgery.

The Green-Anderson method provided the classic approach; the Mosley straight-line graphic method utilizes the Green-Anderson data to allow an elegant graphic prediction. The Melbourne method allows a simple estimation of growth remaining in the distal femoral and proximal tibial physis relying on observational data showing that the distal femoral physis grows 10 mm/year and the proximal tibia approximately 6 mm/year until skeletal maturity (age 16 years in boys, 14 years in girls). Paley and Herzenberg have developed a multiplier method for determining predicted discrepancy with a single time point. This requires a more complex calculation but has been shown to be quite accurate for timing of epiphysiodesis to correct leg-length discrepancies.

Methods to Close the Physis

Once the timing of epiphysiodesis (technically a better term would be physiodesis) has been determined, growth plate closure can be completed in one of many ways. Phemister described removing a 1 × 1 × 1cm rectangle from both the medial and lateral sides of the physis, turning the block 90°, and reinserting it into its bed to permanently stop further growth of the physis (Fig. 13-16). A curet or drill can also be used to methodically disrupt the physis enough to prevent further growth. Some surgeons advised closed, percutaneous image-guided methods to curet the physis; however, these methods require experience and patient volume. One can easily damage the joint cartilage of the distal femur with percutaneous methods. Most of our staff prefer open methods (faster, more certain physeal ablation).

Staples can be used, but they require a second surgery for removal at the time of leg-length equality; they are good to use in younger children if the surgeon prefers only temporary growth arrest instead of the more permanent methods described previously (Fig. 13-17).

SUMMARY

Femur fractures are one of the most common injuries that the pediatric orthopedic surgeon encounters. With adequate understanding of the injury and its possible sequelae including possible leg-length discrepancy and malalignment, femoral shaft fracture treatment will allow predictable return to normal anatomy and function.

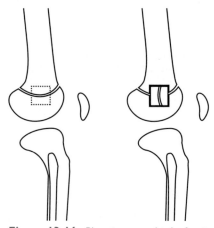

Figure 13-16. Phemister method of epiphysiodesis, rotating a 1 × 1 × 1 cm block 90°.

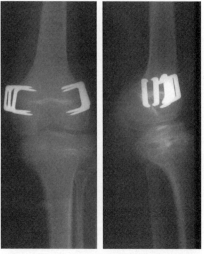

Figure 13-17. Epiphyseal stapling can be used; however, this method requires a second surgery for staple removal at the time of leg-length equality.

Suggested Readings

Beaty, J.H. Femoral shaft fractures in children and adolescents. Journal of American Academy of orthopedic surgeons 3:207–217, 1995.

Blasier, R. D.; Aronson, J.; and Tursky, E. A.: External fixation of pediatric femur fractures. J Pediatr Orthop, 17(3): 342–6, 1997.

Czertak, D. J., and Hennrikus, W. L.: The treatment of pediatric femur fractures with early 90-90 spica casting. J Pediatr Orthop, 19(2): 229–32, 1999.

Flynn, J. M.; Luedtke, L.; Ganley, T. J.; and Pill, S. G.: Titanium elastic nails for pediatric femur fractures: lessons from the learning curve. Am J Orthop, 31(2): 71–4, 2002.

Flynn JM et al. Comparison of titanium elastic nails with traction and a spica cast to treat femoral fractures in children. JBJS Am 2004 86:770–777.

Galpin, R. D.; Willis, R. B.; and Sabano, N.: Intramedullary nailing of pediatric femoral fractures. J Pediatr Orthop, 14(2): 184–9, 1994.

Gustilo, J. Trauma 24:742–6, 1984.

Hedequist, D.; Starr, A. J.; Wilson, P.; and Walker, J.: Early versus delayed stabilization of pediatric femur fractures: analysis of 387 patients. J Orthop Trauma, 13(7): 490–3, 1999.

Heinrich, S. D.; Drvaric, D. M.; Darr, K.; and MacEwen, G. D.: The operative stabilization of pediatric diaphyseal femur fractures with flexible intramedullary nails: a prospective analysis. J Pediatr Orthop, 14(4): 501–7, 1994.

Large TM, Frick SL. Compartment syndrome of the leg after treatment of a femoral fracture with an early sitting spica cast. A report of two cases. J Bone Joint Surg Am. 2003 Nov;85-A(11):2207–10.

Ligier J, Metaizeau J, Prevot J, Lascombes P. Elastic intramedullary nailing of femoral fractures in children. J Bone Joint Surg (Br) 70:74–77, 1988.

Linhart, W. E., and Roposch, A.: Elastic stable intramedullary nailing for unstable femoral fractures in children: preliminary results of a new method. J Trauma, 47(2): 372–8, 1999.

Mazda, K.; Khairouni, A.; Pennecot, G. F.; and Bensahel, H.: Closed flexible intramedullary nailing of the femoral shaft fractures in children. J Pediatr Orthop B, 6(3): 198–202, 1997.

Parsch, K: Modern trends in internal fixation of femoral shaft fractures in children. A critical review. J Pediatr Orthop B, 6:117–125, 1997

Ryan, J. R.: 90-90 skeletal femoral traction for femoral shaft fractures in children. J Trauma, 21(1): 46–8, 1981.

Schwend, R. M.; Werth, C.; and Johnston, A.: Femur shaft fractures in toddlers and young children: rarely from child abuse. J Pediatr Orthop, 20(4): 475–81, 2000.

Staheli, L. T., and Sheridan, G. W.: Early spica cast management of femoral shaft fractures in young children. A technique utilizing bilateral fixed skin traction. Clin Orthop, (126): 162–6, 1977.

Thomas, S. A.; Rosenfield, N. S.; Leventhal, J. M.; and Markowitz, R. I.: Long-bone fractures in young children: distinguishing accidental injuries from child abuse. Pediatrics, 88(3): 471–6, 1991.

Thometz, J. G., and Lamdan, R.: Osteonecrosis of the femoral head after intramedullary nailing of a fracture of the femoral shaft in an adolescent. A case report. J Bone Joint Surg Am, 77(9): 1423–6, 1995.

Weiss A et al. Peroneal nerve palsy after early cast application for femoral fractures in children. J Pediatr Orthop. 1992 Jan; 12(1):25–8.

14

Knee

Maya Pring ❧ *Dennis Wenger*

INTRODUCTION

Acute hemarthrosis of the knee secondary to injury is very common. The knee is a complex hinge joint with minimal capacity for rotation, which is held together by ligaments and cushioned by circular cartilage wedges that are all easily injured. With conditioning, good muscle tone, and good alignment, the knee can last a lifetime. Add a touch of obesity, poor conditioning, poor alignment, (anteversion, valgus), or an unlucky twist in sports and one's knee can quickly become a lifelong liability (Fig. 14-1).

Fractures about the knee in children are common and fortunately heal well if the diagnosis and treatment are correct. At adolescence, the specter of cartilage-ligament injury increases, making results less certain.

Making a clinical diagnosis of an acutely swollen knee may be difficult on the first exam when "everything hurts." Acute patellar dislocation is common and the femur and tibia each have a physis near the joint that can be injured. In the child's knee, the collateral ligaments are stronger than the growth plates; therefore, epiphyseal separation is more common than acute ligamentous tear. The cruciate ligaments attach to the tibial spines and the anterior spine is often avulsed. The physis of the tibial tubercle can be traumatically injured. Although fractures are

"Consistency is contrary to nature, contrary to life. The only completely consistent people are the dead"
—ALDOUS HUXLEY

more common, the child's knee is not immune to adult injuries, such as ligament and meniscus tears, particularly in the adolescent and teenage years.

ASSESSING THE PATIENT

Acute post-traumatic hemarthrosis in childhood is thought to be predictive of intra-articular pathology. Stanitski reported a series of 70 children who presented with acute knee trauma and hemarthrosis; all had arthroscopy. The majority were found to have intra-articular lesions (meniscus tear, ACL tear, and/or osteochondral fracture). For a time, this created a frenzy of arthroscopic evaluation for every child and adolescent with a swollen knee. There has been much debate in the literature, both for and against early arthroscopy for diagnosis; a recent article by Wessel et al. states "in children, compulsory arthroscopy for hemarthrosis after knee trauma is not justified because ligamentous and meniscal damage is rare."

In today's cost conscious medical environment, it may be difficult to decide which patients should have an extensive workup (including MRI and/or arthroscopy) and which patients may do just as well with a more conservative sequence. We lean toward a more conservative approach, saving the big workup for those who do not improve in a timely fashion. Of course, one can never get it just right. Demanding parents, whose child is "on a national travel team," or the soccer player who competes at the junior olympic level may not tolerate a thoughtful, conservative, "lets see how things go" approach. For highly competitive athletes, the Stanitski approach (early MRI or scope for all) is likely correct. On the other hand, high-level insurance and unlimited resources are clearly not available for all. The befuddled surgeon then becomes a pawn of the system, ordering or performing expensive tests on a select few while providing much less for others. We can provide no certain answer to this dilemma; however, it is comforting to know that most children do well with immobilization. They rarely get stiff, and waiting for a few weeks is unlikely to do damage to the joint.

For a child with a large hemarthrosis, aspiration will help symptomatically and may help you determine if there is a fracture: fat in the aspirate suggests bony injury.

There are several clinical tests that will guide you through a differential diagnosis (see Technique Tips); however, these are hard to use if the patient is acutely injured and will not let you touch the knee—a thorough exam becomes more pertinent once the patient and the hemarthrosis have settled down. The opposite may be true if an athlete can be examined immediately (even on the field). Many would agree that this can be the best time to assess for acute ligament injury (the nerve endings may be stunned temporarily by the acute event).

First palpate each area of the knee separately to find areas of point tenderness (femoral physis, tibial physis, tibial tubercle, dorsal aspect of patella medially and laterally, lateral femoral condyle). Then palpate the joint lines; if possible, perform a McMurray (twist) test, and test the cruciate ligaments with the tests described later.

ASPIRATION OF ACUTE HEMARTHROSIS—DOES IT HELP?

A tense, acute knee hemarthrosis in a child (knee full of blood) is easy to aspirate, yet not commonly done. Opinions as to whether it should be done range widely within the orthopedic community. Several guidelines can be provided. If the effusion is tense and the patient in great pain, aspiration may help. A rather firm wrap, plus icing, must follow or it will rapidly reaccumulate.

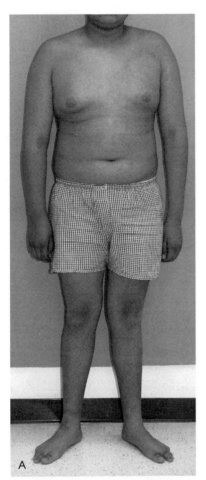

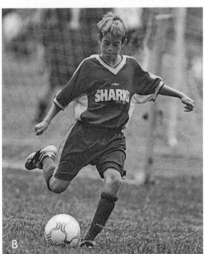

Figure 14-1. There are many factors that can lead to knee injuries. A) Note obesity and genu valgum deformity. B) Athletic children can have an unlucky twist. (Photo courtesy of L. Manhiem.)

On the other hand, if the effusion is less tense, the patient has tolerable pain, and he/she hates needles, aspiration can be avoided. In theory, if one sees fat droplets on the aspirated blood, intra-articular fracture is likely. We advise a case-by-case, individualized approach to the question of aspiration.

RADIOGRAPHIC ISSUES

Standard knee evaluation includes an AP and lateral view of the knee and a Merchant x-ray of both knees (Fig. 14-2). Patellar position is nearly impossible to assess without a comparison to the uninjured side. If the patient has acute hemarthrosis, it may be very difficult to flex the knee enough for a patellar view. Oblique x-rays may help, especially if a physeal fracture is suspected.

If plain x-rays are normal, you are stuck with the question "Do I move the knee or immobilize it?" Some advocate stress x-rays to check for physeal opening; however, this is painful and not very reproducible—we therefore rarely perform stress views. An MRI can answer many questions (physis, ligament, menisci) but is usually not necessary at the time of injury. There are few knee injuries not visible on plain films that will worsen with a short period (1-2 weeks) of immobilization. This gives the soft tissues a chance to heal, the hemarthrosis a chance to resorb, and the bone a chance to begin healing (if there is a nondisplaced fracture) and, more importantly, allows better clinical exam that will direct further studies. If there is concern for ACL, PCL, or meniscal injury, an MRI is the standard for diagnosis.

KNEE DISLOCATION

This is a very rare injury in children because the physis will usually separate before a dislocation occurs, but when it does occur, knee dislocations have a very

Common Abbreviations —Knee
ACL   anterior cruciate ligament
PCL   posterior cruciate ligament
MCL   medial collateral ligament
LCL   lateral collateral ligament

"A tense, acute knee hemarthrosis in a child (knee full of blood) is easy to aspirate, yet not commonly done"

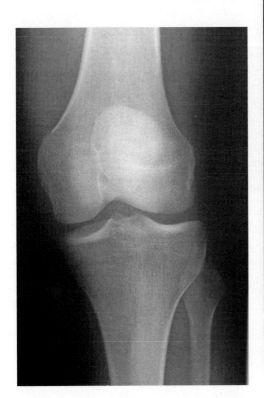
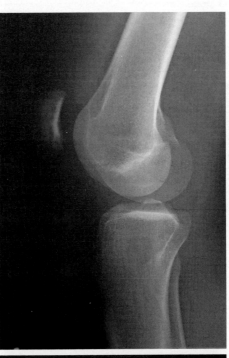

Figure 14-2. The AP, lateral, and Merchant views are a common first step to clarify knee trauma. The Merchant (patellar) view allows one to assess patellar instability, lateralization, and dislocation.

TECHNIQUE TIPS:
Tests Used for Assessing the Injured Knee

Lachman Test

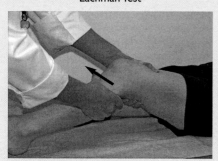

Knee flexed to 30°. Anterior translation of the tibia indicates ACL tear.

Anterior Drawer Test

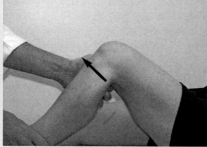

Knee flexed to 90°. Anterior translation of the tibia indicates ACL tear.

Quadriceps Active Test

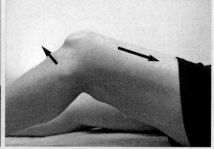

Knee flexed to 45°. Contraction of quads will translate tibia anteriorly if ACL is torn.

Pivot Shift

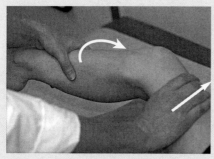

Flex knee while applying valgus stress and internal rotation. If ACL and postero-lateral corner disrupted, tibia will sublux.

Posterior Drawer Test

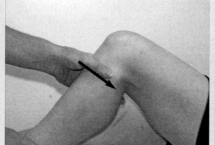

Knee flexed to 90°. Posterior translation of the tibia indicates PCL tear.

McMurray Test

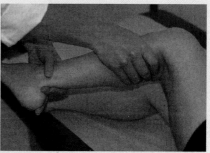

With valgus stress on the knee and external rotation of the tibia, flex and extend the knee. A torn medial meniscus will "pop."

Fairbank Sign

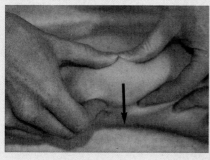

Lateral translation of the patella. Patient aprehension indicates patellar instability.

Varus Stress

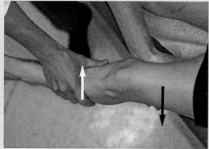

Knee flexed to 10°. Opening of lateral joint space indicates LCL tear.

Valgus Stress

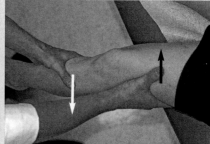

Knee flexed to 10°. Opening of medial joint space indicates MCL tear.

poor prognosis. Initially, as in adult injuries, the major concern is neurovascular injury. An arteriogram should be considered and the patient should be monitored extremely carefully for compartment syndrome. To truly dislocate the femoral-tibial joint, multiple ligaments must be torn. Reconstruction of the ligaments will be required by someone experienced with this type of surgery.

PATELLAR DISLOCATION

This is a very common injury and is what lay people mean when they say, "my knee dislocated." The injury is very common in adolescents and teenagers but less common in early childhood. We see many cases in teenage girls who are somewhat loose-jointed, who have upper range genu valgum (often with increased femoral anteversion), and who are trying sports (but are really not conditioned for it).

Most patellar dislocations are reduced before the patient comes to the hospital, either spontaneously by himself or herself or by a buddy. Diagnosis is not always easy. The signs are hemarthrosis, tenderness along the medial border of the patella, lateral position of the patella, and a positive Fairbanks sign (patient becomes apprehensive when you try to push the patella laterally).

On x-ray, always look for a loose fragment, which can be knocked off the lateral femoral condyle or pulled off the medial edge of the patella (significant for avulsion of the medial patellofemoral ligament—Fig. 14-3). Between 5% and 10% of acute dislocations are complicated by an osteochondral fracture.

Treatment—First Dislocation

There is much argument about the treatment of a first dislocation. Traditionally, they have been immobilized in extension for 3-4 weeks with physical therapy started early. Recent trends include acute surgical intervention, particularly if an acute patellofemoral ligament tear is evident on x-ray or MRI.

If there is no fracture, we typically try conservative management ideally in a cylinder cast (because children tend not to use a knee immobilizer effectively), followed by physical therapy for range of motion and to strengthen the vastus medialis.

For patients with a fracture of the medial patella or lateral femoral condyle, we advise acute arthrotomy plus ligament repair with excision or fixation of the fracture and repair of the medial capsule and patellofemoral ligament (plus possible lateral release).

Reccurent Dislocations

Fifteen percent to 20% of all children will experience recurrent dislocations of the patella (and many more will have patellar alignment problems after their initial injury). This is typically the result of faulty anatomy, including an increased quadriceps angle, increased genu valgum, increased femoral anteversion, femoral condyle hypoplasia, a shallow femoral sulcus, atrophy of the vastus medialis, lateral patellar tilt, and/or general joint laxity. An Install type soft tissue realignment or semitendinosus tendon tenodesis to the patella is often recommended for skeletally immature patients with recurrent patella dislocation. Tibial tubercle transfer procedures (Hauser, Fulkerson) cannot be performed prior to physeal closure because they will produce genu recurvatum owing to growth arrest in the anterior/distal extension of the proximal tibial physis.

"Between 5% and 10% of acute dislocations are complicated by an osteochondral fracture"

At Injury

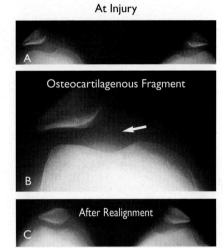

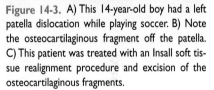

Figure 14-3. A) This 14-year-old boy had a left patella dislocation while playing soccer. B) Note the osteocartilaginous fragment off the patella. C) This patient was treated with an Insall soft tissue realignment procedure and excision of the osteocartilaginous fragments.

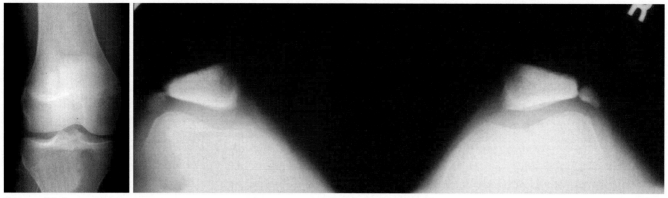

Figure 14-4. This child has bilateral bipartite patellae, which can be a normal finding, but in this case the right was symptomatic and required excision.

PATELLA FRACTURES

The patella is an interesting sesamoid bone designed to improve the lever arm of the quadriceps mechanism. The patella is initially cartilaginous, becoming ossified at age 3-5 years. Some children develop a synchondrosis between embryonic growth centers that have not fused, leading to confusing x-ray findings. A bipartite patella may be mistaken for a fracture of the patella (Fig. 14-4). The typical secondary, bipartite center is located superolaterally. If there is confusion, x-rays of the opposite knee may shed light on the situation, although some cases are unilateral. To add more confusion, it should be noted that, although a bipartite patella is usually a normal variant (and not the cause of pain), in rare cases a fracture may propagate through the synchondrosis causing motion at this junction (and symptoms). In rare cases, the secondary center requires surgical treatment (excision, lateral release, or fusion to main body of patella).

The lower pole of the patella can be avulsed during the course of running, jumping, and kicking. These are often injuries of the take-off leg. Acute injuries result in displaced fracture (sleeve fractures in children), chronic repetitive injuries producing the Sinding-Larsen-Johansson lesion of the patella (a form of repetitive stress injury like Osgood-Schlatter lesion of the tibial tubercle—Table 14-2).

The characteristic lower pole avulsion fracture in childhood was coined as a "sleeve" fracture by Houghton and Ackroyd because a circumferential cartilaginous "sleeve" is plucked off the lower pole with little or no bone (Fig. 14-5). Diagnosis can be difficult, as sometimes there is little or no bone noted in the sep-

"The patella is an interesting sesamoid bone designed to improve the lever arm of the quadriceps mechanism"

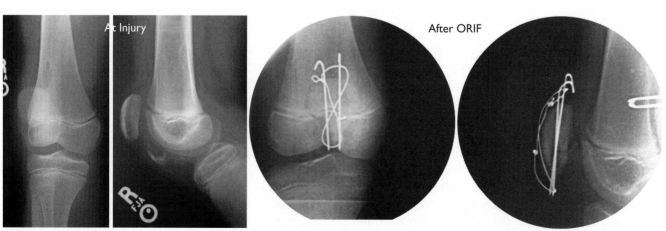

Figure 14-5. A, B) This is classic patellar sleeve fracture with avulsion of the distal pole. C, D) Following open reduction and internal fixation with AO tension band technique.

arated fragment. Contralateral films allow you to compare the position of the patella [the patella will be more proximal (patella alta) on the injured site].

Recognition is important, because some of the articular surface of the patella is displaced with the fragment. Without treatment, an extensor lag will remain with a possible pseudarthrosis. Open reduction, repair of the retinaculum, rigid internal fixation of the fragment, and cast immobilization for 4 weeks are required. If there is little bone present, it is a bit like sewing two rope ends together. If you are not confident of the repair (or you imagine effect of the postanesthetic shakes), insert a temporary wire loop between the patella and the tibial tubercle for protection.

Transverse fractures through the substance of the patella are uncommon, except in older teenagers. When widely separated, they are best treated by the AO technique (parallel Kirschner wires and a tension band) (Fig. 14-6); however, many are not sufficiently displaced to require surgery and can be treated by aspiration of a tense effusion (optional) and a cast. Occasionally, marked patellar overgrowth can occur following patellar injury in infancy.

DISTAL FEMUR FRACTURES

As previously discussed, the physis is a point of weakness in the growing child. The distal femoral physis may be disrupted in several ways as described by Salter and Harris (see Chapter 2). Salter-Harris Type I fractures are often not visible on x-ray but can be suspected by a careful exam (tenderness directly over the physis). True Type I injuries are rarely displaced and are well treated in a long leg cast for 4 weeks. In many cases, with localized physeal pain (and normal x-rays), you are not certain of the diagnosis. One could order an MRI, which is an expensive and impractical route. We advise a long leg cast for 2 weeks and then cast removal with repeat x-rays. If callus is noted at that time, the child is casted for two more weeks.

Salter-Harris II injuries of the distal femur (Fig. 14-7) are common and are concerning because of their tendency to produce physeal closure. Riseborough reported that 11 out of 25 patients with distal femoral Salter-Harris II injuries experienced subsequent physeal closure and leg-length discrepancy >2.4 cm. X-rays often demonstrate a large Thurston-Holland fragment; the fracture often

At Injury   After ORIF

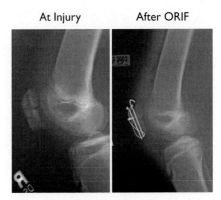

Figure 14-6. Comminuted patellar fractures are a result of a direct blow to the knee. They can be fixed with the AO tension band technique.

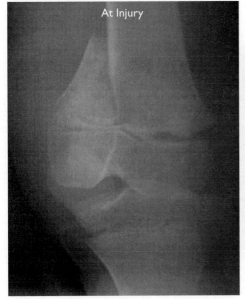

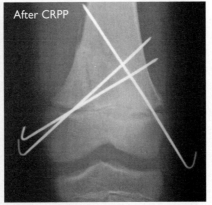

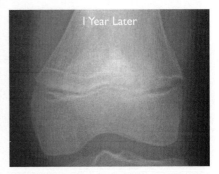

Figure 14-7. Salter-Harris II injuries require anatomic reduction and have a very high risk of physeal arrest. This patient had closed reduction and percutaneous pinning of his fracture. One year following injury, his physis still appeared to be growing appropriately.

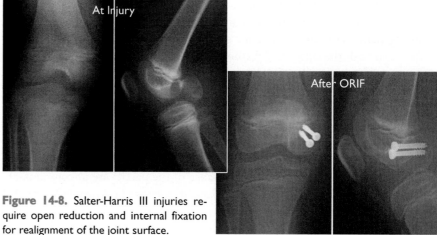

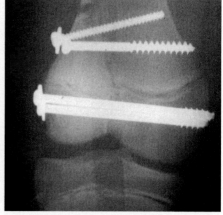

Figure 14-8. Salter-Harris III injuries require open reduction and internal fixation for realignment of the joint surface.

reduces easily with varus or valgus force depending on the injury. Following anatomic reduction, these fractures can be placed in a hip spica or long leg cast. If the reduction is unstable, percutaneous pinning should be performed. A few require open reduction secondary to entrapped soft tissues.

The issue of cast type following closed reduction merits discussion. A long leg cast alone will not ensure maintenance of reduction in a rowdy teenage boy. Bending the knee to 90° and adding a pelvic band provides more certain stability. If K-wires are used, a long leg cast should be enough. Finally, the family must know about the high risk for physeal closure and the patient, followed accordingly.

In Salter-Harris III injuries, the posterior part of a femoral condyle may be displaced (Fig. 14-8). Like most Type III injuries (e.g., Tillaux), these fractures tend to occur as the physis is closing, so the risk of deformity or leg-length discrepancy following this injury is less likely. The fragment must be replaced without devascularizing it. Type III injuries are unusual and should be anatomically reduced with a transepiphyseal screw. The fracture can be reduced and fixed with a compression screw through a posterolateral or posteromedial approach.

Type IV injuries also have a high risk for going on to partial growth arrest (Fig. 14-9). Like any Type IV injury, anatomic reduction is required both to allow subsequent physeal growth and to prevent arthritis (by anatomic joint surface reconstruction).

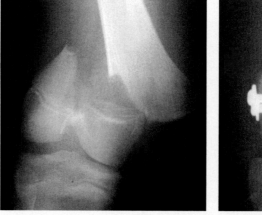

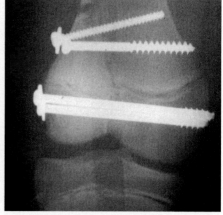

Figure 14-9. This 13-year-old boy was hit by a car and sustained a Salter-Harris IV injury and underwent open reduction and internal fixation.

There are also a variety of osteochondral fragments that can become intra-articular. The most common is a piece sheared off the lateral femoral condyle following patella dislocation.

Osteochondritis (OCD) lesions may be the result of trauma but are more often idiopathic. OCD lesions are most commonly seen in the medial femoral condyle and best visualized on the notch view x-ray or MRI (Fig. 14-10). These should be treated to avoid the osteocartilaginous piece beccoming a loose body, which can damage the joint. We recommend extra-articular drilling if the articular cartilage is still intact. If the articular cartilage is disrupted, the fragment should be fixed or excised.

PROXIMAL TIBIA FRACTURES

Tibial Spine

Injuries that rupture the ACL of an adult typically avulse the anterior tibial spine in a growing child (Table 14-1). The spine repairs by bone when reduced and yields much better results than a complete tear of the cruciate ligament. The majority of fractures are produced in road accidents, particularly falls from bicycles. A child presenting with an acute swollen knee after falling from a bicycle should be presumed to have a fracture of the tibial spine until proven otherwise.

Some children are unaware that anything is seriously wrong until the following day, when the painful hemarthrosis persists. The radiologic findings can be subtle, and the damage is always greater than the x-ray shows. Wide radiolucent wings of articular cartilage from the weight-bearing surface of the tibia are attached to the small ossific fragment. Much more than the spine is lifted up and the fragment is usually partially detached. The anterior part lifts; the posterior part hinges. The femoral condyles can be used to ram the wings of articular cartilage back into position when the knee is extended in an attempt at closed reduction. When the fragment is completely detached, meniscus are interposed, or the fragment is rotated, and open reduction is required.

Type I injuries are treated simply with casting with the knee in slight flexion (10°) for 6-8 weeks. Type II injuries need to be reduced. This can sometimes be accomplished in a closed fashion by extending the knee, but if the meniscus blocks reduction, open reduction and fixation should follow (Fig. 14-11).

Type III injuries almost uniformly require surgery. Be prepared for stiffness following fixation of these injuries. We have had several patients that required

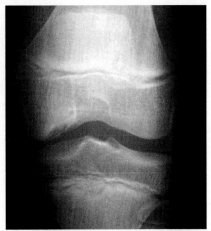

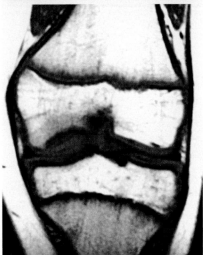

Figure 14-10. OCD lesions are most commonly seen in the medial femoral condyle. If left untreated, this may result in a loose body and cause further damage to the articular surface.

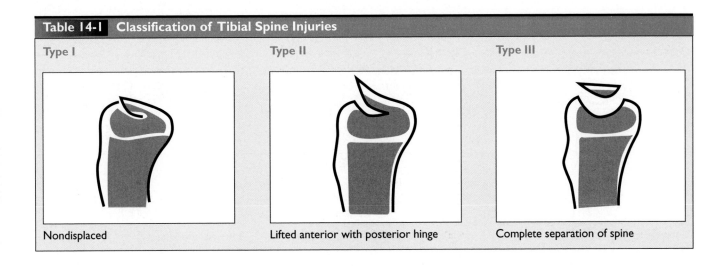

Table 14-1	Classification of Tibial Spine Injuries	
Type I	**Type II**	**Type III**
Nondisplaced	Lifted anterior with posterior hinge	Complete separation of spine

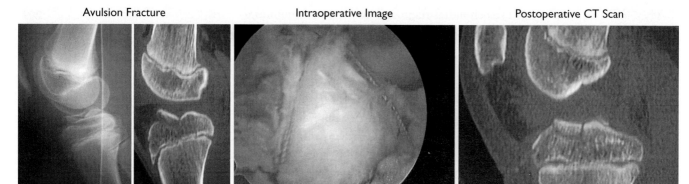

Avulsion Fracture | Intraoperative Image | Postoperative CT Scan

Figure 14-11. Tibial spine avulsion fractures can be fixed arthroscopically with suture fixation.

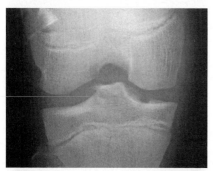

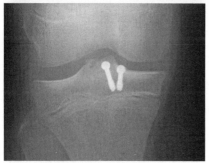

Figure 14-12. Tibial spine fractures can be fixed with epiphyseal screws. This provides more secure fixation and does not injure the physis.

manipulation and lysis of adhesions following both arthroscopic and open fixation of tibial spine fractures. There is always a debate as to when to start moving the patient postoperatively. Every extra day in a cast increases the risk of stiffness, but suture fixation is often not strong enough to hold the fracture until it is healed. Although ACL laxity is a concern, stiffness seems to be a bigger problem. As in multiple children's orthopedic conditions, you will have to pick your poison (too short of immobilization = pseudarthrosis, too long = joint stiffness).

Reduction and fixation of the spine can be accomplished arthroscopically or by an open approach. The knee is opened through a medial parapatellar incision. Two holes are drilled through the epiphysis, and the fragment is tied down. Some have advocated screw fixation of the spine to allow better fixation and earlier motion. The screws must be kept in the epiphysis to prevent injury to the physis (Fig. 14-12).

Tibial Tubercle Fractures

Because the patellar ligament inserts onto the tibial tubercle apophysis, repetitive forceful contraction of the quadriceps (runners, jumpers) can pull this apophysis apart. This can happen slowly or acutely. Chronic stress to the apophysis leads to Osgood-Schlatter disease or inflammation of the tibial tubercle; this condition often precedes acute fracture of the tubercle (Fig. 14-13).

Most proximal tibia fractures can be classified according to the Salter-Harris classification system; however, several attempts have been made to better classify tibial tubercle fractures. Both Watson Jones and later Ogden described three types of acute fracture (Table 14-2).

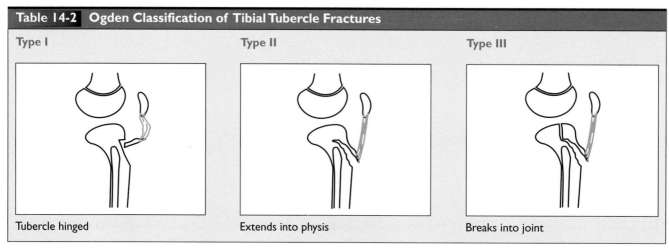

Table 14-2	**Ogden Classification of Tibial Tubercle Fractures**	
Type I	**Type II**	**Type III**
Tubercle hinged	Extends into physis	Breaks into joint

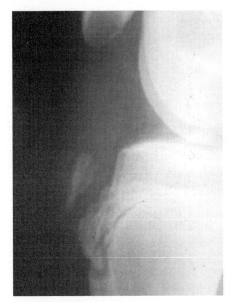

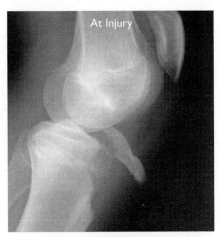

At Injury

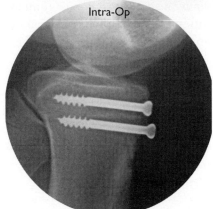

Intra-Op

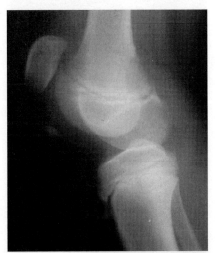

Figure 14-13. Chronic pull of the tibial tubercle apophysis leads to a stress reaction (Osgood-Schlatter disease) and in some instances, leads to fracture.

Figure 14-14. Type III tibial tuberosity fractures are best treated with ORIF to restore the joint surface.

Treatment of tibial tubercle fractures depends on the skeletal maturity of the patient and whether or not the joint is involved (Fig. 14-14). If the child is skeletally immature, it is important not to place screws across the physis to avoid anterior physeal fusion and subsequent recurvatum deformity. In this case, a tension band from the patella to the anterior tibia will allow healing without disrupting growth (Fig. 14-15). Frequently, these injuries occur as the physis is starting to close; in this case, screw fixation is acceptable. If the joint is disrupted, anatomic reduction of the joint surface is mandatory to prevent later arthritis.

MENISCUS TEARS AND LIGAMENT INJURIES

Although seen less commonly in children than in adults, meniscus injuries are relatively common in adolescents. Also, congenital discoid menisci tear easily and are commonly seen in large children's centers. Diagnosis of meniscal injury is more difficult in children because they rarely complain of locking and weakness and may not have a positive McMurray test on clinical exam. Most commonly, a meniscus tear presents with decreased range of motion, tenderness at the joint line, and quadriceps atrophy.

Harvell et al. reported that the accuracy of clinical diagnosis improves with age—it is difficult to get a good exam on a young child with a knee injury. MRI or arthroscopy will provide the definitive diagnosis of a meniscal tear. In times gone by, menisectomy was performed for children with a torn meniscus—this is

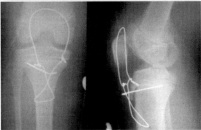

Figure 14-15. In children with open physes, a temporary tension band between the patella and the tibia can be used to fix a tibial tubercle fracture.

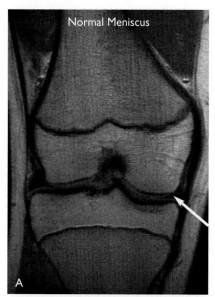

Normal Meniscus

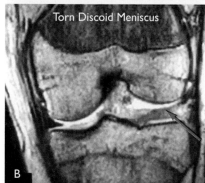

Torn Discoid Meniscus

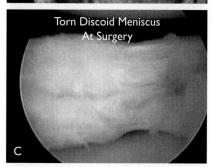

Torn Discoid Meniscus
At Surgery

Figure 14-16. A) MRI of normal meniscus. B) Note the torn lateral discoid meniscus. C) Torn discoid meniscus at time of arthroscopy.

now contraindicated if it is possible to repair or salvage the meniscus. The long-term outcome of patients with menisectomy is dismal, leading to early arthrosis and need for knee replacement. There are now many arthroscopic techniques for repairing torn menisci that properly trained orthopedic surgeons can perform.

The discoid meniscus results from a congenital anomaly that predisposes the cartilage to early tearing and degeneration (Fig. 14-16). The lateral meniscus is most commonly affected, but discoid medial menisci have been reported. A prominent clicking or snapping with knee motion is almost diagnostic of an unstable discoid lateral meniscus in young children. Older children and adolescents are more likely to present with symptoms of a torn meniscus—effusion, joint line tenderness, and quad atrophy. Asymptomatic discoid menisci do not require treatment; however, when these abnormal menisci become torn and symptomatic, they are most commonly treated with arthroscopic saucerization with preservation of enough meniscus to maintain some biomechanical function.

Ligaments

Ligamentous injuries may be the silent partners of femoral and tibial fractures. Always look for a knee effusion if there is a nearby long bone fracture, because the unstable knee may be more memorable than the fracture.

Collateral Ligaments

During the ski season, many children younger than the age of 10 arrive with pain, swelling, and tenderness about the knee. Always consider a physeal injury before a ligamentous injury in the growing child, but don't discard the possibility of torn collateral ligaments. Physeal injuries present with swelling and tenderness circumferentially at the level of the physis and usually no tenderness at the joint line. Collateral ligament injuries present with very localized tenderness along the medial or lateral collateral ligament, which crosses the joint. Stress x-rays or an MRI can differentiate these injuries; however, the treatment is similar, so these tests are usually not necessary.

In equivocal cases, it is best to immobilize the knee in a long leg or cylinder cast for 2-3 weeks. This will give adequate time for most soft tissue injuries to heal and prevent displacement if there is a physeal fracture. Follow-up x-rays will then show callus if a fracture was indeed present. If there is no evidence of fracture at 3 week follow-up, the knee stability is tested. Grade I and II ligamentous injuries will have healed completely and the patient will be asymptomatic. Grade III injuries may still be tender and have varus or valgus instability. These patients should be placed in a hinged knee brace to protect the ligament while it continues to heal for an additional 3-6 weeks. It is very rare that isolated collateral ligament injuries do not heal completely in the child with conservative management. Collateral ligament injuries in combination with ACL and/or meniscus tears may require a more aggressive approach, which is discussed thoroughly in sports medicine texts.

Anterior Cruciate Ligament (ACL)

In the past, it was said that children's ligaments are stronger than the bone, so they do not get ligament injuries. This has been proven untrue by today's aggressive athletic children. Bony avulsions of the ligaments are still more common (tibial spine, distal femoral and proximal tibial physeal injuries); however, we now see more than 50 intra-substance ACL tears a year in our institution. These ligament tears occur during deceleration—often when landing from a jump. A loud pop is often heard followed by immediate hemarthrosis. The patient presents with an acutely swollen knee and instability on exam—the Lachman test is the most sensitive finding in a patient with an acute ACL tear. There is often an associated meniscus tear or osteochondral injury, which is indicated by joint line tenderness. An MRI will clarify the diagnosis (Fig. 14-17).

Initial management of an ACL injury includes immobilization, ice, and crutch use. Once the acute swelling has subsided, range of motion exercises can be begun in a brace that prevents anterior translation of the tibia. Whether one opts for reconstruction or conservative management, therapy is important to regain knee motion. The surgical options are limited in patients with open physes, and many surgeons prefer to wait until close to skeletal maturity to perform the standard bone-tendon-bone reconstruction that is utilized in adults. The bone plugs for this type of reconstruction cross and risk closing the distal femoral and proximal tibial physes, so it is not recommended when the physes are open.

Children that are active in sports are often unwilling to wait and wear a brace with the increased risk of meniscus tear. We see children as young as 10 with ACL tears and it is next to impossible to convince them to wait until their teen years for surgery and a stable knee. Therefore, many techniques have been developed to protect the physes and reconstruct the ACL in skeletally immature patients. We refer you to textbooks directed to sports medicine for children for in depth discussions of these techniques.

Posterior Cruciate Ligament (PCL)

PCL injuries are very rare in children. They usually occur from a direct blow to the anterior tibia when the knee is flexed. In isolated PCL tears, there is often no hemarthrosis as the PCL is extra-synovial. A posterior sag is noted on clinical exam, and a quadriceps active test will show anterior translation of the tibia when the quadriceps are contracted (knee held in 70° of flexion). As in ACL injuries, bony avulsion is more common and, if significantly displaced, can be reduced and fixed (Fig. 14-18). If there is a true intra-substance tear noted on MRI or diagnostic arthroscopy, conservative management with therapy and bracing is usually adequate.

> ### DEFINITIONS
> Strain—a stretching injury of a muscle or its tendinous attachment to bone
> Sprain—an injury limited to a ligament
>   Grade I—a tear of a minimum number of fibers of the ligament with localized tenderness but no instability
>   Grade II—a disruption of more fibers with more generalized tenderness and mild laxity
>   Grade III—a complete disruption of the ligament with resultant instability

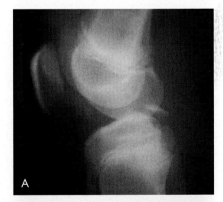

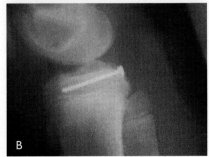

Figure 14-18. A) In children, the PCL is more commonly avulsed with a bony fragment than a true intra-substance tear. B) This can be fixed with open reduction and screw fixation.

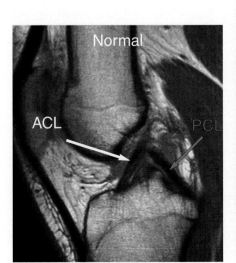

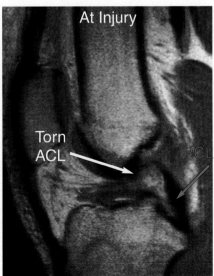

Figure 14-17. A) MRI of normal cruciate ligaments. B) Torn ACL with anterior subluxation of the tibia.

Berg EE. Pediatric tibial eminence fractures: arthroscopic cannulated screw fixation. Arthroscopy. 1995 Jun;11(3):328-31.

Flynn JM, Skaggs DL, Sponseller PD, Ganley TJ, Kay RM, Leitch KK. The surgical management of pediatric fractures of the lower extremity.Instr Course Lect. 2003; 52:647-59.

Harvell JC Jr, Fu FH, Stanitski CL. Diagnostic arthroscopy of the knee in children and adolescents.Orthopedics. 1989 Dec; 12(12):1555-60.

Houghton GR, Ackroyd CE: Sleeve fractures of the patella in children. J Bone Joint Surg 61B:165, 1979

Kocher MS, DiCanzio J, Zurakowski D, Micheli LJ. Diagnostic performance of clinical examination and selective magnetic resonance imaging in the evaluation of intra-articular knee disorders in children and adolescents. Am J Sports Med. 2001 May-Jun;29(3):292-6.

Kocher MS, Saxon HS, Hovis WD, Hawkins RJ. Management and complications of anterior cruciate ligament injuries in skeletally immature patients: survey of the Herodicus Society and The ACL Study Group. J Pediatr Orthop. 2002 Jul-Aug;22(4):452-7.

Matelic TM, Aronsson DD, Boyd DW Jr, LaMont RL. Acute hemarthrosis of the knee in children. Am J Sports Med. 1995 Nov-Dec;23(6):668-71.

Miller, MD, Howard, RF, KD Plancher. Surgical Atlas of Sports Medicine. W.B. Saunders Company; March 7, 2003.

Molander ML, Wallin G, Wikstad I: Fracture of the intercondylar eminence of the tibia. J Bone Joint Surg 63B89, 1981.

Myers MH, McKeever FM: Fracture of the intercondylar eminence of the tibia. J Bone Joint Surg 41A: 209, 1959.

Ogden JA, Tross RB, Murphy MJ: Fractures of the tibial tuberosity in adolescents. J Bone Joint Surg 62A:205, 1980.

Riseborough EJ, Barrett IR, Shapiro F. Growth disturbances following distal femoral physeal fracture-separations. J Bone Joint Surg Am. 1983 Sep;65(7): 885-93

Schenck, RC. Athletic Training and Sports Medicine, 3rd ed. AAOS, 2000.

Stanitski CL, Harvell JC, Fu F. Observations on acute knee hemarthrosis in children and adolescents. J Pediatr Orthop. 1993 Jul-Aug;13(4):506-10.

Thompson JD, Stricker SJ, Williams MM. Fractures of the distal femoral epiphyseal plate. J Pediatr Orthop. 1995 July-Aug;15(4):474-8.

Vocke AK, Vocke AR. Cartilaginous avulsion fracture of the tibial spine.Orthopedics. 2002 Nov;25(11):1293-4.

Wessel LM, Scholz S, Rusch M, Kopke J, Loff S, Duchene W, Waag KL. Hemarthrosis after trauma to the pediatric knee joint: what is the value of magnetic resonance imaging in the diagnostic algorithm? J Pediatr Orthop. 2001 May-Jun;21(3):338-42.

Wiley JJ, Baxter MP. Tibial spine fractures in children. Clin Orthop. 1990 Jun;(255): 54-60.

Willis R, Blokker C, Stoll T. Long term follow-up of anterior tibial eminence fractures. J Pediatr Orthop. 13:361-364, 1993.

15

Tibia

François Lalonde ❧ *Dennis Wenger*

INTRODUCTION

Tibial fractures heal so much more readily in children than in adults that they should be a joy to treat. The majority of children have a cast applied and only require a pair of crutches, a cast shoe, and a note for school outlining their limitations.

Most tibial fractures in children are stable and the child can soon be weight bearing in an above knee (long leg) cast. However, there is more variation to these fractures than is generally realized. If foresight is to be used to prevent problems in treatment, the characteristics of the fracture should be well understood. In this chapter, we will present tibial fractures and discuss common variations according to their anatomic location.

PROXIMAL GROWTH PLATE INJURIES

Growth plate injuries are more common in the distal femur than in the proximal tibia, because of the surrounding anatomy. The medial collateral ligament of the knee is attached to the tibial metaphysis and the femoral epiphysis, protecting the tibial physis from valgus injuries. Laterally, the upper end of the fibula acts as a buttress. In the posteromedial corner, the semimembranosus muscle inserts distal to the physis, and anteriorly, the tubercle projects from the epiphysis over the metaphysis.

"We see what we know"

—GOETHE

"Growth plate injuries are more common in the distal femur than in the proximal tibia, because of the surrounding anatomy"

Fortunately, proximal tibial physeal fractures are rare because injury at this level is often associated with vascular problems owing to the proximity of the popliteal trifurcation into the posterior tibial, anterior tibial, and peroneal arteries. Complete avulsions of the tibial tubercle are considered a specific subgroup of this fracture and are discussed separately in the knee chapter.

The mechanism of injury in proximal tibial physeal injuries is either direct or indirect. A direct injury can result from a child's leg being run over by a vehicle or when it is caught between bumpers of two automobiles. Most injuries are the result of an indirect force such as forced abduction and hyperextension of the lower leg against a fixed knee. Most proximal tibial physeal injuries are Salter-Harris I and II fractures. The frequency of Salter-Harris III fractures varies according to whether displaced avulsion fractures of the tibial tubercle are included.

Up to 50% of type I separations of the proximal tibia are nondisplaced with a tense hemarthrosis usually noted on physical examination. In this situation, stress radiographs can be performed and may reveal widening on the medial or posterior aspect (rarely actually done—very painful for child). For Salter-Harris III and IV fractures, a CT scan is usually recommended to clarify the complexity and thus guide.

Nondisplaced fractures can be treated in a long leg cast with the knee flexed approximately 15° so that the child can walk comfortably. The cast is univalved to allow for swelling, and depending on the clinical exam, consideration should be given to admit the patient overnight to monitor for swelling and/or a compartment syndrome. At 1 week, plain x-rays are repeated to ensure there has been no displacement of the fracture in the cast. The cast is removed 4 to 8 weeks after injury depending on the age of the patient.

Displaced Fractures

"Displaced Salter-Harris II fractures, like proximal metaphyseal fractures, have a high risk for associated vascular injury"

Displaced Salter-Harris II fractures, like proximal metaphyseal fractures, have a high risk for associated vascular injury. Thus when a displaced fracture occurs, assume a vascular injury and potential for a compartment syndrome. The precautions noted in the next segment on proximal metaphyseal fractures must be taken to avoid morbidity.

Displaced Salter-Harris I and II fractures require closed manipulation preferably under general anesthesia. Unless the fracture is very stable, percutaneous crossed Kirschner wires are generally used to secure the reduction. The pins are removed in clinic 3 to 4 weeks after surgery through a window in the cast. Pins left in more than 4 weeks after surgery may increase the risk for infection.

Stress X-ray in Children's Fractures

In the past, stress radiographs were emphasized in the acute setting as part of the routine workup of certain musculoskeletal injuries such as a Salter-Harris I physeal fracture to confirm the diagnosis. If not done under local anesthesia or intravenous sedation, stress radiographs caused significant patient discomfort.

Today, stress radiographs are rarely performed. The information obtained from the clinical exam and routine x-rays are usually sufficient to make an accurate diagnosis. Often, the information gathered from stress radiographs does not change the management of the injury thus justifing the expense and potential discomfort to the child.

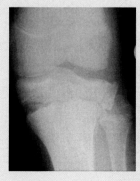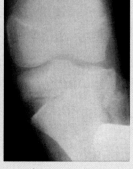

Inability to achieve an adequate closed reduction is often due to soft tissue interposition, most likely perisoteum. In this circumstance, open reduction and internal fixation are indicated.

Salter-Harris III and IV fractures with associated step deformity or displacement of more than 2 mm require open reduction and internal fixation, using screws or wires (Fig. 15-1). If screws are used, care is taken to avoid crossing the physis unless the child is at an age that closure is acceptable (Fig. 15-2). With fractures that extend into this joint or severely disrupt the physis, the patient is kept non-weight bearing for the first 4 to 6 weeks.

Patients with proximal tibial physis fractures are followed for 2 years to watch for signs of angular deformity, shortening (physeal closure), or persistent instability (ligamentous injury).

PROXIMAL METAPHYSEAL FRACTURES

Masquerading as innocent little cracks with no particular reputation for evil, proximal metaphyseal fractures can lead to serious problems. Two distinct types of fracture occur in this region, each with the distinct potential for an almost predictable complication.

Arterial Hazard Fracture

The anterior tibial artery passes over the proximal edge of the interosseous membrane into the anterior compartment and is closely applied to the tibia.

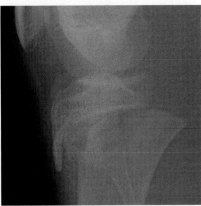

At Inury   **After Reduction**

Figure 15-1. Salter-Harris IV proximal tibia fracture treated operatively and fixed with temporary K-wires. If screws are used for fixation, take care not to cross the physis.

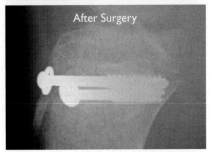

At Injury

After Surgery

Figure 15-2. This type II proximal tibia fracture has a high risk for arterial injury. The patient was near maturity; therefore a fixation method that ensures closure was used. K-wire fixation (and tension band wire) can be used in younger children.

The Hazardous Intersection—Proximal Tibia and Fibula

Nowhere in the body does anatomic configuration provide greater hazard for the pediatric orthopedist. The intersection of two physes (that can be disrupted), three vessels, and associated nerves (peroneal, tibial) create this danger.

At Injury   2 Years Later

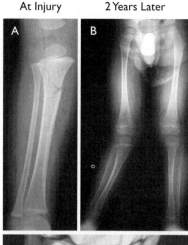

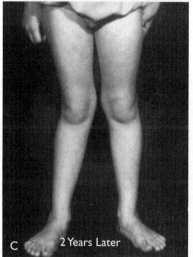

Figure 15-3. Progressive deformity following a proximal tibia fracture. A) At injury. B) Clinical photo 2 years later. C) Standing x-ray 2 years later.

Because of this fixed position, the artery may be compressed, stretched, or torn. If it is stretched, the posterior tibial artery may also be occluded in a displaced type II fracture or in a proximal metaphyseal fracture.

The initial sign of vascular damage may be a cold, pale, pulseless leg that in about an hour becomes anesthetic and paralyzed, but often the findings are more subtle and appear slowly. Muscle ischemia alone is less dramatic; a warm skin has misled many.

With a proximal fibular fracture, the temptation to blame calf and foot neurologic signs of ischemia on local lateral popliteal nerve damage should be resisted. Arterial compromise and/or compartment syndrome must be suspected. Reduction is urgent because correction of the displacement and angulation may restore the circulation. If not, the vessels must be explored because prolonged ischemia increases the risk for compartment syndrome. Ideally, a vascular surgeon and an orthopedic surgeon would collaborate. An angiogram may be helpful but should not overly delay intervention. If an arterial repair is performed or compartment syndrome is diagnosed, four compartment fasciotomies should be performed with internal fixation of the fracture to protect the soft tissues (including the vascular repair) from further trauma.

Valgus Greenstick Fracture

In children between ages of 3 to 10 years, metaphyseal greenstick fractures have attracted much interest. The cortex opens slightly on the medial side of the tibia with the lateral cortex intact. The x-ray angulation is very unimpressive, and most of these fractures are accepted as nondisplaced and are casted in situ following the adage that children's fractures, particularly in younger children, can be expected to remodel and thus don't require exact angular correction.

When the cast is removed, the limb may initially appear in acceptable alignment, but subsequent progressive valgus comes as an unpleasant surprise (Fig. 15-3). This is due to the additive effect of the valgus produced by the fracture to the often exaggerated valgus already present in this age group as well as subsequent asymmetric physeal stimulation due to the asymmetric (incomplete) fracture. Although the valgus attitude may improve over time, it usually does not correct completely and may require subsequent surgery (physeal stapling, rarely osteotomy).

If one takes the trouble to look at the leg itself initially in the fully extended position, comparing it to the opposite limb, the deformity is apparent. Unfortunately, children hold the injured leg flexed, and in the flexed position the deformity is less evident. Proximal tibial metaphyseal greenstick fractures are often best corrected under anesthesia. The reduction can sometimes be improved by first increasing the valgus (to complete the fracture) followed by a varus moment (Fig. 15-4). The leg should be immobilized in extension with varus molding.

Figure 15-4. Five-year-old boy with a proximal tibial metaphyseal fracture—method for reduction illustrated. A) At injury. B) Under anesthesia—further valgus added to complete fracture. C) Now varus applied—fracture is fully reduced. D) In cast with full reduction.

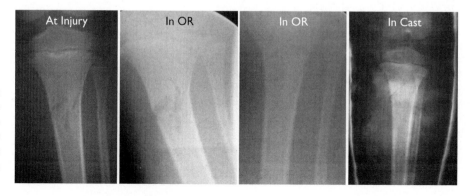

Why Progressive Valgus?

Taylor drew attention to this injury and suggested that valgus was due to overgrowth of the tibia because of fracture hyperemia, whereas the intact fibula acted as a tether. Overgrowth plays a part, but it has been our experience that if the fracture is fully reduced, significant progressive valgus in unlikely. On occasion, the medial gap cannot be reduced by closed manipulation because of soft tissue interposition. Both the lower part of the pes anserinus and the thick periosteum avulsed from the lower fragment can be entrapped (Weber). In this instance, open reduction is needed to ensure an anatomic reduction. Once open reduction is performed, the fracture is usually pinned to maintain reduction.

Aronson found that dividing the periosteum around the medial half of the proximal tibia produced valgus deformity. This may be due to mechanical release of the restraint the periosteum imposes on the growth plate. Likely the mechanism is multifactorial.

An established valgus deformity can be treated either with medial proximal tibia physeal stapling (at age 10-14 years, if the physis remains open) or with corrective osteotomy. If a corrective tibia osteotomy is performed, an osteotomy of the fibula should also be done with anterior compartment fasciotomy plus placement of a drain to minimize the risk of a compartment syndrome. Amazingly, recurrence of valgus deformity has been reported despite corrective osteotomy of both the tibia and fibula.

DIAPHYSEAL FRACTURES

Diaphyseal (midshaft) fractures are common; however, a distinction should be made between low- and high-energy trauma to predict the extent of soft tissue injury. In the majority of cases, the fibula is intact. Often these fractures are stable and minimally displaced because of the more resilient periosteum in children (in the adult, bone is stronger than periosteum, therefore the periosteum is almost always torn when the bone is fractured).

In a child, the recoil of the intact periosteum holds the fracture in good position. Displacement is much more common when both bones are fractured than when the fibula is intact.

Cast Immobilization

Low-energy, nondisplaced fractures are immobilized in a long leg cast applied in two segments with the child's leg hanging over the side of the bed (Fig 15-5). The leg-calf segment should be applied with the limb in a vertical position to ensure the best possible reduction. Casting with the patient supine may lead to posterior angulation (gravity effect). In the "two-segment" application method, good padding is required at the juncture (felt is ideal). The knee is then extended with the remainder of the cast applied.

The knee is flexed 10°-15° and the ankle casted in neutral flexion, if possible, to allow for early weight bearing in stable fractures. It is important to mold the cast at the fracture site and also at the arch and over the Achilles tendon to minimize loosening of the cast, avoid fracture displacement, and prevent heel pressure sores.

If you wish to prevent walking on an unstable fracture, consider flexing the knee beyond 80°. Note that most energetic children will still walk on the cast with less flexion (<45°). There are only two rational choices (15° knee flexion—walking OK and 80° flexion—can't walk). Check x-rays are performed after casting.

"When the cast is removed the limb may initially appear in acceptable alignment but subsequent progressive valgus comes as an unpleasant surprise"

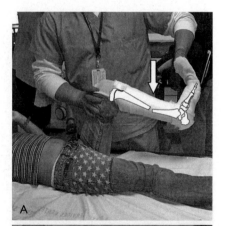

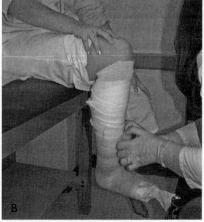

Figure 15-5. A) Casting the patient supine may lead to posterior angulation (gravity effect). B) Casting the patient with the limb hanging over the edge of the table makes anatomic reduction more likely.

At Injury   I Year Post Injury

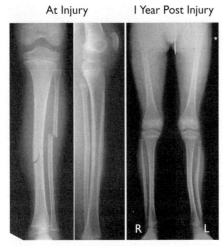
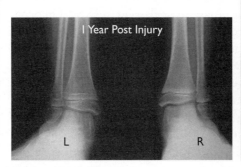
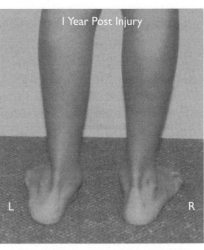

I Year Post Injury

I Year Post Injury

Figure 15-6. This boy had flatfoot and a tibial fracture (distal). The valgus was accepted and 1 year later he had severe ankle valgus. He required an osteotomy. When considering what degree of malalignment to accept, one must consider associated factors (especially knee and ankle valgus).

Fractures Requiring Reduction

Simple fractures may be reduced in the ER; however, many (and perhaps most) significantly displaced tibia fractures are better managed in the peaceful OR setting with ideal analgesia (general anesthesia) and a regular image intensifier. What is an acceptable position? Rotation should be accurate because the knee and ankle are hinge joints and residual will be noted by the patient. The goal is to obtain at least 50% apposition of the tibia and alignment within 5° to 10° of normal in all planes.

Decisions regarding who requires reduction can be difficult. The patient in Figure 15-6 had a 10°-15° valgus angle at his fracture site, which was accepted. Because he also had flatfoot, the combination led to severe ankle symptoms. He required an osteotomy.

The cast is univalved to allow for swelling (bivalved in severe fractures). Most significant tibial fractures are admitted overnight to monitor for swelling and signs of compartment syndrome. The leg should be elevated for 3 to 4 days.

Monitoring Reduction

Fracture alignment must be monitored closely during the first 3 weeks after reduction. Occasionally, a full cast change under general anesthesia is required 2 to 3 weeks after injury to realign the fracture.

Alternatively, corrections can be made by wedging the cast in the clinic during the first 2 to 3 weeks, although this must be done with skill as the wedging can produce complications (skin or muscle necrosis) (Fig 15-7). The cast can be wedged in one of three ways: a closing wedge, an opening wedge, or a combination. We most commonly perform an opening wedge correction at about 2 weeks post fracture when callus has begun to form (this initial stickiness minimizes the chance for recurrence of angulation).

First, a transverse cut is made opposite the apex of the fracture (perpendicular to the long axis of the tibia). A small segment of the cast is left intact directly over the apex of the angulated tibia utilizing two longitudinal stress relief saw cuts. A cast spreader is placed into the cast opposite the apex of the bone, and the cast is opened. A plastic block of appropriate size (usually 1 to 2 cm) is placed into the opened segment and the cast is initially wrapped with tape (for x-ray alignment check) and then overwrapped with casting material.

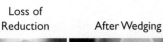

Loss of
Reduction   After Wedging

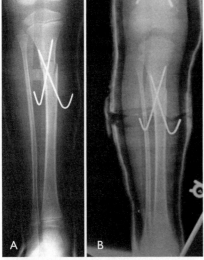

Figure 15-7. A) This patient was treated operatively including cross K-wire stabilization, the fracture began to drift into valgus in the cast. B) Correction of alignment after careful cast wedging. This is an unusual type of cast wedging.

The parents should be made aware of the potential for skin necrosis or compartment syndrome after wedging of casts. Prolonged, intense discomfort after wedging of the cast is often an indicator of problems. In this case, the wedge should be removed and a new cast applied under general anesthesia.

In the presence of a stable, transverse fracture pattern, the patient is allowed to start weight bearing with the help of a cast shoe once the cast is overwrapped (univalve closed 7 to 10 days post fracture). Otherwise, weight bearing is delayed for about 3 weeks until early callus is present with cast change seldom needed.

The cast is usually removed after 6 to 8 weeks. In infants, the bone unites in 3 weeks, whereas in some teenagers it will take 10 to 12 weeks or longer. In such cases, after 6 to 8 weeks, the patient is transitioned into a patellar-tendon-bearing cast, short leg (below knee) cast, or an "off the shelf" plastic cast brace.

When the cast is removed, some children will start to walk unaided immediately, but others need crutches for a week or two. Allow the child to decide when to begin full weight bearing. A limp owing to calf wasting will persist for several months after the cast is removed. Warn the parents about this to save many anxious phone calls.

Operative Treatment

Unstable fractures of the tibia and fibula may require operative reduction and stabilization, especially in older adolescents. Methods of fixation include percutaneous K-wires, external fixation, plates plus screws, flexible nails, and fixed intramedullary nails. Indications for operative treatment include comminuted fractures, irreducible fractures, fractures that cannot be maintained in a reduced position, fractures associated with compartment syndrome, open fractures, multiple system injuries, and the so-called floating knee (fracture of both the tibia and femur in the same limb).

Crossed K-wires

In patients younger than 6 years with open or unstable fractures, we favor crossed percutaneous K-wire fixation followed by immobilization in a long leg cast (Fig. 15-8). The K-wires are usually left outside the skin with felt around and over the pin to protect the skin and prevent movement of the pin inside the cast. The pins are removed through a window in the cast no later than 3 to 4 weeks after surgery. Pins left in longer than this may increase the chance of infection.

Flexible Nails

In patients older than age 6 years, flexible intramedullary nails are the current preferred method for stabilization of fractures requiring operative intervention (Fig 15-9). The nails are inserted from the proximal metaphysis of the tibia below the physis. Two C-shape nails are typically inserted; one from the anteromedial aspect and the other from the anterolateral aspect of the metaphysis. An alternative is to insert one C-shape and one S-shape nail both from the antermedial aspect of the metaphysis. If the fracture cannot be reduced by closed manipulation, the fracture site is exposed through a small incision to facilitate passage of the nails. The nails vary in diameter between 2 and 4 mm.

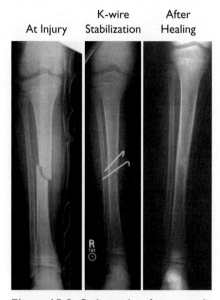

At Injury   K-wire Stabilization   After Healing

Figure 15-8. Radiographs of young pediatric patient treated with a grade I open tibial fracture. After débridement, the fracture was stabilized with K-wires to ensure maintenance of reduction.

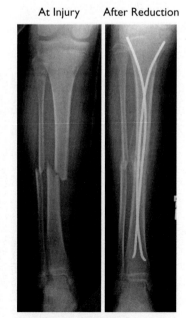

At Injury   After Reduction

Figure 15-9. In patients older than 6 years, flexible intramedullary nails are the current preferred method for stabilization.

In the older adolescent with open physes and wider intramedullary diameter, it may be necessary to stack the nails by using two C-shape nails inserted anteromedially and two C-shape nails inserted anterolaterally to provide sufficient fracture stability. A supplemental long leg cast is usually applied initially to help maintain aligment until there is sufficient callus present.

Rigid Intramedullary Nails

In patients with closed physes, rigid, interlocking nails provide excellent stability and may alleviate the need for postoperative immobilization (Fig 15-10).

COMMON VARIATIONS

The Intact Fibula

The fibula is a bone that will bend without obvious fracture. If you doubt this, take an x-ray of the normal leg in a child with an angulated tibial fracture (with no fibula fracture), and compare the shape of the fibula on each side. Fracture of the tibia in children is more commonly associated with an intact, if bent, fibula.

The intact fibula struts the bone ends apart. Varus deformity with posterior bowing is a common sequela unless the cast is molded into valgus with added posterior molding to prevent recurvatum (Fig. 15-11). The bowing may not be apparent in initial films but commonly develops in the course of 2 or 3 weeks if the cast is not suitably molded. It is a deformity more easily prevented than corrected.

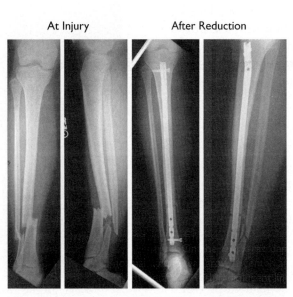

At Injury   After Reduction

Figure 15-10. In adolescents with closed physes, rigid interlocking nails provide excellent stability.

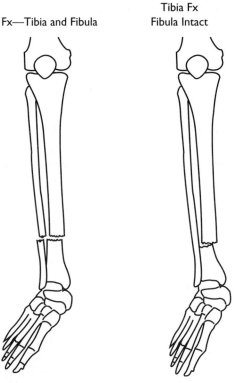

Fx—Tibia and Fibula

Tibia Fx
Fibula Intact

Figure 15-11. The intact fibula struts the bone apart. Varus deformity is a common sequela unless the cast is molded into valgus.

Toddler's Fracture

Children younger than the age of 2 years may present with a painful limp or refusal to walk due to an occult tibia fracture. The injury may or may not have been witnessed. Toddlers often fall and a rotational stress can cause an oblique distal tibia fracture. The presence of fever, constitutional symptoms, or associated illnesses should prompt further workup.

The examination should start on the uninvolved side to provide a comparison for the symptomatic extremity. The examination begins at the hip and proceeds down to the foot. The area of pain is often poorly localized. It is important to note areas with an increase in local temperature and any swelling or bruising.

AP and lateral radiographs of the tibia and fibula should be obtained but are often normal (Fig. 15-12). The fracture may not be visible on the initial radiographs especially if the injury is less than a week old. If a toddler's fracture of the tibia is suspected but the x-ray is normal, we usually get a complete blood count (CBC) with differential, erythrocyte sedimentation rate (ESR), and C-reactive protein (CRP) to rule out infection. If the laboratory studies are normal we then apply a long leg walking cast for 3 weeks. Repeat radiographs in 3 weeks will often show periosteal new bone formation, which helps to confirm the diagnosis.

Open Fractures

Open fractures are usually the result of being hit by a car or some type of motorized vehicle all terrain vehicle (ATV). The wounds are often small and represent a puncture wound from within. They should be treated with thorough débridement of the wound as soon as possible.

In the emergency department, the patient's tetanus status is updated as necessary and antibiotics are started. Antibiotic coverage and duration depends on the grade of the open fracture and presence or absence of gross contamination. Almost all patients are taken to the OR for irrigation and débridement. However, several centers are now studying the concept of treating grade I fractures with ER cleansing plus intravenous antibiotics. Great experience and judgement are required to elect this course.

In the OR, clean grade I and II open fractures can be stabilized with percutaneous pins, intramedullary nails, or plate and screws after the initial irrigation and débridement. External fixation is often used for grade III fractures and grossly contaminated grade II and III fractures. In the presence of more extensive wounds or contaminated wounds, repeat débridement should be performed every 48 hours until the wound is clean.

Fat embolism syndrome occasionally occurs in children and the treating surgeon must be aware of the potential (Limbard, Ruderman—see Suggested Readings). Pulmonary problems following a rather straightforward case should raise suspicion.

Gillespie Fracture—Distal Tibia Diaphysis

Robert Gillespie of the Hospital for Sick Children—Toronto describes this pattern (Fig. 15-13). This little-known fracture is worth recognizing, as it is a potential source of grief. The injury appears to result from landing on a dorsiflexed foot. The anterior border of the tibia is crumpled while the posterior surface opens, producing slight posterior angulation. Seemingly innocent at first, by the time the cast is removed the angulation has increased to an unacceptable degree. Cast the leg with the foot in equinus for the first 4 weeks to

At Injury   3 weeks later

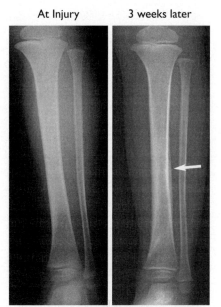

Figure 15-12. Toddler's fracture. The oblique fracture line on the injury film is very hard to see. The child was treated with a long leg cast. Three weeks later the presence of healing callus confirms the diagnosis.

"External fixation is often used for grade III fractures and grossly contaminated grade II and III fractures"

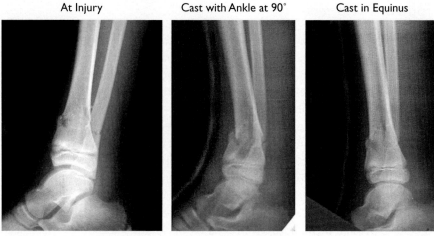

Figure 15-13. The Gillespie fracture is a potential source of grief. Casting the fracture with the ankle at neutral cause unaceptable angulation (recurvatum). To avoid this, the cast must be applied with the foot in equinus.

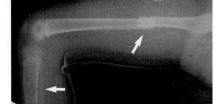

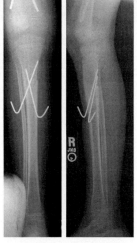

Figure 15-14. The term floating knee has been proposed to describe the very unstable circumstance in which both the tibia and the femur have complete fractures in the same limb.

prevent this problem. The cast can then be changed to one with a more neutral ankle position for remaining healing.

Bicycle Spoke Injuries

Bicycle spoke injuries occur when a bicycle overturns and the child's foot is caught between the spokes of the turning wheel. This causes a severe crushing injury to the soft tissues of the foot and ankle often with an associated laceration. A spiral fracture of the tibia can also occur. The child should be admitted to the hospital when the soft tissue damage is severe. When a tibia fracture is present, initial immobilization should consists of a widely univalved or bivalved non-weight bearing cast to allow for swelling.

The Floating Knee

The term floating knee has been proposed to describe the very unstable circumstance in which both the tibia and femur have complete fractures in the same limb (Fig. 15-14). The usual mechanism of injury involves a pedestrian struck by a car or a motor vehicle accident.

General treatment considerations include age, polytrauma injuries, closed or open fracture, and the physician's experience. Operative intervention is recommended. Depending on the age of the child, both fractures can be treated with flexible intramedullary nails. Alternatively, the femur fracture can be treated with flexible nails and the tibia fracture with crossed percutaneous pins.

Fractures in Paraplegic Children

Tibial fractures are not unusual in children with neurologic conditions (cerebral palsy, muscular dystrophy, spinal bifida, spinal cord injury). In this population, tibia fractures are usually nondisplaced and result from relatively minor trauma (such as a fall from a wheelchair). They are also common after cast immobilization for reconstructive surgery (due to preexisting osteopenia made worse by casting). Displaced fractures are treated with reduction and immobilized for 3 to 4 weeks. In the face of severe osteopenia or repetitive insufficiency fractures, patients should be referred to endocrinology for consideration of medical therapy (sometimes with intravenous biphosphonates).

Stress Fracture with
Delayed Diagnosis

After Cast Immobilization

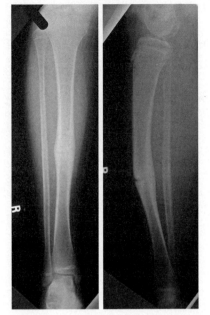
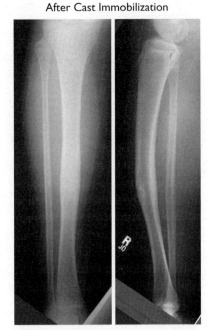

Figure 15-15. Stress fractures occur when normal bone is subjected to repetitive microstresses below the usual threshold needed to cause an acute fracture. In this case, diagnosis was delayed and moderate anterior bowing occured. Often stress fractures can be treated with a decrease in activity.

Stress Fractures

Stress fractures are often associated with poor conditioning prior to sport activity, a sudden change in distance running; and tight heel cords, hamstrings; and quadriceps (Fig. 15-15).

Stress fractures occur when normal bone is subjected to repetitive microstresses below the usual threshold needed to cause an acute fracture. In this setting, osteoclastic bone resorption exceeds osteoblastic activity and bone deposition. Most tibia stress fractures in children occur in the proximal third with a peak age incidence between 10 and 15 years. In contrast, pediatric stress fractures typically occur between the ages of 2 and 8 years and are localized to the distal third of the fibula.

If not readily apparent on plain radiographs, a three-phase bone scan or MRI can facilitate the diagnosis. Treatment can begin with activity restriction only in a very cooperative patient. Other treatment modalities may include protected weight bearing with crutches and immobilization in a walking brace or cast for 4 to 6 weeks.

A gradual return to activities is then recommended with a lower extremity strengthening and stretching program. Although rare, nonunions of stress fractures typically in the middle third of the tibia may occur. This requires use of electromagnetic stimulation or excision of the nonunion, iliac crest grafting and compression plating, or intramedullary fixation.

DISTAL METAPHYSEAL FRACTURES

Distal metaphyseal buckle fractures are common in children and are usually treated with a cast for 3 to 4 weeks.

Distal tibia physeal injuries are also very common and are presented in Chapter 16.

Suggested Readings

Aronson DD, Stewart MC, Crissman JD: Experimental tibial fractures in rabbits simulating proximal tibial metaphyseal fractures in children. Clin Orthop 255:61, 1990.

Balthazar DA, Pappas AM: Acquired valgus deformity of the tibia in children. J Pediatr Orthop 1984;4:538–541.

Briggs TW, Orr MM, Lightowler CD: Isolated tibial fractures in children. Injury 1992;23:308–310.

Buckley SL, Smith G, Sponseller PD, et al: Open fractures of the tibia in children. J Bone Joint Surg 1990;72A:1462–1469.

Burkhart SS, Peterson HA: Fractures of the proximal tibial epiphyses. J Bone Joint Surg 1979;61A:996–1002.

Chow SP, Lam JJ, Leong JC: Fracture of the tibial tubercle in the adolescent. J Bone Joint Surg 1990;72B:231–234.

Hansen BA, Greiff J, Bergmann F: Fractures of the tibia in children. Acta Orthop Scand 1976;47:448–453.

Hope PG, Cole WG: Open fractures of the tibia in children. J Bone and Joint Surg 1992;74B:546–553.

Kreder HJ, Armstrong P: A review of open tibia fractures in children. J Pediatr Orthop 1995;15:482–488.

Limbard T, Ruderman R. Fat embolism in children. Clin Orthop 136:267–268, 1978

Navascués JA, Gonzáles-López JL, López-Valverde S, et al. Premature physeal closure after tibial diaphyseal fractures in adolescents. J Pediatr Orthop 200;20: 193–6.

Ogden JA, Ogden DA, Pugh L, et al: Tibia valga after proximal metaphyseal fractures in childhood: A normal biologic response. J Pediatr Orthop 1995;15: 489–494.

Qidwai MS: Intramedullary kirschner wiring for tibia fractures in children. J pediatr Orthop 2001;21:294–7.

Shannak AO: Tibia fractures in children: Follow-up study. J pediatr Orthop 1988; 8:306–310.

Shelton WR, Canale ST: Fractures of the tibia through the proximal tibial epiphyseal cartilage. J Bone Joint Surg 1979; 61A:167–173.

Taylor SL: Tibial overgrowth: A cause of genu valgum. J Bone Joint Surg 63B:83, 1981

Tuten HR, Keeler KA, Gabos PG, Zionts LE, Mackenzie WG. Posttraumatic tibia valga in children. J Bone Joint Surg 81A: 799, 1999.

Weber BG. Fibrous interposition causing valgus deformity after fractures of the upper tibial metaphysis in children. J Bone Joint Surg (Br) 59:290, 1977.

Yang JP, Letts RM: Isolated fractures of the tibia with intact fibula in children: A review of 95 patients. J Pediatr Orthop 1997;17:347–51.

Zionts LE, MacEwen GD: Spontaneous improvement of post-traumatic tibia valga. J Bone Joint Surg 1986;68A:680–687.

16
Ankle

François Lalonde ❧ *Maya Pring*

INTRODUCTION

In 1898, John Poland made an extensive study of epiphyseal separations about the ankle. He noted that ankle injuries in children differed from those in adults in three important ways:

1. The growth plate forms a plane of weakness directing fracture lines in patterns different from those of adults.
2. Ligaments are stronger than bone so that ligamentous injuries are less common in children.
3. Certain injuries will affect growth.

To Poland's observations the following should be added:

> *"The source for happiness is one of the chief sources of unhappiness"*
> —*ERIC HOFFER*

4. Fractures rarely disturb the talo-tibial relationship, so that persistent disability owing to incongruity is unusual.

5. From the age of 14 to 15 years onward, when the growth plate has closed, the adult pattern of fractures emerges.

APPLIED ANATOMY

The ankle joint is comprised of the talus, which articulates with the ankle mortise. The mortise is formed by the distal tibia and the lateral and medial malleolus. The three major groups of ligaments are each attached to an epiphysis (deltoid, tibio-fibular, tibio-talar) (Fig. 16-1) and provide stability for the articulation.

The distal tibia physis closes around the age of 15 years in girls and 17 in boys. The asymmetric closure of the physis is responsible for many of the fractures that will be discussed in this chapter (Fig. 16-2). Closure proceeds in two directions from an initial site in the near central area. This is followed by fusion of the posteromedial and finally the anterolateral segments of the growth plate. The distal fibula physis closes approximately 1 year later.

When the foot is forced into an abnormal position, tension and compression forces are generated across the ankle. The structure of the ankle appears to permit tension injuries most frequently with the result that avulsion injuries of the epiphyses are common. Compression fractures are unusual.

RADIOGRAPHIC ISSUES

Many people assume that there is no fracture if the x-ray appears normal. However, undisplaced epiphyseal separations show no fracture. The clinical signs

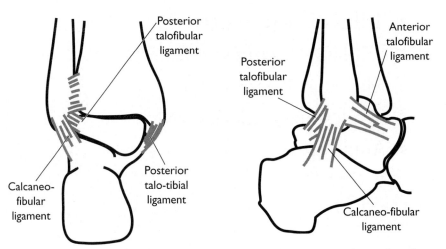

Figure 16–1. Strong ankle ligaments attached to the epiphyses account for epiphyseal separation being more frequent than epiphyseal fractures.

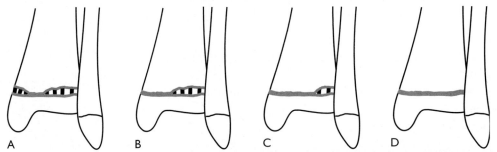

Figure 16-2. Progression of normal distal tibial physeal closure at puberty. A) Begins centrally. B) Spreads medially. C) Then laterally. D) Until complete closure.

and localized soft tissue swelling on the x-ray should be sufficient to sustain the diagnosis. On occasion, there may be widening of the physis when comparison is made with x-rays of the uninjured ankle.

We have missed some fractures about the ankle when we relied on only two views of the ankle (Fig. 16-3). Always take a mortise view (Table 16-1). The mortise x-ray is taken from anterior to posterior with the foot internally rotated 20°; on this view, the outline of the talus is visualized with a symmetric space around it. Asymmetry indicates ligamentous injury and ankle instability.

X-ray measurements of the tibiofibular line, talocrural angle, talar tilt, and medial clear space can be made from the standard mortise view to help determine stability and plan treatment.

CLASSIFICATION

The pattern of injury to the ankle depends on many factors, including the age of the patient; the quality of the bone; the position of the foot at the time of injury; and the direction, magnitude, and rate of the loading forces. In children, the Salter-Harris method still remains the most widely accepted classification scheme for ankle fractures (Table 16-2).

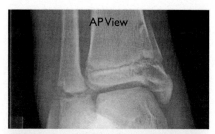

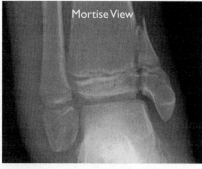

Figure 16-3. This fracture is much more visable in the mortise view than in the AP. The mortise view shows a type IV fracture that will require surgical reduction.

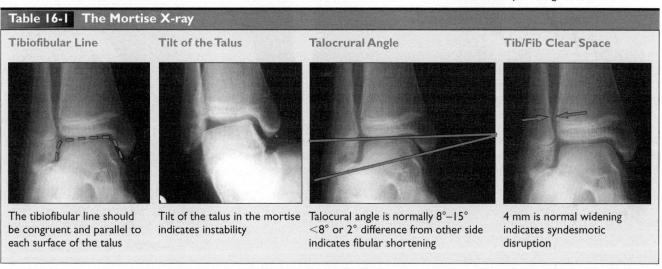

Table 16-1	The Mortise X-ray		
Tibiofibular Line	**Tilt of the Talus**	**Talocrural Angle**	**Tib/Fib Clear Space**
The tibiofibular line should be congruent and parallel to each surface of the talus	Tilt of the talus in the mortise indicates instability	Talocural angle is normally 8°–15° <8° or 2° difference from other side indicates fibular shortening	4 mm is normal widening indicates syndesmotic disruption

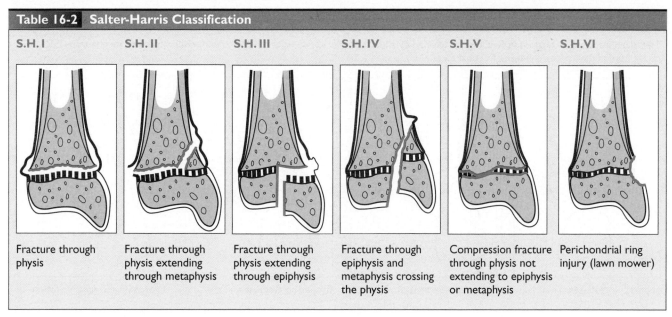

Table 16-2	Salter-Harris Classification				
S.H. I	**S.H. II**	**S.H. III**	**S.H. IV**	**S.H. V**	**S.H. VI**
Fracture through physis	Fracture through physis extending through metaphysis	Fracture through physis extending through epiphysis	Fracture through epiphysis and metaphysis crossing the physis	Compression fracture through physis not extending to epiphysis or metaphysis	Perichondrial ring injury (lawn mower)

Much of our current understanding of the mechanisms of ankle injury (Figs. 16-4, 16-5) is derived from the work of Lauge-Hansen who emphasized the influence that the position of the foot (supination or pronation), and the direction that the deforming forces (adduction, external rotation, or abduction) have on the fracture pattern (Table 16-3). These adult descriptions are often used to describe children's fractures (with only partial success).

Distal fibula fractures and associated syndesmosis injuries are common and can be classified using the Danis-Weber system. The Salter-Harris system suffices for most children's orthopedic descriptions for ankle fractures.

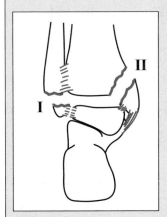

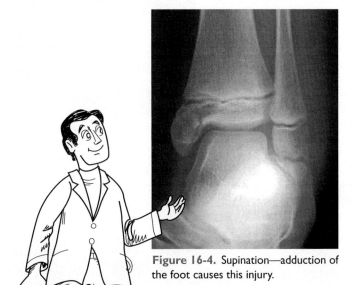

Figure 16-4. Supination—adduction of the foot causes this injury.

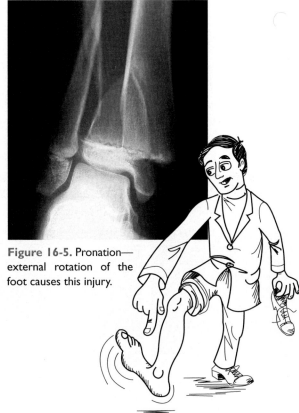

Figure 16-5. Pronation—external rotation of the foot causes this injury.

Table 16-3	Lauge-Hansen Classification

This classification (see Suggested Readings) is learned by all orthopedic surgeons and helps to understand fracture mechanisms but is rarely used in day-to-day children's fracture care.

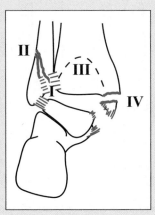

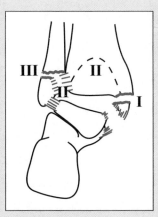

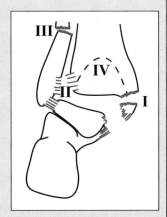

Supination-Adduction	Supination-External Rotation	Pronation-Abduction	Pronation-External Rotation

NONARTICULAR FRACTURES

Salter-Harris Type I and II Fractures of the Fibula

Types I and II are by far the most common injuries to the fibula. They are recognized by swelling and tenderness over the growth plate. In a Type I injury, the radiographs are usually normal (Fig. 16-6). Stress films under anesthesia will demonstrate injury but are unnecessary as a routine, and we neither use nor advocate this technique.

Treatment

The majority of Salter-Harris Type I distal fibular fractures are nondisplaced and can be treated in a walking cast for 3 weeks to allow comfortable healing. If no cast is applied, the injury will heal, but the parents, watching their child hop around on crutches, will be an endless source of trouble to you because of their unrelieved concern and the very small chance that the fracture will displace. When the cast is removed, movement quickly returns, and sequelae are rare.

Displaced Salter-Harris I and II fractures require reduction. Definitive treatment usually depends on the presence of other associated ankle fractures and the quality of the reduction. In widely displaced fractures, there may be soft tissue interposition (peroneal tendons or periosteum) blocking adequate reduction. In this instance, open reduction and internal fixation with cross or longitudinal K-wires is helpful. Fixation of the fracture with a K-wire may be required after closed manipulation if the reduction is unstable.

Salter-Harris Type I Injury of the Tibia

Type I injuries of the tibial physis do occur but are less common. Diagnosis of undisplaced fractures is based on clinical exam—tenderness and swelling directly over the physis. Sometimes, the injury cannot be recognized on radiographs until subperiosteal new bone appears after 3 weeks. These fractures are usually treated in a below knee cast for 3 weeks. The rare displaced fracture requires reduction and a non-weight-bearing cast for a longer period of time (6 weeks).

Salter-Harris Type-II Injury of the Tibia

Type II injuries typically result from higher energy; the force is most commonly supination-plantar flexion or abduction (Fig. 16-7). Gross displacement some-

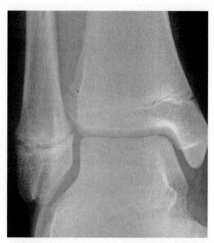

Figure 16-6. Salter-Harris I fractures may be difficult to diagnose on x-ray. The clinical exam is much more telling. This child had focal pain over the distal fibular physis and was assumed to have a type I injury. Standard treatment is a short leg walking cast.

"The majority of Salter-Harris Type I distal fibular fractures are nondisplaced and can be treated in a walking cast for 3 weeks to allow comfortable healing"

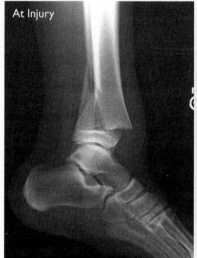
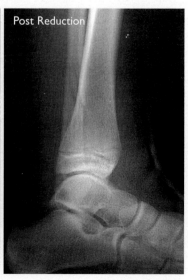

Figure 16-7. The typical Salter-Harris II fracture of the distal tibia was treated with closed reduction and casting.

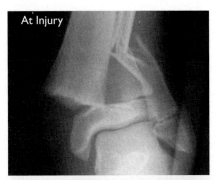

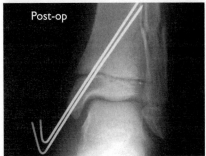

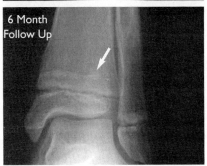

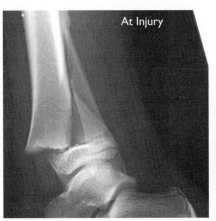

Figure 16-8. This abduction type Salter-Harris II fracture of the distal tibia required open reduction and fixation. The Harris growth line (arrow) on the follow-up x-ray shows that the physis continued to grow normally following the fracture.

times produces ischemia of the foot, which can be relieved prior to transfer or definitive treatment by partially reducing the fracture with the help of longitudinal traction and splinting. Usually, this initial step leads to improved circulation to the foot with palpable pulses by finger or Doppler.

Treatment

The rare nondisplaced fracture can be treated in a below-knee walking cast for 4 to 6 weeks. Patients are followed with x-rays at 6 and 12 months post fracture to rule out physeal arrest.

Closed reduction of Salter-Harris II fractures of the tibia can be done either in the emergency department using conscious sedation or in the operating room under general anesthesia. Greater muscle relaxation with general anesthesia and superior imaging capabilities in the operating room often facilitate the reduction and reduce the number of attempts made at reduction, perhaps decreasing the chance for physeal arrest (Fig. 16-8).

As described for reduction of tibia shaft fractures, reduction of an ankle fracture is often made easier with the knee flexed over the end of the bed. First, the force of injury is recreated with plantar flexion and supination or abduction. Longitudinal traction is then applied to the foot and ankle with an assistant providing counter-traction at the knee. While maintaining traction, the reduction is achieved by bringing the foot around and into a neutral position. Internal rotation will help to keep the fracture reduced. The adequacy of the reduction is checked initially by fluoroscopy and any adjustments are made. Frequently, complete reduction of Salter-Harris II fractures of the tibia is limited by entrapped soft tissues (usually periosteum) at the fracture site; this is identified when the physeal gap is wider than on the contralateral x-ray (Fig. 16-9)

If the reduction is deemed adequate, a long leg cast is applied in two stages, then split to allow for swelling. AP lateral, and mortise x-rays of the ankle are then obtained in cast to document the reduction. Ankle x-rays should be obtained rather than x-rays of the entire tibia/fibula as they demonstrate the reduction more accurately. For comparison, the opposite ankle should also be x-rayed so that precise measurement of the difference in physeal gap or step-off can be evaluated. The length of time in the cast is usually 6 weeks with weight bearing restricted for the first 3 to 4 weeks.

There is current debate regarding whether open reduction of the fracture with removal of entrapped soft tissues and stabilization of the fracture with ei-

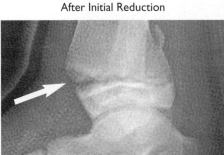

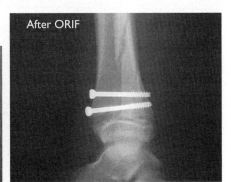

Figure 16-9. This Salter-Harris II fracture could not be reduced completely—a significant amount of periosteum was blocking reduction (arrow). At open reduction, the entrapped periosteum was removed, allowing anatomic reduction. Mubarak and colleagues (see Suggested Readings—Barmada et al.) have found that anatomic reduction reduces the risk of physeal closure.

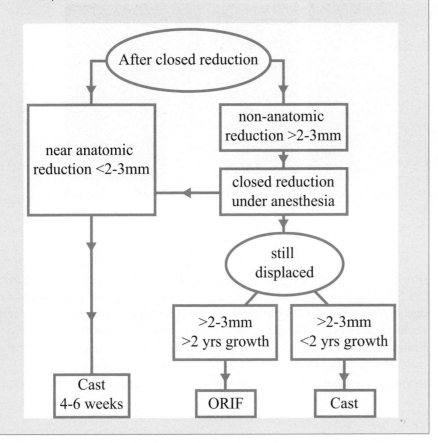

**Distal Tibia Physeal Fractures
Suggested Clinical Pathways**

Salter-Harris I, II and Triplane distal tibia fractures
Mandatory radiographs
- Contralateral films
- Hand for bone age—(younger children—greater risk for deformity if physis closes)

After closed reduction

near anatomic reduction <2-3mm

non-anatomic reduction >2-3mm

closed reduction under anesthesia

still displaced

>2-3mm >2 yrs growth

>2-3mm <2 yrs growth

Cast 4-6 weeks

ORIF

Cast

ther crossed K-wires or screws can decrease the incidence of physeal arrest (Figs. 16-9, 16-10). In patients that are skeletally immature (girls <12; boys <14), advocates of open reduction may intervene surgically in patients with >2 mm difference in physeal gap or translation (compared to the contralateral x-ray) and more than 2 years of growth remaining. The clinical pathway that we follow is presented here.

Pitfalls—Nonarticular Distal Tibial Fractures

Physeal closure occurs more commonly in Salter-Harris I and II fractures of the distal tibia than previously reported. In a recent study of 147 skeletally immature patients with distal tibia Salter-Harris I/II fractures, Mubarak and Rohmiller et al. found a 38% incidence of physeal arrest overall. On further analysis of the direction of the force at the time of injury, it was found that supination-external rotation (SER) injuries have a slightly better prognosis than abduction type injuries. The rate of physeal closure can be affected by surgical intervention in SER injuries; the rate of closure in patients treated without surgery was 56%, whereas those who had open reduction had a physeal closure rate of only 16%.

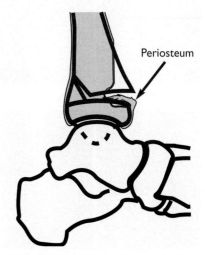

Figure 16-10. The periosteum is firmly attached to the epiphysis—it often pulls off the metaphysis and becomes entrapped in the fracture—preventing complete reduction.

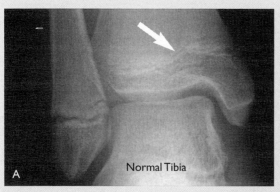 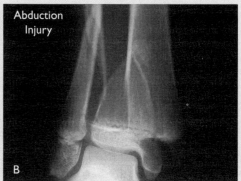
Abduction injuries, however, appear to have a higher rate of closure (52%), which in this study was not changed significantly with surgical intervention (54.5% closure in patients treated closed vs. 50% closure rate in patients treated operatively). One possible explanation for this is that the abduction injuries represent higher energy shearing forces to the physis with probable disruption of Kump's bump at the time of injury (Fig. 16-11). Regardless of type of treatment, patients with Salter-Harris injuries to the distal tibia require close follow-up with x-rays for a minimum of 1 year after injury to follow the growth of the physis.

Extensor Retinaculum Syndrome

The extensor compartment of the ankle, deep to the retinaculum, is vulnerable to increased pressures in association with distal tibia physis fractures. This often occurs when the foot is caught between the ground and the pedal of a bicycle or motorbike causing a distal tibia fracture with apex anterior angulation. Structures that travel within the extensor compartment include the long toe extensors, the anterior tibial artery, and the deep peroneal nerve.

Signs of extensor retinaculum syndrome include severe pain and swelling of the ankle, hypoesthesia or anesthesia in the web space of the great toe, weakness of extensor hallucis longus and extensor digitorum communis, and pain on passive flexion of the toes, especially the great toe. A high index of suspicion is required (Fig. 16-12). If suspected, the extensor compartment pressure should be measured. Interpretation of elevated pressure is similar to that described for compartment syndrome. If the measured pressure is elevated, surgical intervention is warranted with release of the superior extensor retinaculum and stabilization of the fracture.

At Injury

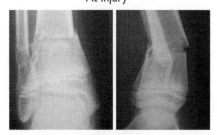

After ORIF

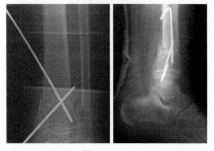

Figure 16-12. This patient has significant swelling and developed an extensor retinaculum syndrome. Release of the extensor retinaculum at the time of surgery relieved his symptoms.

Salter-Harris Type VI Injuries— Ablation of the Perichondrial Ring

Lawn mower and degloving injuries may remove the perichondrial ring. Lipmann Kessel has shown that this permits a callus bridge to form between the epiphysis and metaphysis with resulting varus deformity and failure of growth. The severity of this injury may be missed on initial x-rays.

THE TILLAUX FRACTURE

The Tillaux fracture almost always occurs in the adolescent within a year of complete closure of the distal tibial physis (Fig. 16-13). The central and medial aspects of the physis have closed, leaving the anterolateral aspect open and vulnerable to injury. An external rotation force on the foot may avulse the anterolateral quadrant of the tibial epiphysis, which is bound to the fibula by the strong anterior tibiofibular ligament, resulting in a rectangular or pie-shaped fragment being broken off of the distal tibial epiphyis. A mortise view is essential with this fracture as the fibula may obstruct its visualization. The true amount of displacement is often best appreciated on the lateral view provided the lateral view is taken correctly.

Kleiger and Mankin noted that rotatory instability, detectable by an examination under general anesthetic, is a feature of this fracture. Therefore the fracture may reduce with internal rotation and supination of the foot and thumb pressure over the displaced anterolateral fracture fragment. An above-knee cast is applied in two stages with the foot in supination and internal rotation. Postreduction x-rays (AP, lateral, mortise) are taken to assess the adequacy of the reduction. If the amount of residual displacement remains in question after review of the x-rays, a CT scan of the ankle is helpful. No displacement should be accepted.

Nondisplaced fractures are treated in a non-weight-bearing above-knee cast for 3 weeks, followed by a below-knee walking cast for another 3 weeks. When displacement is present, open reduction and internal fixation is necessary through an anterolateral approach. After reduction, fixation is achieved using one or two cancellous screws, crossing the fracture line in a perpendicular fashion; the screw can cross the physis because the physis is in the process of closing.

THE TRIPLANE FRACTURE

The tibial triplane fracture is a complex fracture defined by sagittal, transverse, and coronal components that courses in part along and in part through the physis and enters the ankle joint (Fig. 16-14). As pointed out by Von Laer, these

"Regardless of type of treatment, patients with Salter-Harris injuries to the distal tibia require close follow-up with x-rays for a minimum of one year after injury to follow the growth of the physis"

At Injury

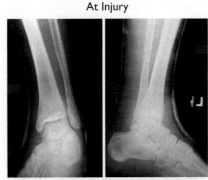

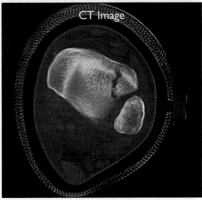

CT Image

Figure 16-13. A minimally displaced Tillaux fracture is better visualized with CT. This fracture was treated with a cast, often analyzing the amount of displacement of the CT scan.

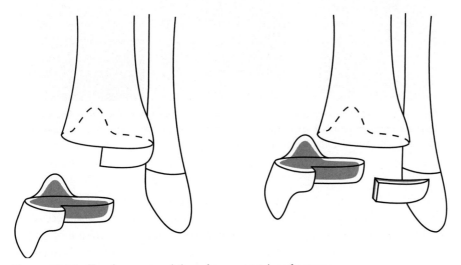

Figure 16-14. Two fragment and three fragment triplane fractures.

"The Tillaux fracture almost always occurs in the adolescent within a year of complete closure of the distal tibial physis"

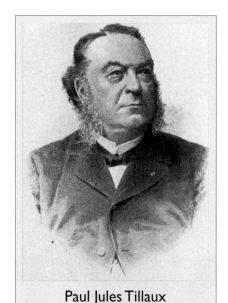

Paul Jules Tillaux
1834–1904

Tillaux, a Parisian surgeon, is credited with first understanding this fracture. His description was originally drawn on a scrap of paper. The drawing was found after he died by Chaput, who made the best of the ambiguous sketch.

The Tillaux Fracture

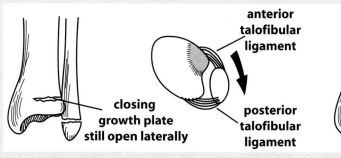

Anatomy of the Tillaux fracture. Characteristically, the fracture is difficult to see.

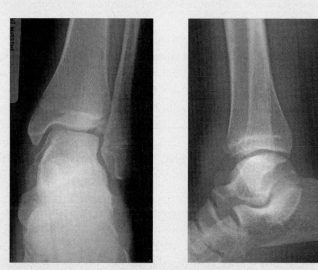

Frequently the fracture line is overlaid by the fibula.

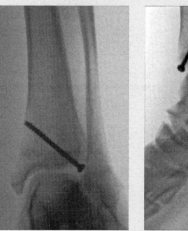
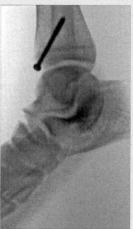
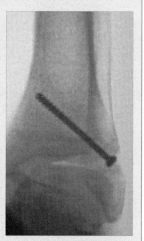

Open reduction and fixation allows restoration of the joint space. The young fibula is pliable and rarely fractures. In the usual Tillaux fracture, the fibula probably bends and then springs back, returning the fragment into place.

"...these fractures with their complicated course of fracture lines in different planes, challenge the imagination of the surgeon"

fractures with their complicated course of fracture lines in different planes, challenge the imagination of the surgeon. The triplane fracture also occurs as a result of the special anatomic circumstances surrounding the nature of closure of the distal tibial growth plate. Most fractures are the result of an external rotation of the foot on the leg. Less commonly, an internal rotation force can produce a medial triplane fracture.

Classically, this fracture appears as a type III injury in the AP x-ray and as a type II injury on the lateral view. Radiographs are hard to interpret. A CT scan is an invaluable tool in defining the fracture configuration and the amount of intra-articular displacement (Fig. 16-15).

It is the lateral part of the epiphysis that tends to be involved more commonly, as in the Tillaux fracture. Medial triplane fractures can occur in children prior to fusion of the medial physis. Most classification systems are based on three factors: (1) medial or lateral, (2) number of parts, and (3) intra- or extra-articular. Fractures of the fibula may be seen with any triplane fracture. Not uncommonly, triplane fractures can be seen in conjunction with ipsilateral tibial shaft fractures. Three-part fractures have a propensity for intra-articular incongruity. These types of fractures often leave a posterior metaphyseal-epiphyseal fragment that behaves like a Salter-Harris IV fracture. This fragment may migrate proximally leaving a residual step in the joint surface.

Neurovascular compromise is rare. Occasionally, in widely displaced fractures, tenting of the skin over the fracture fragment may lead to skin necrosis if reduction is not carried out expediently. Accurate closed reduction is the usual mainstay of treatment. Reduction is performed either under conscious sedation or general anesthesia for optimal relaxation and is achieved by traction and internal rotation of the foot, usually with the foot in plantar flexion. The exception is the rare medial fracture, which may require external rotation. Overly aggressive internal rotation and forceful dorsiflexion before the distal fragment is reduced can fracture the anterolateral beak of the epiphysis, which then converts a two-part fracture into a three-part fracture.

Once closed reduction is achieved, a long leg cast is applied with the foot in internal rotation (not varus). The patient is kept non-weight-bearing for about 3 weeks, then transitioned into a short leg or patellar tendon weight-bearing cast for an additional 2 to 4 weeks.

Maximum acceptable residual displacement is 2 mm at the articular surface. For the extra-articular variant, less stringent requirements may apply. Open reduction is often necessary for medial fractures and some three-part fractures (Fig. 16-16). CT scans are extremely helpful in planning operative intervention.

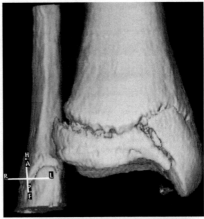

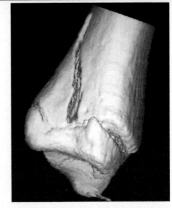

Figure 16-15. A 3-D CT scan often helps to understand the pattern of a triplane fracture and helps to plan surgical correction.

At Injury   Additional Film   After ORIF

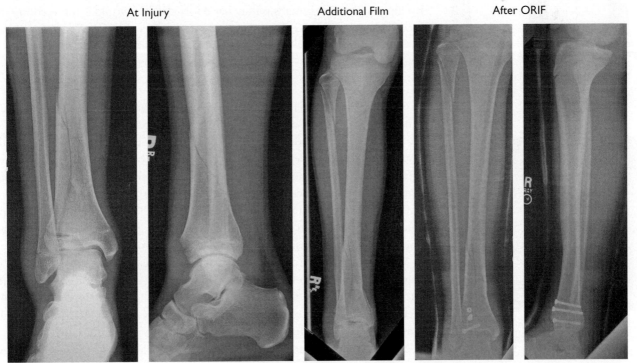

Figure 16-16. Triplane fractures may have more proximal associated fractures. In this case, initial films showed a triplane fracture with extension to the tibial shaft. The proximal fibular fracture was missed on the initial x-rays, because the entire tibia-fibula was not included on the film. The triplane fracture required ORIF.

"In a young child, the lateral cartilaginous model can be avulsed by a ligament. Initially there is just swelling, and radiographs are normal. After a month or more, the cartilage model forms an ossicle"

Normal   Original Injury   Later

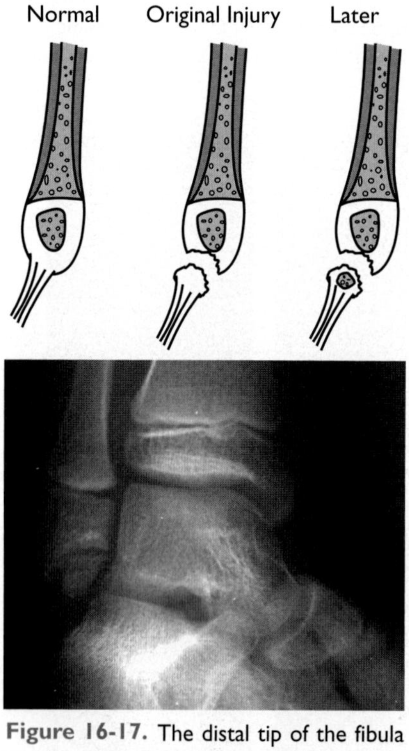

Figure 16-17. The distal tip of the fibula may be avulsed by the attached ligament. Note the well-rounded ossical distal to the fibular tip—this is the late consequence of an earlier avulsion fracture.

Typically, the lateral triplane fracture is approached using an anterolateral incision for the free anterolateral epiphyseal fragment. A second posterior incision may be medial or lateral depending on the fracture configuration. Interfragmentary screws are usually used for fixation with occasional plating of displaced fibular fractures.

MALLEOLAR FRACTURES

Provided one has a good understanding of the mechanism of injury and inherent stability of the injury, closed reduction can be attempted under oral or intravenous analgesia and/or sedation. Closed reduction is obtained by reversing the mechanism of injury to the ankle and then bringing it into a reduced position while maintaining traction on the foot. Post-reduction x-rays are essential to assess stability and the quality of the reduction. The majority of pediatric malleolar fractures can be treated with casting.

Operative treatment of ankle fractures is recommended when:

- Closed reduction fails
- Maintaining closed reduction requires forced, abnormal positioning of the foot, such as forced plantar flexion and inversion
- There is displacement of the talus or widening of the mortise greater than 1 to 2 mm
- Displaced fractures involve the articular surface
- The fracture is open

The surgical procedure is carried out as soon as possible but is dependent on evaluation of the entire patient, the condition of the soft tissues, and the amount of swelling present. Initially, the ankle should be gently reduced and immobilized in a padded splint to prevent further soft tissue injury and to decrease swelling. Ice and elevation are used to reduce swelling until operative treatment can be safely performed. Ankle swelling usually peaks between day one and seven, and operative treatment is best done before the period of maximal swelling or after the initial swelling has resolved. The "wrinkle" test is commonly used to determine if swelling is likely to prevent skin closure following surgery.

Lateral Malleolus

In a young child, the lateral cartilaginous model can be avulsed by a ligament. Initially, there is just swelling, and radiographs are normal. After a month or more, the cartilage model forms an ossicle (Fig. 16-17). The anterior talofibular ligament pulls a fragment off the anterior fibula; this is the adolescent equivalent to an adult ligament rupture. Occasionally, the ossicle remains symptomatic and can be excised with relief.

Often, the original injury occurs at a young age (age 4-10 years) and the patient appears later with symptoms (now ossified). This condition is often confused with a normal ossification variation (os subfibulare).

Most avulsion fractures of the lateral malleolus can be treated closed by everting the ankle to relax the lateral collateral ligaments prior to reducing the fracture. The fracture is then immobilized in a short leg cast for 4-6 weeks. Weight bearing is started once the initial symptoms subside. An associated fracture of the medial malleolus makes closed treatment more difficult.

External rotation fractures at the level of the syndesmosis (SER) are reduced by gentle distraction, internal rotation, and varus stress (Fig. 16-18). A cast is then applied with the foot in this position. Residual shortening and external rotation of the fibula may be difficult to appreciate on post-reduction films. More severe injuries requires surgical reduction (Fig. 16-19).

The lateral malleolus is approached through an anterolateral or posterolateral approach. Depending on the skeletal maturity of the patient, there are many options for fixation. In young children, a longitudinal or crossed K-wire is sufficient. An oblique fracture that is longer than two times the diameter of the bone can be fixed with lag screws alone. An external rotation oblique fracture of the distal fibula at the level of the syndesmosis can be stabilized with lag screws alone or more commonly a plate to neutralize the rotational and axial forces on the fibula. The one-third tubular plate conforms better to the fibula and has a lower profile than the thicker compression plate. Fractures above the syndesmosis are stabilized with a one-third tubular plate with or without lag screws.

In treating deltoid ligament injuries in association with a fracture of the lateral malleolus, it is generally accepted that an anatomic reduction of the fibula and talus restores the medial anatomy and will allow the medial ligamentous structures to heal without need for operative repair. Anatomic restoration of the fibula usually restores the talus to its normal position. If, however, the medial clear space remains widened by more than 2 mm after reduction of the fibula, or the reduction of the fibula is blocked, then the medial side should be explored.

Medial Malleolus

Avulsion fractures of the medial malleolus are rare and must be distinguished from variations of ossification. True displaced medial malleolus avulsion fractures require open reduction and internal fixation.

Isolated medial malleolus fractures are uncommon and the possibility of an undisplaced lateral injury such as a Maisonneueve proximal fibula fracture should be considered. Isolated fractures are treated closed if they are nondisplaced, involve the distal portion of the malleolus, or can be anatomically reduced by manipulation. A CT scan may be necessary to ensure that the joint surface is not disrupted if closed management is chosen.

Fixation for displaced medial malleolus fractures depends on the fracture pattern and the patient's age. In skeletally immature patients, reasonable efforts should be undertaken not to cross the open physis. This can often be accomplished with two transepiphyseal cannulated or cancellous screws (Fig 16.20).

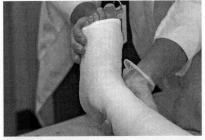
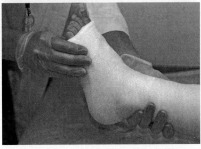

Figure 16-18. Closed reduction of a distal fibular (lateral malleolar) fracture is best maintained with the application of an internal rotation and varus moment to the ankle-foot.

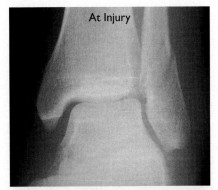
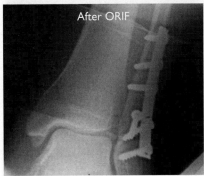

Figure 16-19. An external rotation oblique fracture of the distal fibula at the level of the syndesmosis can be stabilized with lag screws alone or more commonly a plate to neutralize the rotational and axial forces on the fibula.

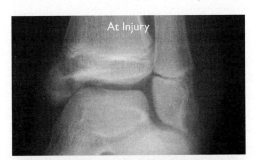
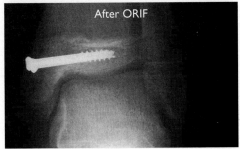

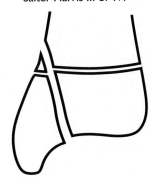

Salter-Harris III or IV?

Figure 16-20. Displaced intra-articular fractures of the medial malleolus require ORIF. Often it is difficult to determine whether this is a type III or IV injury. The Thurston-Holland fragment may be very small. Care should be taken not to put screws across an open growth plate.

At Injury   6 Months Later

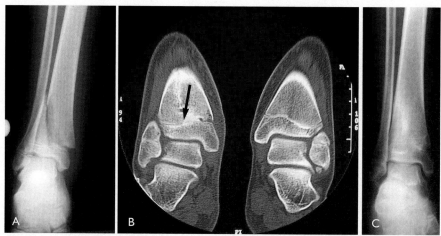

Figure 16-21. A) This Salter-Harris II injury underwent closed reduction and cast treatment. B) CT scan 6 months later shows physeal arrrest of the right distal tibia. C) The x-rays show valgus deformity, a physeal bar, and assymmetric Harris growth lines.

"Asymmetry of the Harris growth line is often an important indicator of early premature physeal closure"

On occasion, the metaphyseal portion of the fracture is large enough to accommodate a transmetaphyseal screw.

When transepiphyseal fixation is not possible because of the location of the fracture, it may necessary to use smooth K-wires across the physis with or without tension-band wiring. Reduction may be hindered by trapped, loose fragments that will require removal. In skeletally mature patients, medial malleolus fractures are stabilized using two cancellous or cannulated screws inserted perpendicular to the fracture in the classic adult fashion.

Pitfalls—Physeal Fractures of the Distal Tibia

In skeletally immature patients, premature physeal closure is common after distal tibia fractures (Fig. 16-21), especially those involving with the medial malleolus. The potential impact of distal tibia physeal arrest on limb-length inequality and angular deformity at the ankle depends on the growth remaining.

Patients are usually followed at 6 months and 1 year post injury with radiographs of the involved ankle. If the patient is close to skeletal maturity, or to assist in interpretation of possible physeal closure, x-rays of the non-injured ankle may be helpful.

Asymmetry of the Harris growth line is often an important indicator of early premature physeal closure. If premature physeal closure is documented by x-rays, one should obtain a left hand x-ray for bone age and either an MRI or CT scan to document more precisely the extent and location of the physeal arrest. Depending on the growth remaining, treatment of premature physeal arrest may consist of close observation with serial x-rays, excision of the physeal bar with interposition material; epiphysiodesis of the remaining open tibia physis, ipsilateral distal fibula, and/or contralateral tibia and fibula; or corrective osteotomy.

At Injury   After ORIF

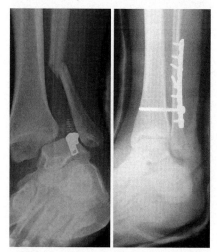

Figure 16-22. Syndesmotic disruption requires fixation of the syndesmosis. The syndesmotic screw should be removed after adequate healing (usually 3 months).

SYNDESMOSIS INJURIES

Fractures associated with syndesmotic disruption (pronation-abduction/external rotation) are usually unstable and most require operative stabilization (Fig. 16-22). The decision to use syndesmotic fixation is based on the fracture pattern and intraoperative assessment of stability. Fixation is recommended when:

- There is medial ligamentous injury, syndesmotic disruption, and talar shift without a fracture of the fibula (tibiofibular diastasis)
- When the treatment of a high fibula fracture (Maisonneuve fracture) is directed primarily at stabilization of the syndesmosis and ankle mortise
- When there is continued evidence of syndesmotic instability after fixation of the fibula and any avulsion fracture(s) of the tubercles or medial malleolus

Intraoperative assessment of stability involves placing a hook around the fibula at the level of the syndesmosis and applying lateral traction. Lateral movement of the intact or internally fixed fibula or widening of the mortise on intraoperative x-rays are indications for a syndesmotic screw.

If indicated, one or two (3.5 or 4.5 mm) cortical screws are used to hold but not compress the syndesmosis. The screw is inserted just above the level of the tibiofibular ligaments. It is recommended that the foot be placed in dorsiflexion at the time of screw insertion to bring the widest portion of the talus into the mortise. Both cortices of the fibula and the lateral cortex of the tibia are drilled, tapped, and engaged by the screw(s). Patients with syndesmotic injuries should be kept non-weight-bearing for 6 to 8 weeks. Although controversy exists, we favor removal of the syndesmosis screw(s) prior to weight bearing.

ANKLE SPRAINS

Ankle sprains are very common injuries that result from an inversion stress to the ankle. The ligaments most commonly affected are the anterior talofibular ligament and the calcaneo-fibular ligament. In skeletally immature patients, this injury must be differentiated from the Salter-Harris I or II distal fibula fracture. Both present with swelling and ecchymosis over the anterolateral aspect of the ankle but the point of maximum tenderness helps to differentiate these two injuries.

Ankle sprains are commonly graded according to severity. A grade I sprain indicates that the ligaments are in continuity, grade II refers to a partial tear of the ligaments, and grade III denotes a complete tear of the ligaments with gross instability. Ankle sprains can be treated in a number of ways including an elastic bandage, an aircast, a posterior splint, or a short leg cast. With mild and moderate sprains, the patient is allowed to weight-bear as tolerated with or without the help of crutches depending on the method of immobilization.

Recurrent ankle sprains may be due to residual ankle weakness, ligamentous instability, or unsuspected tarsal coalition. In the non-acute setting, ligament instability can be assessed on exam by the drawer test and inversion stress (Fig. 16-23) and by imaging such as stress radiographs and/or MRI.

If subsequent examination of the foot and ankle after injury reveals decreased subtalar range of motion, one should suspect a tarsal coalition and AP, lateral, oblique, and axial (Harris) x-rays of the foot should be obtained (Fig. 16-24). A talo-calcaneal coalition may be difficult to visualize on x-rays and a CT scan may be helpful to make the diagnosis.

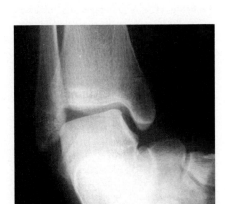

Figure 16-23. Stress view indicating ankle sprain.

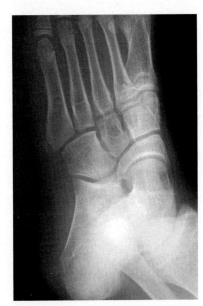

Figure 16-24. Recurrent ankle sprains may be due to residual ankle weakness, ligamentous instability, or unsuspected tarsal coalition.

Barmada A, Gaynor T, Mubarak SJ: Premature physeal closure following distal tibia physeal fractures. A new radiographic predictor. J Pediatr Orthop 2003;23:733-9.

Cameron HU: A radiologic sign of lateral subluxation of the distal tibial epiphysis. J Trauma 15: 1030, 1975

Canale ST, Belding RH: Osteochondral lesions of the talus. J Bone Joint Surg 1980;62A:97-102.

Danielsson LG: Avulsion fracture of the lateral malleolus in children. Injury 12:165, 1980

Dias LS, Tachdjian MO: Physeal injuries of the ankle in children: Classification. Clin Orthop 1978; 136:230-3.

Ertl JP, Barrack RL, Alexander AH, et al: Triplane fracture of the distal tibial epiphysis: Long-term follow-up. J Bone Joint Surg 1988;70A:967-76.

Horn D, Crisci K, Krug M, Pizzutillo PD, MacEwen GD: Radiologic evaluation of junvenile Tillaux fractures of the distal tibia. J Pediatr Orthop 2001;21: 162-4.

Jarvis J: Tibial triplane fractures In: Pediatric Fractures, Letts M ed.: 735-49, 1994

Kleiger B, Mankin HJ: Fracture of the lateral portion of the distal tibial epiphysis. J Bone Joint Surg 1964;46A:25-32.

Kling TF Jr: Operative treatment of ankle fractures in children. Orthop Clin North Am 1990;21: 381-92.

Kump WL. Vertical fractures of the distal tibial epiphysis. Am J Roentgenol Radium Ther Nucl Med. 1966 Jul;97(3):676-81.

Lauge-Hansen N. Fractures of the ankle: analytic historic survey as basis of new experimental, roentgenologic, and clinical investigations. Arch Surg 1948;56: 259-317.

Mooney J, Charlton M, Costello R, Podeszwa D. Ankle joint contact pressures after transepiphyseal screw fixation of the distal tibia. POSNA 2004

Mubarak S: Extensor retinaculum syndrome of the ankle after injury to the distal tibial physis. J Bone Joint Surg 2002;84B:11-4.

Mubarak S: Salter Harris I/II fractures of the distal tibia: Does operative treatment decrease the incidence of premature physeal closure? (POSNA 2004)

Quigley TB: A simple aid to the reduction of abduction-rotation fractures of the ankle. Am J Surg 97:488, 1959.

Spiegel PG, Cooperman DR, Laros GS: Epiphyseal fractures of the distal ends of the tibia and fibula: A retrospective study of two hundred and thirty-seven cases in children. J Bone Joint Surg 1978; 60A:1046-50.

Vahvanen V, Aalto K: Classification of ankle fractures in children. Acta Orthop Traumat Surg 97:1, 1980

Von Laer L: Classification, diagnosis, and treatment of transitional fractures of the distal part of the tibia. J Bone Joint Surg 67A:687, 1985.

Foot

François Lalonde ❧ *Dennis Wenger*

INTRODUCTION

Injuries to children's feet, despite all the little bones and joints, are usually simple and easily managed. Most fractures are straightforward with no subtleties or tricks and few are even displaced. On the other hand, a missed midfoot fracture-dislocation could lead to disability. In many cases, the magnitude of the soft tissue injury may be more significant than the fracture.

In contrast to the traditional presentation of many fracture texts that begin with the hindfoot, we will start the chapter by discussing the more common phalangeal and metatarsal fractures, followed by the less common talar and calcaneal fractures.

PHALANGEAL FRACTURES

Modern culture provides a variety of opportunities for toe fractures ranging from a television falling on a toe to kicking a sibling (Fig. 17-1). The pain is severe, the x-rays may be uncertain, and the patient requires your care and attention even though the problem may seem small to you.

> "The happiest people seem to be those who have no particular cause for being happy except that they are so"
> —DEAN INGE

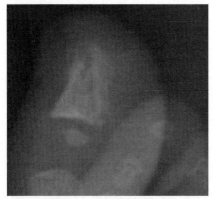

Figure 17-1. Longitudinal fracture of distal phalanx great toe was treated with a hard-soled shoe.

"For toe fractures the choice of immobilization methods (tape vs. hard shoe vs. cast) is often determined by the patient and family's temperament and response to pain"

Simple phalangeal fractures require protection to allow healing. This protection may range from simple taping, taping plus a hard-sole shoe (wooden-sole style-"post-op" shoe) versus a well-molded short leg (below knee) cast. For toe fractures the choice of immobilization methods (tape vs. hard shoe vs. cast) is often determined by the patient and family's temperament and the child's response to pain. For simple taping treatment, follow-up may not be required, because post-healing x-rays are rarely needed.

On occasion, the toe fracture is significantly angulated (especially Salter-Harris II fracture—proximal phalanx) and requires reduction. The digital block plus pencil as fulcrum reduction method used for fingers also works well for toe fractures.

In cases requiring surgery, reduction can often be achieved by closed manipulation with the help of a reduction clamp followed by percutaneous K-wire fixation. Small, fine K-wires are used to stabilize the fracture in its reduced position. If the fracture cannot be reduced by closed means, open reduction is indicated followed by fixation with fine K-wires or a small screw. The open reduction may be associated with joint stiffness.

Growth arrest is occasionally seen as a late consequence after stubbing of the great toe, likely due to an occult Salter-Harris V physeal injury. In other circumstances, a stubbed great toe may sustain an open Salter-Harris I fracture of the distal phalanx with damage to the nail bed and matrix. Infection may follow without adequate care. These fractures should be recognized as open injuries and carefully cleaned and kept well-dressed, and the patient should be treated with oral antibiotics.

Problem Fractures—Great Toe

Displaced, intra-articular fractures of the big toe proximal phalanx, a common injury in soccer and other sports, are often undertreated. These fractures require accurate reduction. All intra-articular fractures have a risk for nonunion and this important joint is no exception. As in any intra-articular fracture, a gap of <2 mm may allow cast treatment only (cast to tip of great toe, dorsal and plantar, to optimize immobilization—non-weight-bearing for 3 weeks, then weight-bearing—Fig. 17-2). Interim x-ray checks are required to rule out loss of reduction. Fractures within the gray zone of 2-3 mm of displacement may need a fine-cut CT scan to make a final decision regarding operative treatment. With significant displacement, internal fixation is required (Fig. 17-3).

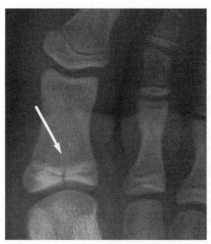

Figure 17-2. This Salter-Harris III fracture is a common soccer injury that can be treated in a cast if minimally displaced.

At Injury   After ORIF

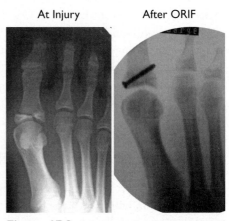

Figure 17-3. Intra-articular fractures need to be anatomically reduced to minimize the risk of arthritis. A step off or gap >2 mm should not be accepted at any joint.

Old nonunions often persist with symptoms and a relatively smooth longitudinal line crossing the proximal phalanx epiphysis. A cast can be tried but internal fixation likely will be needed to achieve union. A similar smooth longitudinal line crossing the epiphysis of the distal phalanx (so-called fissuring is considered a normal anatomic variation.

METATARSAL FRACTURES

Current childhood culture that includes aggressive skateboarding, dirt-bike racing, and television-inspired jumps often from dizzying heights, makes foot fractures common, especially metatarsal fractures.

Shaft and Neck Fractures

The often severe nature of these injuries (as well as the foot being naturally dependent) often leads to marked swelling with metatarsal fractures. Compartment syndrome can involve the interossei and short plantar muscles. X-rays may need to include oblique views to clarify the injury (especially important if a tarsal-metatarsal fracture-dislocation is suspected).

Most metatarsal fractures, even with moderate displacement can be treated simply by immobilization in a short-leg walking cast for 3 to 6 weeks depending on the child's age and activity level (Fig. 17-4). The cast is split widely for the first week to allow for swelling. In cases with severe swelling, a well-padded (bulky Jones) splint may be needed for the first week.

Multiple Fractures

Multiple, displaced, metatarsal fractures may require reduction depending on the age of the patient and whether the first and fifth metatarsals are involved. A fair amount of displacement of the middle metatarsals is acceptable as is angulation of the metatarsal necks (often up to 45°) because significant remodeling can be expected in younger children.

In the child nearing skeletal maturity, much less angulation can be accepted, because abnormal weight bearing will result with little potential for adequate remodeling. Thus in the older age group, the foot should be aligned, not only to prevent splayfoot deformity but also to prevent asymmetric loading of the metatarsal heads (Fig. 17-5).

At Injury   After ORIF

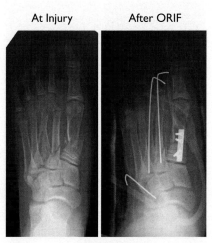

Figure 17-5. Multiple metatarsal fractures with displacement can be treated with closed reduction and pinning (metatarsal 2 and 3 in this patient) or ORIF (1st metatarsal). This patient also had a cuboid fracture that required ORIF.

I Year After Cast Treatment

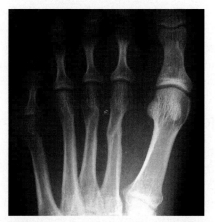

At Injury

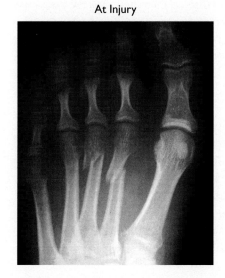

Figure 17-4. Initial and 1-year follow-up AP x-rays in a teenage boy with 2nd and 3rd metatarsal neck fractures treated in a short leg cast with toe plate. Remodeling of the fractures has allowed normal function.

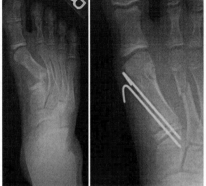

At Injury	After Closed Reduction and Pinning

Figure 17-6. First and 5th metatarsal fractures need to be reasonably well aligned to maintain the borders of the foot.

"Unfortunately, this distinction is clouded by the fact that the apophysis can be traumatically avulsed"

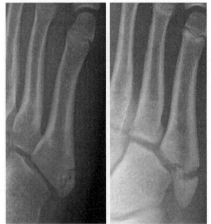

Normal Apophysis	Avulsion Fracture

Figure 17-7. On the left, x-ray depicts a normal apophyseal growth center at base of 5th metatarsal with radiolucent line parallel to shaft. In contrast, the x-ray on the right shows a transverse fracture at the base of the 5th metatarsal.

In cases requiring reduction, manipulation can be attempted with traction applied to the corresponding toes of the fractured metatarsals and countertraction applied to the distal tibia. Percutaneous K-wire fixation may be necessary if the reduction is unstable. In this instance, K-wire fixation may also prevent a nonunion from developing, which can result in a short toe and in asymmetric metatarsal head position with painful metatarsalgia. K-wire fixation of the first and fifth metatarsal fractures maintains metatarsal length and assists in preserving reduction of the other metatarsals.

Occasionally, open reduction is necessary for unreducible fractures. This is performed through a dorsal longitudinal approach. The K-wire is passed through the medullary canal of the distal fragment, exiting in a plantar direction after passing across the metatarsal head. The wire is pulled through distally to the level of the fracture, and after reduction, the wire is drilled retrograde into the proximal fragment and into the midfoot if necessary.

Compartment syndromes of the foot can occur with severe fractures and must be recognized with proper monitoring and treatment (Silas et al.—Suggested Readings).

First Metatarsal Fractures

Proximal fractures (Fig. 17-6) may damage the physis resulting in shortening of the medial side of the foot. Johnson described a variation of the Lisfranc injury (in children younger than the age of 10 years), which causes a fracture of the proximal first metatarsal physis with associated medial cuneiform injury.

Crush injuries of the first metatarsal may affect its length. Length can be restored by closed reduction and percutaneous pinning to adjacent metatarsals.

Fifth Metatarsal Base Fractures

Soccer, football, baseball, and basketball inversion injuries commonly produce avulsion fractures of the base of the fifth metatarsal. The avulsion is thought to occur because of the pull of the peroneus brevis or the tendinous portion of the abductor digiti minimi.

The fracture is distinguished from the apophyseal growth center (os vesalianum) by the direction of the radiolucent line. The long axis of the apophysis is parallel with the shaft (a normal finding), whereas a true fracture line is transverse (Fig. 17-7). The apophysis appears around age 8 and unites to the shaft by age 12 years in girls and 15 in boys.

Unfortunately, this distinction is clouded by the fact that the apophysis can be traumatically avulsed, often with little or no displacement and thus the x-ray may seem normal (longitudinal line), yet the patient has severe pain and requires treatment. In both true fractures and apophyseal separation, treatment includes a short-leg weight-bearing cast worn for 3 to 6 weeks, depending on the child's age.

Jones Fracture

Because of Robert Jones' intricate description of his own fifth metatarsal injury, fractures of the proximal diaphysis of this bone are known as "Jones fractures." It is important to differentiate this fracture from a fracture of the tuberosity, as the two differ considerably in prognosis and management. Jones fractures are much more likely to go on to nonunion and cause long-term difficulties. Metaphyseal fractures on the other hand heal quickly and uneventfully.

The mechanism of injury of a Jones fracture is not thought to be an avulsion but rather the result of vertical or mediolateral ground forces on the weight-

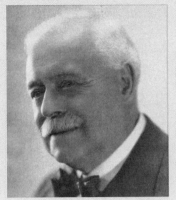
bearing foot. Because the blood supply of the proximal diaphysis is limited compared to that of the tuberosity, healing will be delayed, especially in athletes (Fig. 17-8). Non-weight-bearing immobilization is therefore recommended. Repeat fractures or nonunion are usually treated with intramedullary screw fixation with or without bone grafting. In athletes, regardless of age, there has been a recent trend toward immediate intramedullary screw fixation.

Stress Fractures

Metatarsal shaft stress fractures are commonly referred to as "march fractures" because of their high incidence in military recruits. Athletes frequently sustain these fractures, but they also can occur after procedures to correct clubfoot, hallux valgus, and hallux rigidus, in which the weight-bearing distribution to the lesser metatarsal heads is affected. Repetitive microstresses cumulatively lead to fatigue fractures of the bone.

Many patients with this injury present with foot pain but normal x-rays. If there is a high degree of suspicion, a bone scan or MRI should be obtained to clarify the diagnosis. The second and third metatarsals are most commonly involved.

Treatment involves activity restrictions and usually immobilization in a short leg cast for 3 to 6 weeks. Subsequent x-rays will show the periosteal new bone that typifies the fracture (Fig. 17-9).

TARSOMETATARSAL INJURIES (Lisfranc Injury)

The tarsometatarsal joints can be injured directly or indirectly with the indirect method being by far the more common. Forces producing an indirect injury include violent abduction or forced plantarflexion of the forefoot, either alone or in combination. Hardcastle and associates proposed an anatomic method of classifying tarsometatarsal injuries (Table 17-1).

Although swelling of the midfoot is usual, there may be no obvious deformity because spontaneous reduction of the injury to a near-anatomic position commonly occurs. A fracture of the base of the second metatarsal should raise suspicion of an associated tarsometatarsal dislocation. The combination of a fracture of the cuboid with a fracture of the second metatarsal base also indicates a tarsometatarsal dislocation.

Radiographic documentation of this injury is difficult and oblique views are mandatory. Although stress views have been suggested, a CT study is more commonly used.

Jones Fracture

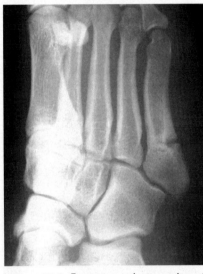

Figure 17-8. Fractures at the metaphyseal diaphyseal junction of the 5th metatarsal are at higher risk of nonunion.

Initial X-ray   3 Weeks Later

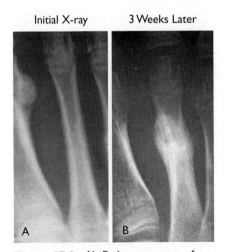

Figure 17-9. A) Early on, x-rays of patients with stress fractures often appear normal. B) X-ray of same patient several weeks later after immobilization in cast showing healing 2nd metatarsal stress fracture.

247

Table 17-1 **Lisfranc Injury Patterns**

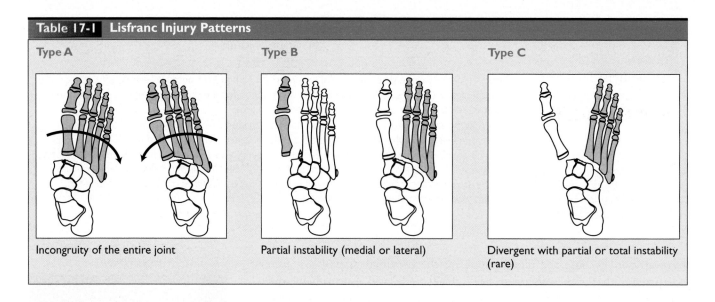

Type A	Type B	Type C
Incongruity of the entire joint	Partial instability (medial or lateral)	Divergent with partial or total instability (rare)

At Injury   After ORIF

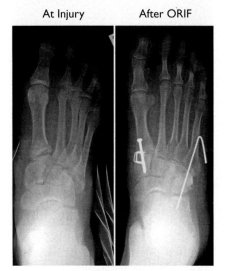

Figure 17-10. Initial and postoperative AP radiograph of teenager with type C Lisfranc injury treated with open reduction and internal fixation.

Nondisplaced tarsometatarsal dislocations can be treated with elevation and an initial compression dressing initially followed by a short leg cast to complete 4 to 6 weeks of immobilization. Displaced fractures require reduction. Manipulative closed reduction is often successful, but supplemental Kirshner wire fixation is almost always added to ensure stability (Fig. 17-10). The key to reduction is to stabilize the second metatarsal base fracture.

A posterior splint is usually applied for the first week to allow for postoperative swelling, with the child then placed in a short leg non-weight-bearing cast to complete 4 to 6 weeks of immobilization. At the end of 4 weeks, the Kirshner wires are removed often through a window in the cast (less stressful for the patient). Weight bearing in a walking cast or in a hard-sole shoe continues for another 2 to 3 weeks.

MIDFOOT (LESSER TARSAL BONES) FRACTURES (Navicular, Cuneiforms, Cuboid)

Isolated fractures of the lesser tarsal bones are usually the result of direct trauma such as an object falling from a height. More often, these fractures are seen in association with a more severe injury to the foot.

A simple compression fracture of the cuboid bone due to a jumping injury is actually more common than was traditionally thought (Fig. 17-11). Often diag-

Cuboid Compression Fracture

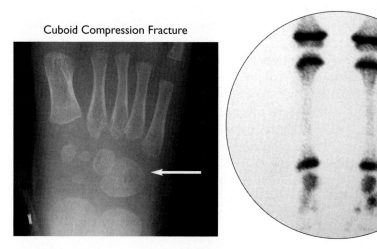

Figure 17-11. AP x-ray of a child afebrile, who presented with a limp after a fall. The x-ray suggests a subtle compression fracture of the cuboid (arrow). A three-phase bone scan shows increased uptake at the fracture site. After 2 weeks in a walking cast he had no symptoms.

nosed as a sprain, very careful x-ray analysis will show a subtle buckle of the cortex (early) or a radiodense healing line after several weeks.

Treatment of isolated nondisplaced fractures consists of immobilization in a weight-bearing cast for approximately 3 weeks.

CALCANEAL FRACTURES

Children seldom fracture the os calcis, but when they do, most are caused by a fall from a height. Schmidt and Weiner reported on compression fractures of the spine in association with calcaneal fractures in children when the mechanism involved a fall from a height. Lateral radiographs of the spine are therefore recommended in this setting. Open fractures resulting from a lawn mower injury are also relatively common in parts of North America where children participate in lawn care activities.

Sagittal plane calcaneus fractures are easily missed if axial (Harris) views of the os calcis are not taken. On the lateral view, Bohler's angle (angle formed by a line parallel to the articular surfaces of the calcaneus with a line drawn along the superior border of the tuberosity—Fig. 17-12) is measured. Depression of the subtalar joint decreases this angle.

As in other complex fractures, a CT scan is often required for a clear understanding of the injury pattern. For intra-articular fractures, the CT scan clarifies the degree of subtalar joint incongruity.

Most fractures of the calcaneus in children involve the tuberosity and heal uneventfully. Nondisplaced fractures can be treated in short leg cast, which is initially split widely to allow for swelling. At the end of a week, once the initial swelling is decreased, the cast is overwrapped and weight bearing is allowed. The cast is discontinued once sufficient healing is present, usually after 4 to 6 weeks. With avulsions of the tuberosity or significant displacement, open reduction and internal fixation is necessary.

Given the remodeling potential of the talus and calcaneus in a growing child, and the favorable results reported after non-operative management, most of these fractures in children can be managed without surgery (Fig. 17-13). Treatment involves non-weight-bearing immobilization for 6 weeks.

In cases with severe intra-articular involvement and loss of Bohler's angle, difficult decisions may be required. Some surgeons may elect conservative treatment (cast only) even in relatively severe injuries because they are not certain that the natural history would be improved on by an operation. Open reduction is appropriate for certain cases. Because of the rarity of such an injury in a child, one should likely seek the help of a surgeon who has experience with these injuries in adults.

Extra-articular fractures seem to do well regardless of treatment, with the possible exception of fractures involving the anterior process. The anterior process of the calcaneus is not well seen on radiographs until age 10 and varies in shape. The distal portion of the fracture fragment articulates with the calcaneocuboid joint. If severe articular displacement and joint depression are evident, open reduction is indicated.

Open fractures should be treated with standard irrigation, débridement, and fixation. Lawn mower injuries are a common cause of open foot fractures (Fig. 17-14).

SUBTALAR DISLOCATION

Subtalar dislocations are extremely rare in children and can be associated with talar neck fractures or other fractures around the foot and ankle. Reduction can usually be accomplished by closed methods.

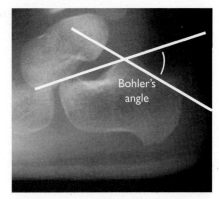

Figure 17-12. Lateral x-ray of the foot illustrating landmarks used to measure Bohler's angle—Normal = 20°-40°. This angle will be decreased in compression type calcaneus fractures.

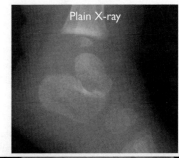

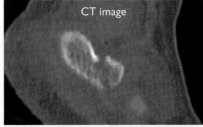

Figure 17-13. Minimally displaced fractures of the calcaneus in young children can be treated with immobilization.

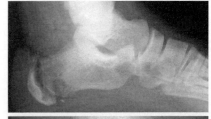

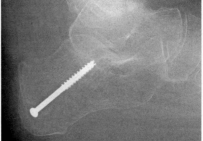

Figure 17-14. This lawn mower injury with open fracture of the calcaneal tuberosity was treated with irrigation, débridement and ORIF.

TALAR FRACTURES

Fractures of the talus are unusual in children. The talus, entirely articular and saddle shaped, is divided into three parts—the neck, body, and head. Because so much of the talus is articular, it has a precarious blood supply with few sites for blood vessel entry. The arterial source enters the bone on the dorsum of the talar neck in the sinus tarsi and medially deep to the deltoid ligament (Fig. 17-15).

The most common mechanism of injury is forced dorsiflexion of the foot. AP, lateral, and oblique radiographs centered on the hindfoot should be taken. If the nature and extent of the talus injury remain difficult to define by x-ray, a CT scan is recommended.

"Because so much of the talus is articular, it has a precarious blood supply with few sites for blood vessel entry"

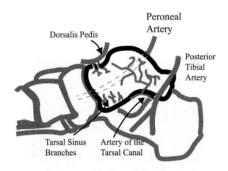

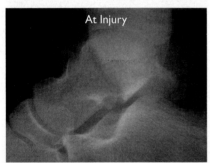

Figure 17-15. Blood supply to the talus is limited and can be interrupted by fractures, resulting in AVN—especially of the talar body.

Talar Neck

The majority of talar fractures are nondisplaced neck fractures, which can be treated with immobilization for 6 to 8 weeks in a long leg cast with the knee flexed to prevent weight bearing. At this time, the fracture is usually united, and the child can be changed to a short leg walking cast for another 2 to 3 weeks. Nondisplaced fractures of the talar neck are rarely associated with osteonecrosis. However, more severe injuries can result in avascular necrosis (AVN) of the talar dome due to vessel damage (Fig. 17-15).

The amount of acceptable displacement of talar neck fractures in children is not well defined. Canale and Kelly considered a reduction with less than 5 mm of displacement and less than 5° of malalignment on the AP view to be adequate.

Minimally displaced fractures can usually be treated by closed reduction with the foot in plantarflexion. Depending on the direction of instability the hindfoot is either inverted or everted. With a stable reduction, the foot can be dorsiflexed during immobilization. Otherwise, the foot is immobilized in plantarflexion for 6 to 8 weeks. If the reduction remains unstable despite plantarflexion of the foot, fixation can be achieved by percutaneous K-wires. Patients with more displaced fractures should have urgent reduction in the operating room.

If the ankle joint is disrupted because of displacement of the talar body, open reduction is necessary. The posterior approach just lateral to the Achilles tendon is preferred, if possible, because it avoids dissection around the neck with its vulnerable blood supply. A minimal anterior exposure may be added if necessary to obtain a satisfactory reduction.

The traditional open reduction has been performed through a dorsomedial approach staying on the medial side of the extensor hallucis longus. Care must be taken to avoid removing any soft tissue attachments from the bony fragements. Two 4-mm canulated screws, a single larger screw, or multiple K-wires can be used for fixation.

The child should be monitored monthly for the first 6 months to assess the vascular status of the talus as most cases of osteonecrosis occur during this time interval in children. In the absence of complications, talar neck fractures should be followed for 1 to 2 years after injury.

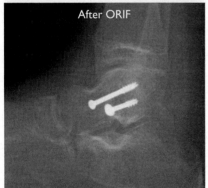

Figure 17-16. Initial and postoperative lateral x-rays of patient with displaced talar body fracture treated with open reduction and internal fixation through combined medial and lateral approach. There is a significant risk for osteonecrosis.

Body

Displaced fractures through the body are rare and require open reduction and internal fixation using a combination of approaches listed previously (Figure 17-16).

Lateral Wall

Lateral wall fracture, probably representing an osteochondral fragment avulsed by the anterior talofibular ligament, is rare and seldom recognized initially. The mechanism of injury is dorsiflexion of the inverted foot. Persistent pain and point tenderness just in front of the lateral malleolus should indicate the need for oblique radiographs or a CT scan to show the small, loose body. Open reduction and internal fixation versus excision may be needed.

Os Trigonum

The os trigonum is a normal variant, which can sometimes be confused with a fracture of the posterior process of the talus (Fig. 17-17). It is an accessory center of ossification that appears around the age of 8 to 10 in girls and 11 to 13 in boys. Unlike a fracture with sharp, jagged edges, the os trigonum appears rounded and smooth. In rare cases, this center is injured and chronic movement through the fibrous union attachment can cause symptoms (especially in ballet dancers). The workup is difficult and, in rare cases, the os trigonum must be surgically removed.

PUNCTURE WOUNDS OF THE FOOT AND PSEUDOMONAS OSTEOMYELITIS

The smell of socks and shoes is due to *Pseudomonas*. Puncture wounds, as a result of a nail penetrating the shoe, can inoculate *Pseudomonas* and produce osteomyelitis (Fig. 17-18). Puncture wounds are common but this is rare—perhaps 0.6% of puncture wounds will get a *Pseudomonas* abscess.

Pseudomonas infection becomes apparent a week or two after the puncture because of increasing pain, swelling, and erythema. If the joint was punctured, a septic arthritis may be produced. This is common at the metatarsophalangeal joint. Radiographic changes may take 3 to 4 weeks to appear. A three-phase bone scan or MRI can help make the diagnosis of osteomyelitis earlier.

Débridement of the area under general anesthetic is recommended. Antibiotic coverage should initially include a cephalosporin to cover for *Staphylococcus Aureus* and an antipseudomonas drug such as gentamicin until the organism is identified and the sensitivities are known. With late presentation, the joint and physis may be permanently damaged by the infection, although chronic infection is rare.

"Patients with displaced fractures should have urgent reduction in the operating room"

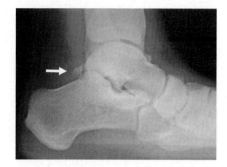

Figure 17-17. Os trigonum is a normal variant that may be mistaken for a fracture.

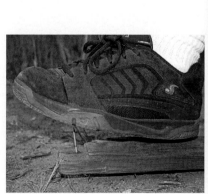
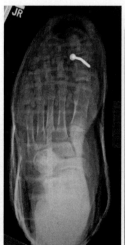
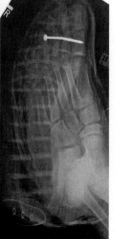

Figure 17-18. Puncture wounds through a tennis shoe may lead to a *Pseudomonas* osteomyelitis.

Suggested Readings

Brunet JA. Calcaneal fractures in children. Long-term results of treatment. J Bone Joint Surg Br. 2000 Mar;82(2):211-6.

Buoncristiani AM, Manos RE, Mills WJ. Plantar-flexion tarsometatarsal joint injuries in children. J Pediatr Orthop. 2001 May-Jun;21(3):324-7.

Dameron TB Jr: Fractures of the proximal fifth metatarsal: Selecting the best treatment option. J Am Acad Orth Surg 3:2:110, 1995.

D'Souza LG, Hynes DE, McManus F, O'Brien TM, Stephens MM, Waide V. The bicycle spoke injury: an avoidable accident? Foot Ankle Int. 1996 Mar; 17(3):170-3.

Fitzgerald RH, Cowan JDE: Puncture wounds of the foot. Orthop Clin North Am 6:965, 1975.

Horowitz JH, Nichter LS, Kenney JG, Morgan RF. Lawnmower injuries in children: lower extremity reconstruction. J Trauma. 1985 Dec;25(12):1138-46.

Inokuchi S, Usami N, Hiraishi E, Hashimoto T. Calcaneal fractures in children. J Pediatr Orthop. 1998 Jul-Aug; 18(4):469-74.

Jensen I, Wester JU, Rasmussen F, et al: Prognosis of fracture of the talus in children: 21(7-34)-year follow-up of 14 cases. Acta Orthop Scand 1994;65: 398-400.

Kay RM, Tang CW. Pediatric foot fractures: evaluation and treatment. J Am Acad Orthop Surg. 2001 Sep-Oct;9(5):308-19.

Laliotis N, Pennie BH, Carty H, et al: Toddler's fracture of the calcaneum. Injury 1993;24:169-170.

Maffulli N. Epiphyseal injuries of the proximal phalanx of the hallux. Clin J Sport Med. 2001 Apr;11(2):121-3.

Mora S, Thordarson DB, Zionts LE, Reynolds RA. Pediatric calcaneal fractures. Foot Ankle Int. 2001 Jun;22(6): 471-7.

Schmidt TL, Weiner DS: Calcaneal fractures in children: an evaluation of the nature of the injury in 56 children. Clin Orthop 171:150, 1982.

Silas S, Hertzenberg J, Myerson M, Sponseller D. Compartment syndrome of the foot in children. J Bone Joint Surg (Am) 77:356-361, 1995.

Wiley JJ. Tarso-metatarsal joint injuries in children. J Pediatr Orthop. 1981;1(3): 255-60.

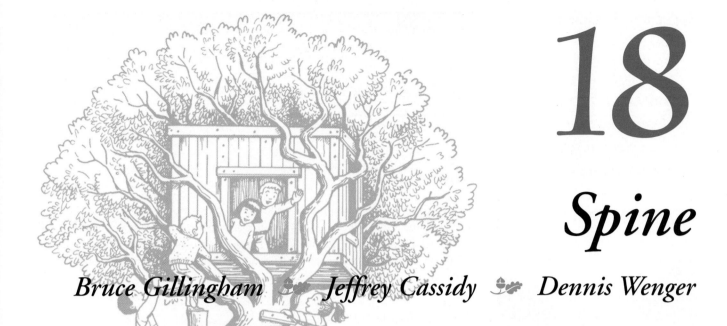

18
Spine

Bruce Gillingham ❦ *Jeffrey Cassidy* ❦ *Dennis Wenger*

INTRODUCTION

Perhaps no injury to the developing skeleton incites as much anxiety in patient and doctor as trauma to the spine. Fortunately, pediatric spine fractures are rare with only 5% of all spinal cord and vertebral column injuries affecting children age 16 and younger. Although uncommon, spine fractures in children can lead to chronic instability, deformity, neurologic sequelae, and posttraumatic stenosis. An extra measure of vigilance is called for in evaluating these injuries because they can often be subtle or even absent on initial radiographs. Successful treatment is based on knowledge of the radiographic, anatomic, and developmental differences between the pediatric and adult spine.

Etiology

The location, pattern, and etiology of a child's spine fracture is primarily dependent on the patient's age at the time of injury (Table 18-1). Birth trauma is the major cause of spinal trauma in children younger than age 2. In patients between the ages of 3 and 8, the most frequent mechanisms of injury are falls, motor vehicle accidents, and child abuse. Children older than 8 years are more commonly injured in motor vehicle accidents, gunshot wounds, or sports including swimming, diving, and surfing.

> *"What people want is not knowledge but certainty"*
> —BERTRAND RUSSELL

Table 18-1	Spine Fractures in Children (United States)	
Age	**Most Common Causes**	
0–2 years	Birth trauma	
3–8 years	Falls, MVA, child abuse	
8 years and older	MVA, sports (swimming, diving, surfing), gunshot wounds	

MVA = Motor vehicle accident.

"Perhaps no injury to the developing skeleton incites as much anxiety in patient and doctor as trauma to the spine"

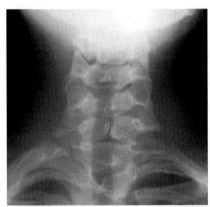

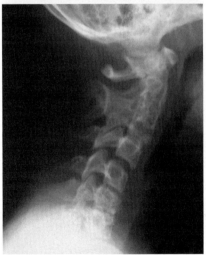

Figure 18-1. Klippel-Feil syndrome includes congenital fusion of two or more cervical vertebrae. The AP view is less diagnostic in this case but does show spina bifida occulta at the C7 level.

"The patterns and types of spine injuries seen in children reflect unique age-related features of the developing spine"

Level of Injury

The majority of spinal column fractures in childhood occur in the thoraco-lumbar spine. Cervical spine fractures in patients 8 years old or younger involve the upper cervical spine (above C4). These most often include the occiput or C1-C2 complex and are more likely to be fatal. Patients older than 8 more typically sustain injures below C4 with a much lower fatality rate.

Applied Anatomy

The patterns and types of spine injuries seen in children reflect unique age-related features of the developing spine.

In children younger than 8 years of age, a number of anatomic factors place the upper cervical spine at greater risk for injury. These include the relatively large head size compared to the body, increased ligamentous laxity, relative strap muscle weakness, and horizontal, shallow facet joints.

In addition, there is increased spinal column elasticity relative to older children and adults. Injuring forces are dissipated over several adjacent motion segments exceeding the elasticity of the spinal cord itself.

Spinal cord injury without associated plain radiographic evidence of bony trauma can occur resulting in the phenomenon known as spinal cord injury without radiographic abnormality (SCIWORA).

Equally perplexing to the uninitiated are several normal developmental features that can be misconstrued as evidence of injury to the spine. Lateral C-spine views in children younger than age 2 years may be hard to interpret because the anterior ring of the C1 vertebra has not yet ossified. Thus the dens-C1 interval cannot be measured. The dento-central synchondrosis of C2, appearing as a lucent line below the level of the body-dens interface, does not usually fuse until about age 6 years and is often confused with an odontoid fracture.

Further complicating matters include congenital and genetic conditions that have cervical spine manifestations. Klippel-Feil syndrome is characterized by congenital fusion of two or more vertebrae (Fig. 18-1). Given the relative lack of motion segments and resultant longer lever arm within the cervical spine, these patients are felt to be at greater risk for fracture. A higher level of scrutiny be given to these patients following trauma.

This is equally true of patients with trisomy 21 (Down's syndrome) whose inherent ligamentous laxity may result in symptomatic atlanto-axial instability and cervical myelopathy. A careful instability assessment with lateral flexion-extension radiographs should be performed. Absence of the characteristic cervical lordosis is seen in up to 14% of patients younger than age 8 and can be misinterpreted as representing injury-related muscle spasm.

Os odontoideum, thought to represent either a failure of fusion of the top of the dens to the body of C2 or a nonunion of an occult fracture, can be difficult to distinguish from an acute fracture. Further evaluation of these patients with advanced imaging should be undertaken if this condition is identified on screening trauma radiographs, as fixation or upper cervical fusion may be required.

After age 8, the spine begins to mature. The ligaments and facet capsules strengthen, the facets become more vertically oriented, and the vertebral bodies become more rectangular. By late childhood the patterns of spinal injury and healing become similar to the adult.

The presence of the vertebral body ring apophysis also presents a challenge in diagnosing spinal column fractures because the injuring force can traverse this cartilaginous growth plate, producing deformity that is unrecognizable on plain films.

In infancy, notching of the anterior and posterior vertebral bodies by vascular channels is common and is easily confused with a vertebral body fracture. The anterior channel generally disappears by age 1, whereas the posterior notch persists throughout life. Many issues make reading infant neck films problematic (Figs. 18-2, 18-3)

Wedge-shaped vertebrae are common up to age 8 and are distinguished from a compression fracture by similar appearance to their neighbors and absence of associated soft tissue findings.

Initial Evaluation

Evaluation of the child with a suspected spinal fracture or spinal cord injury (SCI) depends largely on the setting in which the child is seen. The vast majority of pediatric spinal fractures and SCIs are due to motor vehicle accidents, sports-related injuries, and falls.

The first orthopedic evaluation for most children will occur in the emergency room. Given the increased participation of children in organized sports, a physician may, on occasion, be required to perform an evaluation on the athletic field and to coordinate the safe handling and transport of the potentially spine-injured child to a medical facility.

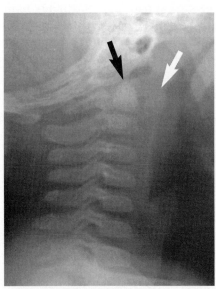

Figure 18-2. Lateral C-spine view in a 3-month-old child. The odontoid or dens (black arrow) is identified, but there is no bone noted anterior to it (white arrow). This is because the anterior ring of C1 has not yet ossified.

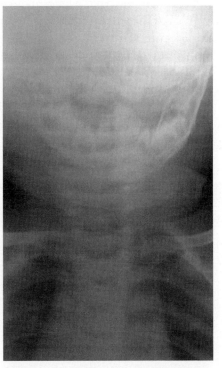

Figure 18-3. Moderate head tilt and rotation seen in an AP view of the C-spine in an infant with torticollis.

On the field, or at the scene of an accident, any children complaining of neck or back pain or transient/prolonged neurologic symptoms must be treated as though they have a spinal injury. Once the airway, breathing, and circulation have been secured, a brief secondary survey can be performed. Early immobilization will help to prevent propagation of a SCI. Because the child's head is relatively large in relation to the body, a spine board with an occipital recess is ideal for transport to ensure proper spinal alignment (Table 18-2). If one is unavailable, any rigid platform with blankets placed beneath the shoulders and trunk will suffice. A pediatric cervical orthosis and sandbags or towels placed on each side of the head will limit further motion. Until the cervical spine is cleared, movement of the patient should only be performed with in-line traction using a logroll technique.

A brief history in the awake, alert, and cooperative child may be very helpful. Any history of numbness, tingling, or brief paralysis or complaint of neck or back pain should alert the physician to the possibility of a SCI. Physical examination begins with inspection of the body for signs of possible trauma to the spine including obvious or subtle deformity, abrasions, edema, or bruising.

Inspection for abdominal wall ecchymosis suggestive of a lap belt injury are important when evaluating a child involved in a motor vehicle accident. Pain or step-off along the spinous processes should raise suspicion. Range of motion of the spine should only be attempted in the awake and cooperative child in which there is no suspicion of an unstable injury.

RADIOGRAPHIC ISSUES

For minor spine trauma, often an AP and lateral view of the affected area will be the only x-rays ordered. For more severe trauma, a more in-depth analysis is required.

Great care should be taken in the evaluation of children who are incapable of verbal communication, who cannot cooperate with the clinical examination, or who have other injuries that may divert their attention from concomitant neck or back pain. These patients must be considered as having a spine injury until proven otherwise. A diligent clinical and radiographic search for injury to the axial spine is required.

The essential first study in these patients is a screening cross-table lateral x-ray of the spine (Figs. 18-4, 18-5). This study, in addition to the AP pelvis and chest x-rays, are considered standard in the evaluation of all trauma patients. It

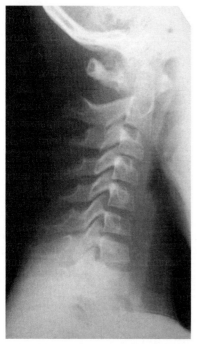

Figure 18-4. Loss of lordosis of the cervical spine may indicate occult injury.

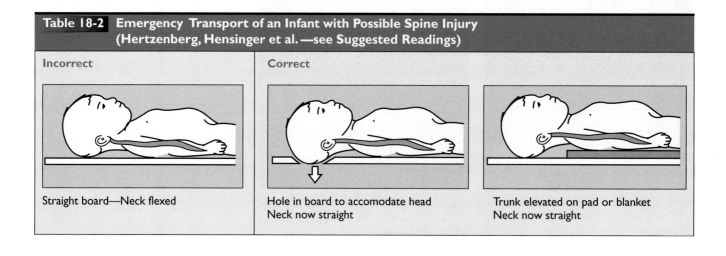

Table 18-2	Emergency Transport of an Infant with Possible Spine Injury (Hertzenberg, Hensinger et al. —see Suggested Readings)

Incorrect	Correct	
Straight board—Neck flexed	Hole in board to accomodate head Neck now straight	Trunk elevated on pad or blanket Neck now straight

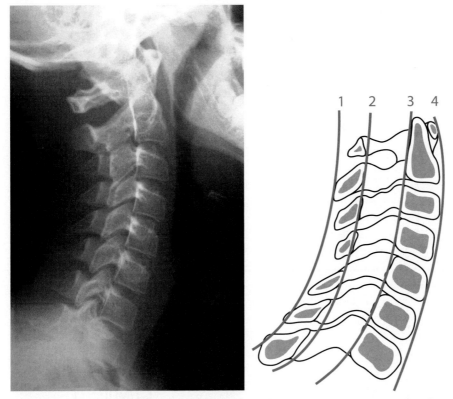

Figure 18-5. Normal alignment of the lateral cervical spine. 1 = spinous process line, 2 = spinolaminar line, 3 = posterior vertebral body line, 4 = anterior vertebral body line. Space available for the cord is the distance between 2 and 3 at the level of C1.

is important to personally review this x-ray for technical adequacy, ensuring that the top of the first thoracic vertebrae is visible. A systematic evaluation of bony alignment (Fig. 18-5), soft tissue parameters, and relationships between key landmarks is then performed (Table 18-3).

Any high-risk patient should have x-rays taken of all symptomatic areas or have a complete spine series if the examiner is unable to focus the evaluation clinically. In the obtunded patient, the spine should be cleared as early as possible to facilitate ICU services. A cervical orthosis and spine board precautions should be maintained until definitive x-ray or clinical clearance is obtained (see flow chart—Simple Algorithm for an Awake Patient).

Table 18-3 Normal Parameters of the Pediatric Cervical Spine	
Parameter	Normal Value
C1 facet-occipital condyle distance	≤ 5 mm
Atlanto-dens interval	≤ 4 mm
Pseudosubluxation of C2 on C3	≤ 4 mm
Pseudosubluxation of C3 on C4	≤ 3 mm
Retropharyngeal space	≤ 8 mm (at C2)
Retrotracheal space	≤ 14 mm (at C6, under age 15)
Torg ratio (canal to vertebral body)	≥ 0.8
Space available for cord	≥ 14 mm

Modified from Black BE. Spine Trauma—see Suggested Readings.

Simple Algorithm for an Awake Patient with C-spine Injury
(neurologically intact)

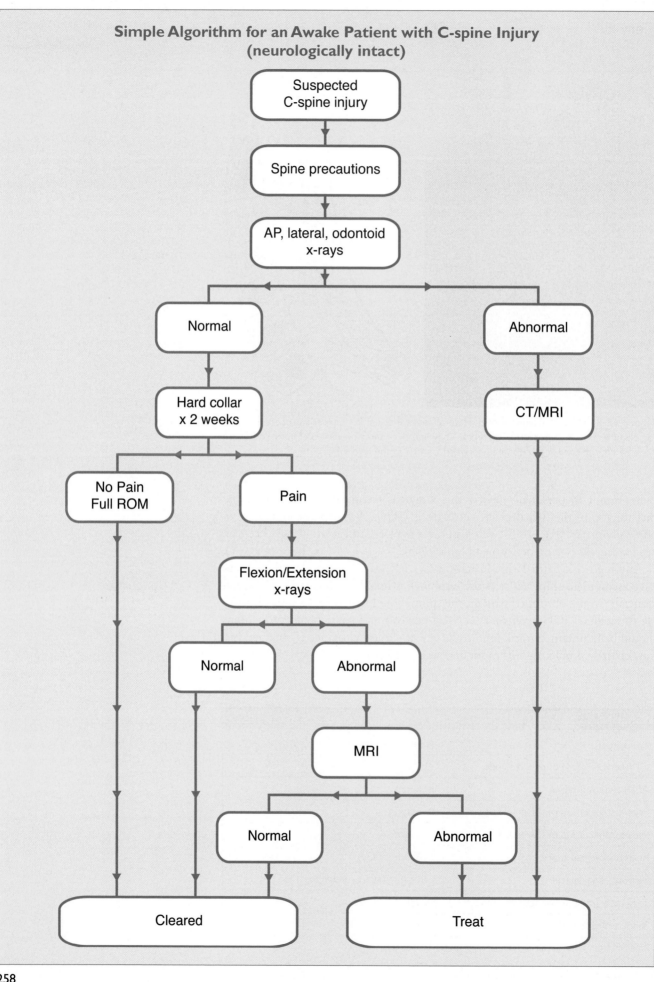

Cervical Spine Imaging

AP and lateral x-rays of the cervical spine will detect greater than 95% of fractures. The open-mouth odontoid view may be a helpful adjunct to detect odontoid and atlas ring fractures (Fig. 18-6), although its usefulness and safety has been questioned. As mentioned previously, the treating physician should be aware of anatomic and physiologic variants unique to the developing cervical spine in order to correctly interpret the images (Fig. 18-7).

If the child is alert and cooperative in the face of negative x-rays and complains of neck pains, flexion/extension views may be used to identify ligamentous injuries (see flow chart). In cases with a high index of suspicion, the physician can personally supervise this study with only active range of motion by the patient assessed. No attempt to "assist" the patient to passively increase the range of motion should be attempted. It is frequently necessary to delay flexion-extension films until the first outpatient visit when muscular soreness has

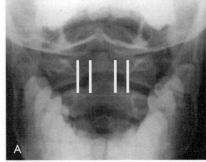
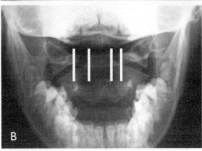

Figure 18-6. Odontoid views. A) Space lateral to the odontoid is symmetric (normal). B) Assymetry of the space lateral to the odontoid can indicate C1-C2 instability. In this case, the child had only muscle spasms.

Common Methods to Immobilize the C-Spine

Soft Collar

"Just do something"

Philidelphia Collar

More immobilization

Aspen Collar

More immoblization

Minerva Type Brace

A serious brace

Braces courtesy of Bluebird Orthotics and Prosthetics—San Diego

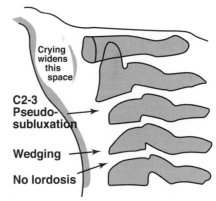

Figure 18-7. Normal findings on a pediatric C-spine film that may be mistaken for pathology.

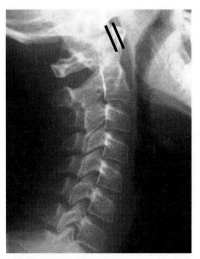
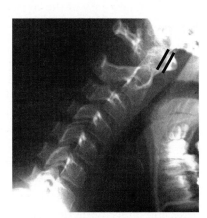

Figure 18-8. X-rays with the C-spine flexed are used to evaluate ligamentous instability. Maintainence of a normal interval between the dens (odontoid) and the ring of C1, as well as no change in vertebral body or posterior element alignment from C1-C7, suggests that the ligaments are intact.

abated (Fig. 18-8). The patient is maintained in a Philadelphia type cervical orthosis for comfort and safety until then.

CT can help to identify occult fractures or to fully characterize fractures that have been identified on plain films. MRI should be obtained to assess the degree of cord injury in any child, with or without fracture, who has neurologic complaints or symptoms, particularly those suspected of having SCIWORA. MRI is also useful in assessing the extent of soft tissue damage in purely ligamentous and cartilaginous injuries.

Thoracic/Lumbar Spine Imaging

AP and lateral views of the thoracic and/or lumbar spine should be obtained in the initial evaluation of any patient suspected of having a thoracic or lumbar spine fracture. CT is the study of choice to evaluate bony architecture or to evaluate suspected injuries to the ring apophysis. As in the cervical spine, an MRI should be obtained in the face of any neurologic signs or symptoms to assess the degree of cord injury and is the imaging modality of choice for suspected cartilaginous and ligamentous injuries.

TREATMENT

With a few exceptions that will be highlighted, the majority of fractures in the pediatric spine can be treated non-operatively. Surgical stabilization should be undertaken in unstable injuries or injuries associated with SCI.

Most cervical injuries are simple strains and require generic treatment (cervical collars are often used and come in a variety of types with varying capacity for immobilization. A halo may be required for a very serious injury.

Antiinflammatories are also used and the patient is followed. Most are greatly improved or asymptomatic within a few weeks. A few have more severe injuries that will take weeks or even months to get well. Confusing the issue are legal cases in which the patient, parents, and attorneys are monitoring the outcome. Children often have a hard time recovering while these stressful events are ongoing.

CERVICAL SPINE INJURIES

Atlanto-occipital Dislocations

Atlanto-occipital dislocations occur almost exclusively in younger children and are associated with the highest rates of closed head injury and mortality in pediatric spine injuries (Fig. 18-9). These injuries were traditionally immediately fatal but modern rapid rescue methods have led to a few survivors. Occipital condyle fracture in association with this injury has been described and should not be overlooked. If the child is neurologically intact, halo immobilization for 2-3 months will be successful in a majority of patients. For children with persistent instability an occiput-to-C1 fusion may be necessary. Children with atlanto-axial dislocation associated with SCI require fusion from occiput to C2.

Atlanto-axial (C1-C2) Injury

C1-C2 is the most common level of injury in the pediatric and adolescent spine (Fig. 18-10). Either a fracture of the odontoid or atlanto-axial dislocation without fracture may occur. Atlanto-axial dislocation without fracture is most likely to occur in children younger than the age of 13. Fracture is more common in children older than 13. Dislocations may be treated with halo immobilization for 3 months, but posterior C1-C2 fusion may be required for those with persistent instability.

Atlas Fractures (C1 Ring)

Fractures in the "ring" of the C1 vertebra (atlas) are uncommon in children and are usually the result of a high-energy mechanism. For stable fractures, immobilization in a rigid cervical collar for 10-12 weeks allows healing. For more severe injuries, or for families who do not have good internal discipline (for brace wear), immobilization in a Minerva jacket or halo for 2-3 months will usually result in complete healing. Immobilization up to 6 months is sometimes required, and surgery is rarely indicated.

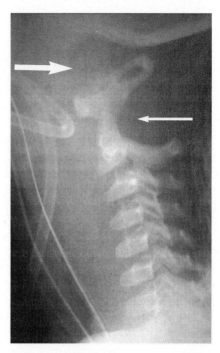

Figure 18-9. Atlanto-occipital dislocations occur almost exclusively in younger children and are associated with the highest rates of closed head injury and mortality in pediatric spine injuries. In this case (fatal), the skull is dissociated from C1 (large arrow) and C1 and C2 are distracted (small arrow).

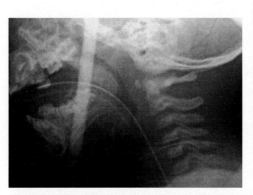 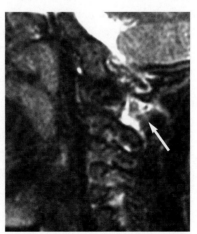

Figure 18-10. This toddler suffered a flexion injury to the C-spine. The MRI study shows posterior ligamentous injury (white arrow) at the C1-C2 level. She was treated with prolonged immobilization.

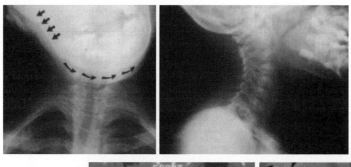
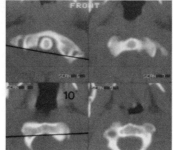
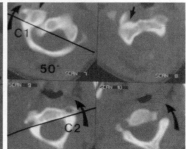

Figure 18-11. Fixed rotary subluxation—C1 on C2. This 6 year old developed a fixed rotary subluxation documented by CT scans. The problem eventually resolved with conservative treatment.

Grisel Syndrome

Trauma versus inflammation or infection as the cause of sudden change in use of the spine may confuse the physician faced with cervical spine pain. Grisel was the first to clarify the relationship between acute torticollis and pharyngitis.

Grisel P. Enucleation des l'atlas et torticollis nasopharyngien. Presse Med 38:50-53, 1930.

Atlanto-axial Rotary Subluxation

The onset of C1-2 rotary subluxation is often spontaneous and manifested by pain, torticollis, and diminished range of motion. Often the result of only minor trauma, Grisel (1930) first noted that the condition often is associated with pharyngitis. In the current era, it often follows ear, nose, and throat procedures and dental procedures in which the patient's head was maintained in an unusual position for a sustained period of time.

Radiographs, particularly the open-mouth odontoid view, will reveal a persistent asymmetry of the odontoid in relation to the atlas. Dynamic CT studies provide the best method for confirming the diagnosis (Fig. 18-11).

For minor cases, treatment consists of a brief period of immobilization in a soft collar, rest, and analgesics. For more significant degrees of subluxation, a brief period of head halter traction accompanied by systemic muscle relaxants such as diazepam may be needed until reduction is achieved. For more severe or longstanding cases in which a fixed subluxation has developed, halo traction or, in extreme cases, surgical reduction with fusion may be needed.

Odontoid Fracture

Fractures of the odontoid process are rare in children and the incidence of associated SCI is low. Treatment should consist of reduction and external immobilization in a halo or Minerva jacket for 3 to 4 months. Surgical intervention is rarely required and has been associated with a high rate of complications.

Hangman Fracture

This morbid terminology follows the understanding that the cause of death in successful hanging is not strangulation but instead traumatic fracture of C2 with associated SCI (Fig. 18-12). The diagnosis of traumatic spondylolisthesis

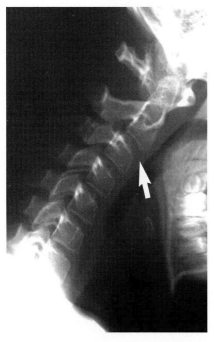

Figure 18-12. Pseudosubluxation C2-C3. Many patients have a normal slight forward positioning of C2 on C3.

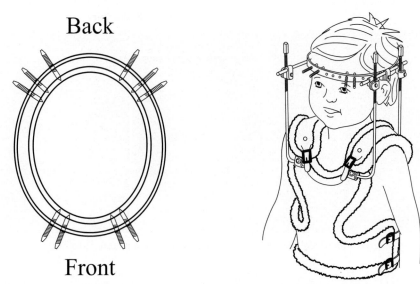

Back

Front

Figure 18-13. Halo application in an infant. Because the skull is soft, multiple pins are required and are tightened with a low torque (initially finger tightened)—then with a torque wrench but not to exceed 4 to 5 inch-pounds of torque. (Mubarak et al.—see Suggested Readings.)

of the axis (C2) may be confounded in children by persistence of a synchondroses until the age of 7.

Additionally, "pseudosubluxation" of C2 on C3 may be mistaken for injury. Anterior subluxation of C2 on C3 of 2 mm or more implies pathologic subluxation and suggests fracture although a CT scan will be needed for confirmation. Treatment should consist of reduction and application of a rigid cervical collar for 2-3 months. For more significant injuries or for poorly disciplined families, immobilization in a halo device (Fig. 18-13) or a Minerva jacket may be necessary.

Middle to Lower Cervical Spine Injuries

Similar to fractures in the upper cervical spine, unstable ligamentous injuries in the middle to lower cervical spine can be successfully treated with external immobilization in either a halo device or Minerva jacket for 3 months. Injuries that remain unstable after 3 months require a posterior fusion. For acute, unstable fractures, as well as fractures associated with SCIs, posterior fusion is required.

THORACIC AND LUMBAR FRACTURES

Compression and Burst Fractures

In general, the inherent elasticity and mobility of the pediatric spine protects children from compression and burst type fracture patterns. As the pediatric spine matures and becomes more adultlike the pattern of injury in adolescents and older children begins to mirror that seen in adults, with an increasing incidence of compression and burst fractures. The patient's relative maturity, degree of deformity, instability, and the presence of SCI are all factors that must be considered in planning treatment.

A working knowledge of the three-column concept of spinal stability developed by Francis Denis is essential to correctly identify and treat thoraco-lumbar spinal instability. He defined three categories of instability (Fig. 18-14, Table 18-4).

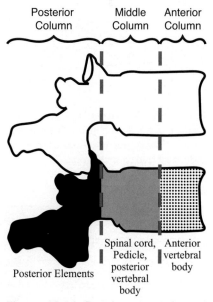

Posterior Column   Middle Column   Anterior Column

Spinal cord, Pedicle, posterior vertebral body

Posterior Elements   Anterior vertebral body

Figure 18-14. Denis' concept of spinal columns. If more then one column is disrupted, stability is compromised.

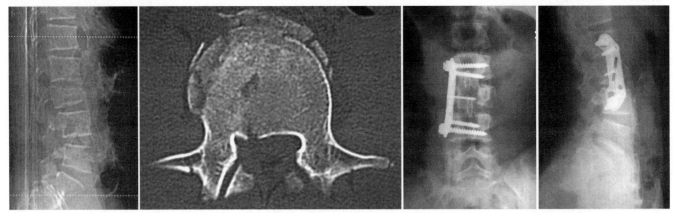

Figure 18-15. L3 burst fracture in a motorcycle racer. Treated with partial corpectomy and anterior instrumentation L2 to L4.

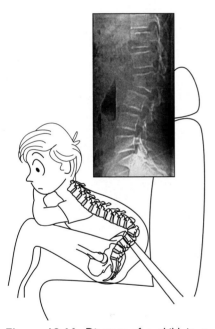

Figure 18-16. Diagram of a child in a seatbelt with a flexion injury that can produce a Chance fracture. Associated intra-abdominal trauma is common.

Bed rest and immobilization are better tolerated in children than in adults. Consequently, stable burst fractures and compression fractures with less than 10° of kyphosis and less than 50% loss of anterior column height can be treated symptomatically. Most children do not require external immobilization and are symptom free in 1-2 weeks but should refrain from sports for at least a month to prevent re-injury. Children with more significant injuries or symptoms may be treated with a brief period of bed rest followed by 4-6 weeks in a cast, a thoraco-lumbo-sacral orthosis (TLSO) for thoracic fractures or a Jewett hyperextension orthosis for lumbar fractures.

With increasing skeletal maturity, the likelihood of improving sagittal alignment by subsequent vertebral growth decreases. For children beyond Risser stage 2 with greater than 10° of kyphosis, the development of progressive deformity in both the sagittal and coronal planes is more likely. For these patients, posterior instrumented fusion should be considered. In addition, it has been shown that children with compression fractures are more likely to develop evidence of disc degeneration on MRI. The role of this phenomenon in guiding treatment is unclear at this time.

As with injuries in the cervical spine, unstable fractures and fractures associated with SCI should be treated with a posterior instrumented fusion (Fig. 18-15). The role of decompression in neurologically compromised patients remains controversial. Patients with incomplete return of neurological status or degrading neurologic function are candidates for decompression. Evidence suggests that early decompression may enhance neurologic recovery. In centers with skilled spine surgeons, decompression and stabilization (even though classic predictors would not suggest neurologic recovery) should be considered. "Miracle" recoveries or partial recoveries are occasionally seen in adults and more often in children.

Table 18-4	Denis Classification of Spinal Column Instability			
Type	**Instability Pattern**	**Example**	**Risk**	**Treatment**
1st degree	Mechanical	Severe compression fracture	Progressive kyphosis	Brace in extension
2nd degree	Neurologic	Ligamentously stable burst fracture susceptible to collapse from axial load	Neurologic injury	Operative stabilization
3rd degree	Mechanical and neurological	Unstable burst fracture, fracture-dislocation	Progressive displacement and neurologic injury	Operative stabilization decompression

Adapted from Denis F. Spinal instability as defined by the 3 column spine concept—see Suggested Readings.

Chance Fractures

Chance fractures, or Chance fracture equivalents, are flexion-distraction injuries. As in adults, they may be purely ligamentous, exclusively bony, or a combination of both types (Table 18-5). Unique to children is the vertebral apophysis in the anterior column, through which the fracture frequently traverses. The association between Chance fractures and lap belt injuries (Fig. 18-16) in motor vehicle accidents has been well documented. Once associated intra-abdominal injuries have been ruled out or treated, treatment of the spinal injury may be planned.

As with compression fractures, stable injuries may be treated in a cast or TLSO as long as an adequate reduction can be obtained and maintained. Purely soft tissue injuries are less likely to respond to conservative treatment. These injuries as well as those associated with a SCI are best treated with a posterior instrumented fusion from one level above to one level below the injury (Fig. 18-17).

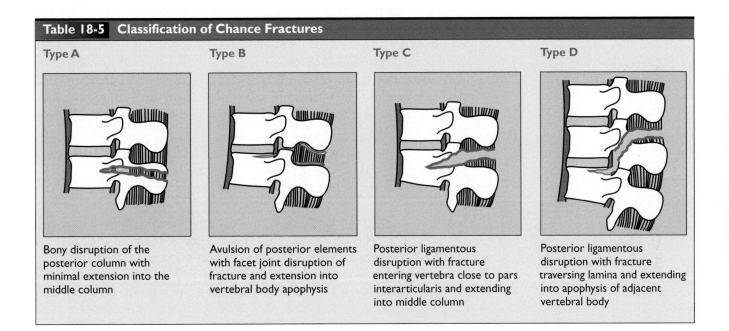

Table 18-5	Classification of Chance Fractures		
Type A	**Type B**	**Type C**	**Type D**
Bony disruption of the posterior column with minimal extension into the middle column	Avulsion of posterior elements with facet joint disruption of fracture and extension into vertebral body apophysis	Posterior ligamentous disruption with fracture entering vertebra close to pars interarticularis and extending into middle column	Posterior ligamentous disruption with fracture traversing lamina and extending into apophysis of adjacent vertebral body

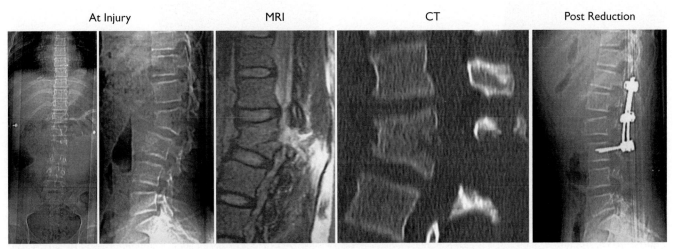

At Injury   MRI   CT   Post Reduction

Figure 18-17. Chance fracture of the L2 vertebra in a teenager. Surgical reduction and stabilization was performed.

Table 18-6	Radiographic Classification of Lumbar Apophyseal Injury	
Type	Age Group	Radiographic Findings
I	11–13 years	Separation of the posterior vertebral rim. Arcuate fragment without osseous defect
II	13–18 years	Avulsion fracture of vertebral body, annular rim, and cartilage
III	≥ 18 years	Localized fracture posterior to end plate irregularity
IV	≥ 18 years	Defect spans entire length and breadth of posterior vertebral margin between endplates

Adapted from Epstein N et al.—see Suggested Readings.

"Fractures of the vertebral ring apophysis are unique to the adolescent spine"

Fractures of the Ring Apophysis

Fractures of the vertebral ring apophysis are unique to the adolescent spine. Typically, a portion of the ring apophysis will be retropulsed into the spinal canal along with herniated disc material. Four age-associated patterns have been described (Table 18-6). Patients will typically present with back and or leg pain after minor injury. Plain films and MRI are often inconclusive, and CT must be used to confirm the diagnosis. Ring apophyseal fracture must be considered in any adolescent presenting with symptoms of lumbar disc herniation. Conservative treatment may consist of rest, analgesics, and physical therapy and bracing but is often ineffective in children. Surgical treatment includes decompression of all herniated material including excision of the bony and cartilaginous fragments and is felt to prevent healing of the lesion to the posterior vertebral body with resultant spinal stenosis.

SPONDYLOLYSIS AND SPONDYLOLISTHESIS

Sudden acute lumbar back pain in an athlete is a common presentation in an ER. The "spondy" conditions are often the cause. A form of "fracture," the condition is really developmental. Spondylolysis and spondylolisthesis, conditions related to weakness and then separation (stress fracture) of the pars interarticularis, most commonly occurs at the L5 level (Fig. 18-18). Symptoms usually develop gradu-

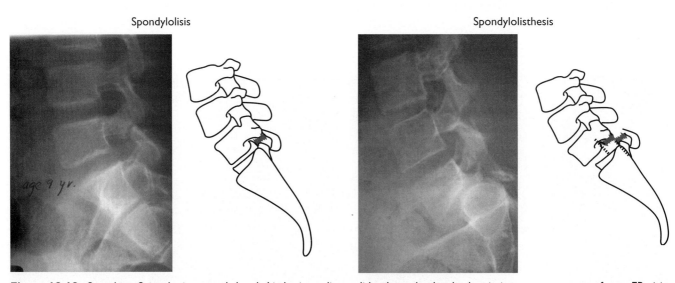

Spondylolisis

Spondylolisthesis

Figure 18-18. Spondy = Spine. Lysis = crack, break. Listhesis = slip or slide. Acute lumbar back pain is a common reason for an ER visit. The "spondy" conditions are a common culprit.

ally and the diagnosis is most common in vigorous young athletes (especially gymnasts). In rare instances, a child can have an acute injury (or acute onset of pain) and present as an emergency. Oblique views of the lumbosacral spine or a CT scan can clarify the diagnosis. Treatment will not be described here.

SPECIAL CONDITIONS

Nonaccidental Trauma—Spine Injuries

Although child abuse is frequently thought of in terms of long bone injury, injury to the axial skeleton and spinal cord is well described in this setting. SCIWORA can be seen as a component of the aptly named "shaken baby syndrome." The infant's large head-to-body ratio and relatively weak cervical musculature likely predispose the defenseless child to this injury as a result of repetitive hyperextension and flexion forces. Evidence of neurologic deficit should be carefully sought in infants evaluated for nonaccidental trauma, as this condition can be easily unappreciated in this age group.

A team approach is essential to thoroughly evaluate these patients in a comprehensive, systematic manner, with Child Protective Services notified immediately. A thorough orthopedic evaluation, including a skeletal survey that includes a lateral spine x-ray is essential in this setting. Consideration should also be given to obtaining MRI images of the spinal cord at the time of intra-cranial imaging if indicated by the clinical circumstances.

Thoraco-lumbar and lumbar injuries are most common in mid-childhood. As with long bone fractures, spine fractures at different stages of healing are highly specific for nonaccidental trauma. Fracture-dislocations and multiple compression fractures may also be seen. Specific treatment is based on the injury pattern present.

Spinal Cord Injury

The characteristic patterns of SCI in children are fundamentally different than that seen in adults. Children sustain a disproportionately higher incidence of upper cervical and thoracic spine injuries, a higher proportion of complete neurologic injuries, and a much higher incidence of spinal cord injury without plain film evidence of spinal column injury (SCIWORA). In addition, when an injury to the spinal column occurs in association with SCI it is often difficult to detect on plain x-ray. Most SCI in children younger than age 16 years results from falls and motor vehicle accidents.

Following the initial trauma assessment and identification and resolution of life-threatening conditions, a meticulous baseline neurologic evaluation is performed and documented. Serial examinations should then be planned in order to identify neurologic deterioration should it occur. In those patients capable of understanding and communicating with the examiner, a history of transient paresthesia, numbness, or paralysis should be sought, as this may be the only clue to an occult SCI. Immobilization of the spinal column should be maintained until clinical and radiographic clearance is obtained.

The use of methylprednisolone should be considered if the patient arrives less than 8 hours following injury, although the efficacy of this treatment is unproven in children younger than 13 years of age. GM-1 ganglioside, a glycolipid found at high levels in the cell membranes of mammalian nervous system cells with known neuroprotective and neuro-functional restorative properties, has also demonstrated the potential to enhance functional recovery in SCI patients.

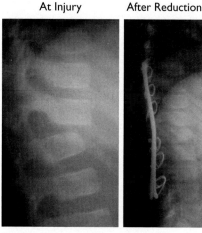

At Injury After Reduction

Figure 18-19. This 8-year-old boy presented with complete paralysis distal to T12 due to fracture dislocation. He was emergently reduced and stabilized and was walking (with Fott orthosis) by 4 months. It is best to err on the side of overtreatment (surgical reduction) in children who have great potential for recovery from spinal cord injury.

"The mechanism of spinal cord injury presumably occurs due to the inherent immaturity and elasticity of the spinal column relative to the relatively fixed spinal cord"

The prognosis for children with a SCI is better for incomplete lesions, although up to 20% of patients with a complete SCI experience significant recovery.

Three patterns of MRI signal in acute SCI have been described (Table 18-7). In general, laminectomy alone should be avoided as this contributes to increased instability with the subsequent development of localized kyphosis. Laminectomy, cord decompression, and instrumented fusion can be considered in cases with potential for neurologic recovery (Fig. 18-19).

Children who are preadolescents at the time of injury are at significant risk for developing scoliosis following SCI, irrespective of the level of neurologic injury, and are more likely to develop a severe scoliosis (Fig. 18-20). The presence of spasticity is also a significant risk factor. The development of sagittal plane deformity, especially lumbar kyphosis, is also common. Initial treatment should consist of bracing and fabrication of a wheel chair seating system. The primary goal of treatment is maintenance of sitting balance in order to prevent decubitus ulcers and to preserve independent upper extremity use. Vigilant skin care is essential to avoid pressure sores from the brace. Instrumentation and fusion are often needed but ideally should be delayed until the child is mature enough to allow for posterior segmental instrumentation alone (no longer at risk for postfusion progressive deformity due to the crank-shaft phenomenon.

Late neurologic deterioration has been reported in children who sustain a SCI. Posttraumatic syrinx should be searched for with an MRI and, if present, surgically corrected.

Spinal Cord Injury Without Radiographic Abnormality

As originally described, the syndrome of SCIWORA is diagnosed in patients with objective findings of myelopathy following trauma without evidence of skeletal injury or subluxation on plain films, tomography, or myelography. The syndrome was described prior to the use of MRI for diagnosis.

The mechanism of SCI presumably occurs due to the inherent immaturity and elasticity of the spinal column relative to the relatively fixed spinal cord. Significant but self-reducing intersegmental displacements of the spine due to flexion, extension, or distraction forces cause SCI without associated vertebral column disruption.

The condition is most common in children younger than 8 years of age. These younger patients sustain more serious neurologic damage and suffer a larger number of upper cervical cord lesions than children over the age of eight. Up to half of the patients have delayed onset of paralysis, occurring as long as 4 days after injury. Of particular importance to the initial treating physician,

Table 18-7	MRI Patterns on T2 Weighted Images of Acute Spinal Cord Injuries	
Type	Findings	
I	Decreased signal due to intraspinal hemorrhage	
II	Bright signal due to spinal cord edema	
III	Mixed signal: central hypointensity and peripheral hyperintensity due to contusion	

Adapted from Bondurant FJ et al.—see Suggested Readings.

most of these children experienced transient paresthesia, numbness, or subjective paralysis at the time of injury. Occult instability with subsequent repetitive insults is one possible explanation for this phenomenon. Careful evaluation is therefore critical in this setting to identify the underlying cord injury and source of instability and to provide appropriate spinal stabilization to avoid preventable progression.

Further evidence for occult instability as a cause of delayed SCIWORA is the phenomenon of recurrent injury. In one series, a trivial injury after an initial mild SCIWORA resulted in a second episode of the condition several weeks later.

Radiographic evaluation includes initial plain films and an MRI. The MRI, which allows assessment for occult ligamentous and disc injury and the status of the spinal cord, has served to invalidate the SCIWORA terminology.

Clinically, the most reliable predictor of neurologic outcome is the initial neurologic status. An initial severe neural injury is almost always associated with a poor prognosis, whereas an initially mild to moderate injury is compatible with good recovery. MRI findings are also highly correlated with prognosis. A poor outcome is predictable if there is evidence of cord transection and major hemorrhage, a moderate to good recovery is observed when minor hemorrhage or edema only is present, and a complete recovery occurs in those patients without abnormal cord signal.

The orthopedist's role is to rule out occult fractures and subluxation requiring surgical fusion, identifying patients likely to have delayed deterioration and preventing recurrent cord trauma by initiating and rigidly enforcing a strict neck immobilization program. It is recommended that a well-fitted custom cervical orthosis that is difficult for the child to remove by him/herself be worn for up to 12 weeks in patients who have sustained a mild to moderate form of this injury. These patients are inclined to discontinue bracing and attempt to return to their usual activities prior to complete healing. They are therefore at greatest risk for recurrent injury. Late instability should be ruled out with dynamic cervical spine x-rays prior to clearing a patient for return to regular activities, especially sports.

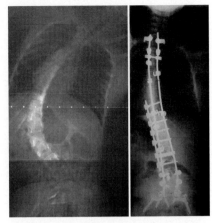

Figure 18-20. Progressive scoliosis has been reported in children who sustain a spinal cord injury. This child went on to require anterior/posterior spinal fusion.

CONCLUSION

A thorough knowledge of the developmental characteristics of the pediatric spine will greatly assist the treating physician. An understanding of the differences between the immature spine and that of the adult is fundamental to correctly diagnosing and treating pediatric spinal trauma. Fortunately, childhood spinal trauma is rare and good outcomes are the rule in these resilient patients.

The views expressed in this chapter are those of the authors and do not reflect the official policy or position of the Department of the Navy, Department of Defense, or the United States Government.

Suggested Reading

Bondurant, F.J.; Cotler, H.B.; Kulkarni, M.V.; McArdle, C.B.; and Harris, J.H.: Acute Spinal Imaging. Spine, 15:161-168, 1990.

Brown, R.L.; Brunn, M.A.; and Garcia, V.F.: Cervical spine injuries in children: a review of 103 patients treated consecutively at a level 1 pediatric trauma center. J Pediatric Surg, 36(8): 1107-14, 2001.

Cattell, H.S.; and Filtzer, D.L.: Pseudosubluxation and other normal variations in the cervical spine in children. J Bone Joint Surg, 47:1295-1309, 1965.

Copley, L.A.; and Dormans, J.P.: Cervical spine disorders in infants and children. J Am Acad Orthop Surg, 6: 204-214, 1998.

Cullen, J.C.: Spinal Lesions in Battered Babies. J Bone Joint Surg, 57-B:364-366, 1975.

Dearolf, W.W.; Betz, R.R.; Vogel, L.C.; Levin, J.; Clancy, M.; and Steel, H.H.: Scoliosis in Pediatric Spinal Cord—Injured patients. J Pediatric Orthop, 10: 214-218, 1990.

Denis, F.: Spinal Instability as Defined by the Three-column Spine Concept in Acute Spinal Trauma. Clin Orthop, 189: 65-76, 1984.

Grabb, P.A.; and Pang, D.: Magnetic Resonance Imaging in the Evaluation of Spinal Cord Injury without Radiographic Abnormality in Children. Neurosurgery, 35: 406-414, 1994.

Herzenberg J, Hensinger R, Dedrick D, Phillips W. Emergency transport and positioning of young children who have an injury of the cervical spine: the standard backboard may be hazardous. J Bone Joint Surg 1989;71:15-22.

Lalonde, F.; Letts, M.; Yang J.P.; and Thomas, K.: Analysis of burst fractures of the spine in adolescents. Am J Orthop, 30(2): 115-21, 2001.

Mubarak SJ, Camp JF, Vuletich W, Wenger DR, Garfin SR. Technique: Halo application in the infant. J Pediatric Orthop, 9:612-614.

Odent, T.; Langlais, J.; Glorion, C.; Kassas, B.; et al.: Fractures of the odontoid process: a report of 15 cases in children younger than 6 years. J Pediatr Orthop, 19(1): 51-4, 1999.

Reid, A.B.; Letts, R.M.; and Black, G.B.: Pediatric Chance fractures: association with intra-abdominal injuries and seatbelt use. J Trauma, 30(4): 384-91, 1990.

Takata K, Inoue S-I, Takahashi K, Ohtsuka Y. Fracture of the Posterior Margin of a Lumbar Vertebral Body. J Bone Joint Surg 1988;70(4):589-594.

19

Fractures in Special Circumstances

(Vascular-Compartment Problems, Nonaccidental Trauma, Pathologic Fractures)

Mercer Rang ❧ *Dennis Wenger* ❧ *Scott Mubarak*

VASCULAR AND COMPARTMENT PROBLEMS

On the battlefield, arterial injuries are transported, and the decision to expose the artery is already partly made. The amputation rate is only 13% because of prompt expert repair. For closed fractures with arterial damage, the amputation rate is up to 50% because of late diagnosis.

In fractures with arterial injury, the maximal permissible interval between injury and repair is about 6-8 hours, depending on the degree of arterial occlusion, the state of the collaterals, and shock. These 6-8 hours may pass quickly while the patient is given narcotics and a doctor is found to split the cast. The doctor always realizes there is trouble but seems unable to act immediately and decisively, hoping that the situation will miraculously improve.

Slowly, the doctor comes to appreciate that hope is not enough and calls for an arteriogram or transfers the case to another hospital. Every minute should

> *"Every great mistake has a halfway moment, a split second when it can be recalled and perhaps remedied"*
> —*PEARL BUCK*

"Unfortunately, in the emergency room, a child with a fracture with ischemia is not startlingly different from a child with a simple fracture"

count, because invisible changes are taking place in the muscles and nerves of the limb. Yet in almost all the patients we have cared for, hours have been frittered away. Successful care comes from a high index of suspicion and early arterial repair. Successful care produces a normal limb; delay produces a Volkmann's contracture or gangrenous limb.

Physical Signs

Unfortunately, in the emergency room, a child with a fracture with ischemia is not startlingly different from a child with a simple fracture. A crying child, with a limb swathed in splints and bandage, and surrounded by distraught relatives, is not easily viewed with cool, clinical detachment. A quick squeeze of a protruding digit or nail bed for capillary filling is often considered sufficient to demonstrate an intact circulation. Demonstrate the fallacy of this sign next time you operate. Inflate the tourniquet before the limb is exsanguinated. Squeeze the digit: capillary return is still present. This test only indicates that blood is present in the limb and not that it is circulating.

In recent years, the guesswork has been taking from these problems by direct measurement of compartment tissue pressure and by the use of Doppler pulse meters.

The Three Faces of Arterial Occlusion

If occlusion is not recognized on admission, there is usually a considerable delay before anyone notices it. A child's ischemic pain may be borne stoically by the staff and attributed to fracture pain or be clouded by opiate. Pulses are hidden by a cast or traction so that observation is difficult. Remember that a splinted limb should be relatively painless. Pain after reduction should be attributed to ischemia until proven otherwise. A special trap is painless ischemia in a child with a nerve palsy.

Complete Arterial Occlusion

The pulse is absent, the veins are empty, and in the course of an hour or two the limb becomes white and cold. Failure of nerve conduction produces glove and stocking anesthesia and paralysis. After a few more hours, rigor mortis results in the muscles shortening, and attempts to overcome this are painful. Pain is extreme. Later, the skin becomes marbled, and gangrene follows.

ISCHEMIC MUSCULAR PARALYSES AND CONTRACTURES

Richard Volkmann, 1881
(Halle, Saxony, Germany)

"For many years I have been drawing attention to the fact that the paralyses and contractures of the limbs which sometimes follow bandages applied too tightly, do not arise, as was assumed, through paralysis of the nerves by pressure, but through wholesale and swift disintegration of the contractile substance and the resultant reaction and regeneration. The paralysis and contracture should be understood to have their origin in the muscle."

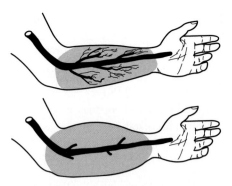

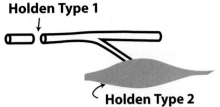

Holden Type 1

Holden Type 2

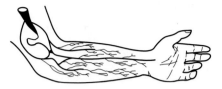

Figure 19-1. Volkmann's ischemia. A) Normally the pressure in the brachial artery is 120 torr. Muscle is perfused at a pressure of 30 torr. B) Muscle ischemia. If the pressure within the muscle compartment is raised about 30 torr, muscle will not be perfused, but the radial pulse is not necessarily occluded.

Figure 19-2. Compartment ischemia may be due to arterial injury or to increased compartment pressure.

Figure 19-3. Compensated occlusion. Anastomotic channels maintain perfusion at low pressure and sufficient to sustain the tissue but insufficient to produce a pulse at the wrist. The pulsations have been abolished, but the flow remains. If an eponym had been attached to this condition it would be diagnosed infrequently.

Incomplete Occlusion—Compartment Ischemia

Ischemia of muscle, called Volkmann's ischemia (Fig. 19-1), is compatible with an intact pulse and adequate peripheral circulation. The first signs are pain in the muscle and pain on stretching the muscle. For this reason, we do not give strong analgesics to children with fractures that have a reputation for vascular problems. Compartment ischemia may be a sequel to an arterial injury (Holden Type I) or to direct compartment injury (Holden Type II) (Fig. 19-2). Frequently, there is sufficient arterial flow to maintain a pulse and distal circulation, but the muscles and nerves become hypoxic and damaged. The outcome of muscular ischemia is a Volkmann's contracture. Compartment syndromes will be described in more detail later.

Compensated Occlusion

This is most often seen in the child with a supracondylar fracture who has an adequate distal circulation but no pulse (Fig. 19-3). The extremity may be a little cool, but there are no signs of nerve or muscle ischemia. Despite occlusion of the major artery, the collaterals maintain an adequate circulation. The best treatment is immediate reduction. Apart from worrying and ordering an hourly check on sensation and movement, there is nothing special to do. A Doppler can be used to detect a faint pulse. Arteriography and exploration are meddlesome. Within a few weeks the pulse returns, and we have yet to see a child with claudication in this circumstance.

Sites of Fracture Associated with Vascular Damage

Although any fracture carries the hazard of vascular damage, the problem is most likely in supracondylar fractures, elbow dislocations, fractures of the shaft of the femur, especially the distal one-third (Fig. 19-4), dislocation of the knee, fractures of the proximal tibia physis, grossly displaced fractures of the ankle and talus, and midtarsal dislocations.

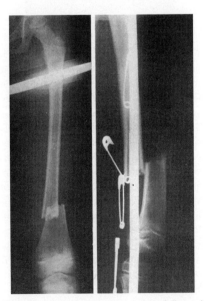

Figure 19-4. In the hour that followed this injury, the leg became cold, white, anesthetic, and weak. The pulse was absent. After the fracture was reduced under general anesthesia, the veins became full and the foot warm and pink. The pulse did not return for several weeks. The femoral artery passes through the adductor opening at this site, where it is liable to injury.

The Nature of the Arterial Lesion

The incidence of arterial damage, as distinct from ischemia, in fractures is not known.

Lesions in Discontinuity. There is completely transsection of the vessel.

Lesions in Continuity: Intimal Lesions. Intimal tears and contusions can only be diagnosed with confidence by arteriotomy. The distal part of the vessel is empty and stringlike. The condition is indistinguishable from spasm until the intima is inspected.

Spasm. Traction has been shown experimentally to produce spasm. Application of this observation has reduced the incidence of Volkmann's ischemia in fractures of the femoral shaft. However, in the past, the importance of "temporary spasm" has been greatly overplayed at the cost of many limbs.

Compression. The most common causes of ischemia are undoubtedly tight casts and deformity at the fracture site. Release the cast or align the limb, and the circulation comes bounding back. Kinking and stretching of vessels has been convincingly demonstrated after high tibial osteotomy.

Thrombosis. Prolonged occlusion owing to any cause will produce propagating thrombosis.

Aneurysm. After a few days or weeks, the site of the fracture becomes painful, red, swollen, and warm—like an infection—but when it is drained, there is a gush of blood. The aneurysm may be caused by a partial tear of the artery at the time of fracture; by the end of a pin, drill, or screw; or by a mycotic infection. Small vessels may be tied off, but major vessels require a graft (Fig. 19-5).

Whenever you embark on releasing a hematoma, bear in mind that it may be a false aneurysm. Listen for a bruit; consider an arteriogram. Check on the whereabouts of your vascular surgeon before you start, just in case you will need help.

Management

Prevention

Traction, tight casts, excessive flexion of a swollen elbow, and hypotension all produce ischemia in the absence of an arterial injury at the time of fracture. Be vigilant, be quick, and be decisive. If you are lucky, removing bandages, bivalving the cast, and placing the limb in a dependent position may be enough to improve circulation. If you are the resident, get on and do this; don't call your chief first, however precious the patient or the reduction.

Treatment of Limb Ischemia

If the circulation does not improve rapidly, you must make preparations to take the child to the operating room immediately. As soon as diagnosis of ischemia is reached, it is obviously a matter of extreme urgency, and you must not be put off by any other service commitments or by anesthetists telling you that the child has a full stomach. You should carry out surgery with the help of a vascular surgeon. However, in civilian practice, vascular surgeons do not have much experience with the problem, and you cannot look to him or her to make all the decisions. His or her greatest experience is in the treatment of vascular disease in the elderly. The new group of microvascular surgeons may be your best ally.

Treatment Steps—Limb Ischemia

Arteriography. Arteriography is only of value if it can be carried out immediately: do not waste time rounding up staff. Arteriography always takes at least

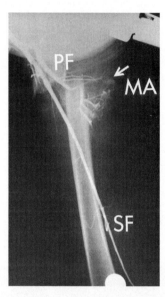

Figure 19-5. Mycotic aneurysm of profundus femoris. This 7-year-old girl was hit by a truck. She sustained a fracture of the femur (treated by 90-90 traction) and a severe head injury, which resulted in her being unconscious for a month. During this time she was pyrexial at times and then developed multiple staphylococcal abscesses, which required drainage. The mycotic aneurysm attracted attention because of swelling and repeated hemorrhages. Embolization failed and the vessel was tied off. Infection is a risk in multiple injuries because of poor nutrition and a plethora of needles and tubes. Antibiotics are wise. PF, profunda femoris; MA, mycotic aneurysm; SF, superficial femoral artery.

an hour, whatever you are told, and in most cases this time could be better spent relieving ischemia. It will demonstrate the site of occlusion, although it will probably not disclose the type of lesion. The site of occlusion is usually opposite the fracture site. In one case, we suspected that the cause of ischemia may have been tight bandaging; however, the arteriogram showed an intimal tear opposite the fracture site.

Jim, aged 8, went down the hill on his friend's bike so quickly that he was unable to use the brakes on the handlebars and hit a truck, fracturing the left femur. The circulation was unremarkable and he was placed in traction. The following morning the leg was found to be white, anesthetic, and cold. An arteriogram showed obstruction of the superficial femoral artery (Fig. 19-6A). At a later phase, the distal part of the artery filled slowly through collaterals (Fig. 19-6B). The appearances indicated a block in the femoral artery with a distal compartment syndrome.

A femoral arteriotomy in the groin was carried out; Fogarty catheters were passed the popliteal artery, and the clot was removed. Subcutaneous fasciotomy of three compartments of the leg was carried out. The skin became warm and pink, but the pulse did not return.

Thirty-six hours later the circulation deteriorated and the leg looked like white marble. It looked like the end. Another arteriogram (Fig. 19-6C) showed an intimal tear at the fracture site and a block at the popliteal trifurcation (Fig. 19-6D). The leg was laid open through a Henry approach from groin to ankle. After excision of the damaged section of the femoral artery, Fogarty catheters were passed under vision to the ankle through the anterior and posterior tibial arteries.

"Ideally arterial damage should be recognized early and repaired before irreversible complications occur"

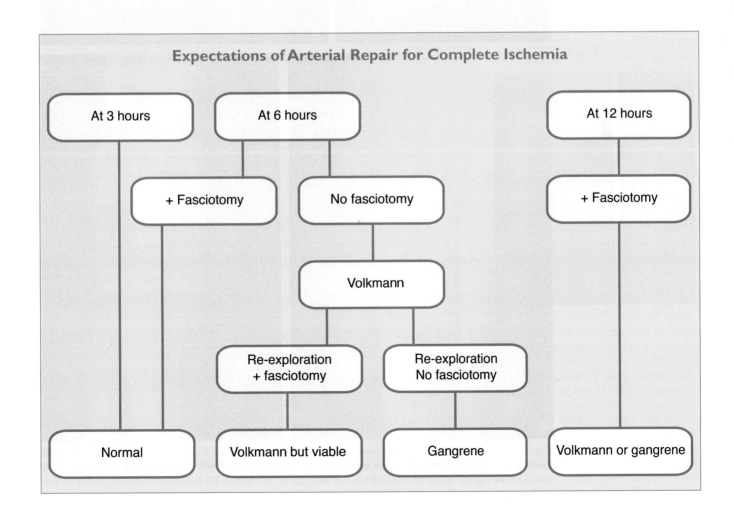

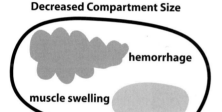

Decreased Compartment Size

hemorrhage

muscle swelling

Increased Volume of Contents

Figure 19-8. Mechanisms of compartment hypertension.

Note-Keeping and Public Relations. Parents of children in whom ischemia is noticed late usually believes that this catastrophe is somebody's fault, and often they are right. These cases usually go to litigation. Keep scrupulous notes; every time you see the child, record your findings and note the time. Put down everything; nothing is too insignificant. In all probability, you will rely on these notes in court. You or your colleague will need all the help that only pages and pages of notes will provide.

Request Your Colleagues' Advice, As Needed. Not only may this be helpful, but their written notes may be useful as well. If the case is referred to you, you should keep in touch with the original doctor. Do not jump to the conclusion that it is all his or her fault. Do not write inspired opinions about the quality of prior care. If you do, you will usually be wrong, and certainly damage not only to your colleagues' reputation but also your own.

The Aftermath. In a few days, you will know whether a normal limb may be expected or whether amputation or reconstruction will be required. The reward of early repair will be a normal limb. Wet gangrene usually requires early amputation and secondary suture. In children, it is worth skin grafting a stump in order to preserve length, particularly if it allows you to save the knee joint.

COMPARTMENT SYNDROMES

A rise in the pressure within a closed compartment may tamponade the muscles and nerves so that they become ischemic. Muscles are normally perfused by blood at a pressure of about 30 torr in a compartment with a tissue pressure of 3 torr to 4 torr. If the compartment pressure exceeds 30 torr, the muscle will receive no blood, but the main arteries will not be compressed, the pulse will get through (Fig. 19-8).

In everyday life, compartment pressure often exceeds 30 torr for a few minutes at a time. When making a fist, the muscle becomes hard, the pressure rises, and the muscle loses its circulation for a time.

You may have noticed the effects when applying a cast on a leg. Have you noticed how your assistant, who is grasping the toes, always drops the leg just before you have finished? This is because your assistant's forearm muscles are ischemic all the time he or she grips; when the limit is reached, the leg is dropped.

The science of compartment syndromes has been much advanced by experimental models. The anterior compartment of a dog's leg can be injected with blood to raise the pressure. Studies of nerve and muscle show that irreversible changes begin after 6-8 hours of ischemia. After 24 hours, the muscle shows only slight histologic changes, despite the fact that it is dead and will undergo necrosis later. Muscle damage is related to the duration of ischemia. Nerve damage is related to the compartment pressure. At first there is loss of conduction, which quickly returns when the pressure is lowered, but prolonged compression causes nerve degeneration.

Compartment pressures may be measured by several techniques (Fig. 19-9). The wick or slit catheter is very satisfactory; however, special catheters are not always available. A very suitable replacement is an epidural catheter (from the anesthesia department), which has holes in the sidewall at the tip. Special patented bedside units have been developed but are expensive and fragile. We no longer use them. With a suspected compartment syndrome, we prefer to have the help of the anesthesia department who routinely monitors arterial and venous pressures. They have the equipment. We do this in the ER, OR, or ICU with a large bone needle inserted into the compartment and an epidural catheter then inserted within the needle. Anesthesia then hands you the fluid-filled line, which is attached to their pressure monitors. You can manually com-

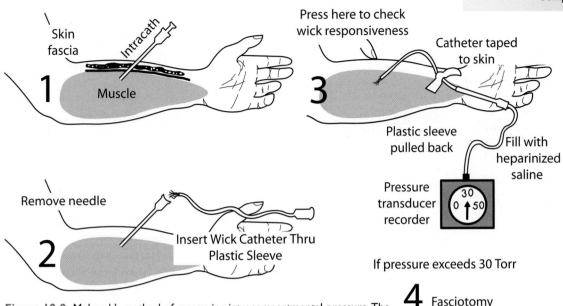

Figure 19-9. Mubarak's method of measuring intracompartmental pressure. The "wick" or "slit" end may not be available. The anesthesia department can provide an epidural catheter, which has many small holes in the side wall of the distal tip of the catheter.

press the compartment, with the catheter in place, to show a fluid wave on the monitoring screen, to assume that you are in the compartment and that the equipment is functioning

However, whichever you choose, you should become familiar with one technique before you are confronted by a problem case. We usually measure pressure in children under general anesthesia, but it can be done using local anesthesia. Do not inject a local anesthetic into the muscle.

Why measure the pressure? If you rely on clinical signs alone, you will do fasciotomies too late and too infrequently. Numbers galvanize you into action and will carry weight in your struggle to get into the operating room quickly.

What should you do if you believe that a child has a compartment syndrome, but the pressure in both deep and superficial compartments are normal? Check the equipment. Repeat the test in an hour or two. If technology continues to contradict common sense, do a fasciotomy despite the pressure numbers.

Differential Diagnosis of a Compartment Syndrome

Fracture pain, a lonely child, an arterial injury, and a nerve palsy may each resemble a compartment syndrome. A Doppler pulse measurement and a pressure measurement will distinguish these.

Care of Compartment Syndrome

On suspicion of a compartment syndrome, the cast and padding should be split to the skin and spread apart widely (bivalved). There is a lot to be said for taking the front of the cast off to be 100% certain that there are no edges digging in. An acutely flexed elbow should be straightened. This is a time to forget the reduction. Contact the parents so that that you do not have to hang around waiting for a consent for the next stage. Elevate the part to the level of the heart

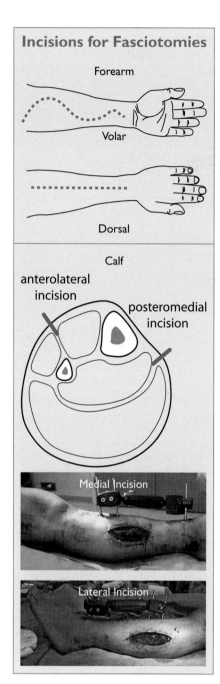

Incisions for Fasciotomies

Forearm

Volar

Dorsal

Calf

anterolateral incision

posteromedial incision

Medial Incision

Lateral Incision

but not above. Does the compartment feel hard? If after 30 minutes decreased sensation or pain on stretching muscles remains, plan to measure the pressure preferably under general anesthesia.

Carry out a fasciotomy if the pressure measured by wick catheter extends 30 torr.

Upper Limb

The deep flexor compartment is usually affected. The extensor compartment is affected in 20% of cases. Measure the pressure in the extensor as well as the deep flexor compartment. The fasciotomy should extend above the elbow into the palm; always open the carpal tunnel. Expose the median nerve and the radial artery. Open the fascia over profundus and flexor pollicis longus.

Do not try to close the wound—little stitches just cut in. The edges can be drawn together with Steri-strips or a skin staple—rubber band weave method. With Steri-strips, the edges can be pulled further together at 1, 2, and 3 weeks, by which time closure succeeds. Stitches cut out or leave railway-track scars; the strips are much better. In some cases, the patient can be taken to the OR for delayed primary closure. Skin grafts are sometimes needed.

Lower Limb

Use the catheter to decide which compartments need opening—peroneal, anterior, superficial posterior, or deep posterior. There are several techniques available. We prefer a medial and lateral incision; the medial incision opens the posterior compartments between the tibia and the gastrocsoleus; the lateral incision opens the anterior tibial and peroneal compartments. They should be opened widely.

NON-ACCIDENTAL TRAUMA

Although assault has been a criminal offense for centuries when directed toward adults, it has only in the last hundred years been considered an offense when directed against children. The first action brought on behalf of a battered child took place in New York City in 1870. Mary Ellen was being beaten daily by her parents. Attempts to correct this situation by appeals to the police and to the District Attorney's office were unsuccessful. Eventually, an action was brought by the American Society for Prevention of Cruelty to Animals, which succeeded because Mary Ellen was certainly a member of the animal kingdom and was being cruelly abused.

Today, child abuse is a major pediatric problem. Physical abuse affects about 225 children per million of population. Two percent to 3% of abused children die; the mortality rate of battering is equal to or greater than that of leukemia. Why a parent should want to injure or kill their own offspring remains a deep philosophical question. Much thinking has been devoted to the topic. Interestingly, animals (dogs, lions, domestic cats) sometimes willfully abandon or kill their offspring. Thus parental, imposed injury may represent a poorly understood innate biological element. In most cases, simple explanations can be found (high family stress, poverty, poor family support, separation of parents, psychological or psychiatric disorders).

The gradual recognition that the cause of unexplained multiple fractures in children was the result of abuse was slow to penetrate the medical conscience. Prior to 1950, children with multiple fractures and a subdural hematoma were thought to perhaps have a metabolic bone disorder (Caffey). Reading these early descriptions, in the light of modern understanding, is frightening. In

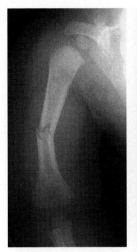
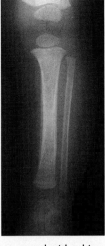
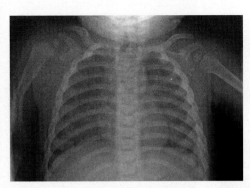
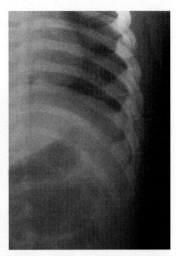

Figure 19-10. This infant presented with a history that she slipped off a bathroom counter while having a bath. She had a humeral fracture, a tibial fracture (in a later stage of healing), and multiple rib fractures. This is diagnostic of nonaccidental trauma.

1954, Kempe coined the term "the battered child syndrome," and received wide medical and lay press exposure, leading to our understanding of the disorder.

Each year, each of our institutions (The Hospital for Sick Children, Toronto, Children's Hospital—San Diego) treats several hundred abused children. The incidence of child battering is three times as great as that of congenital dislocation of the hip or of clubfoot. Failure to recognize that a fracture in a young child is due to abuse can be fatal. If the child is treated as a straightforward fracture and sent home, he/she may be killed (by the abuser). Each of our orthopedic departments has suffered through this tragic sequence in our early years.

Recognition of Abuse

Battered children may come to the hospital with head injuries; with visceral injuries, fractures, or bruises; or with all of these (Fig. 19-10). Twenty-five percent to 50% of abused children have fractures. The humerus, femur, and tibia are the most commonly fractured long bones. The corner or bucket-handle type fracture was thought to be the most common pattern, but recent studies suggest a transverse fracture as the most common (King et al). In King's series, spiral fractures (26%) were much less common than transverse fractures (48%).

In many cases, a "normal fracture" plus a suspicious social history is all that you have as a lead. If you do not inquire, for instance, the nature of the injury etc., you may miss the pattern. The typical patterns of child abuse include:

Multiple Injuries Over a Period of Time. Some fractures are new and some are old. Infants commonly sustain Type I epiphyseal separations. If these are manipulated every day, a characteristic appearance is produced. A skeletal survey is mandatory; it may show healed rib fractures with more recent limb injuries. "Corner" fractures (Fig. 19-11) or "bucket-handle" fractures (Fig. 19-12) are commonly seen. Transphyseal distal humerus fractures are a "classic" child abuse injury (Fig. 19-13).

Although these radiographic appearances are diagnostic and much used as illustrations, it should be realized that they are unusual. Most battered children have fractures indistinguishable from those produced in everyday life (Fig. 19-14).

Evasive Explanations. "He must have fallen out of his crib." "He fell down three days ago." Considerate parents bring their children right away when they are hurt, and they are sure of the cause of injury. In fact, few children who fall do themselves any harm. Levin studied 100 infants who fell (and these were only the falls that alarmed mother) and not one gave cause for concern.

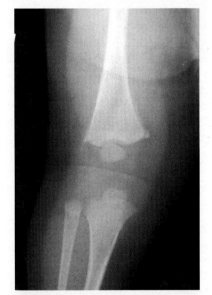
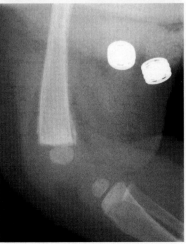

Figure 19-11. Typical "corner fracture" of the distal femur. This is due to repetitive stress and is almost always diagnostic of child abuse.

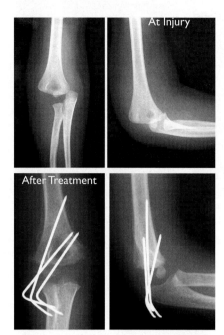

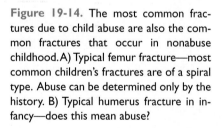

Figure 19-13. Transphyseal fracture of distal humerus in a very young child. One must think of child abuse in such a case. A) At injury. B) After reduction plus K-wire fixation.

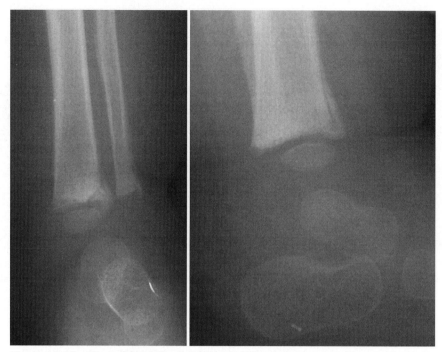

Figure 19-12. Classic "bucket handle" fracture of the distal tibia in a very young child. This fracture is common in child abuse.

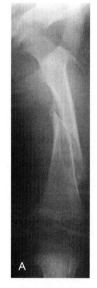

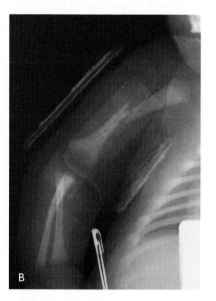

Figure 19-14. The most common fractures due to child abuse are also the common fractures that occur in nonabuse childhood. A) Typical femur fracture—most common children's fractures are of a spiral type. Abuse can be determined only by the history. B) Typical humerus fracture in infancy—does this mean abuse?

On the other hand, recent experience with large immigrant families in crowded housing contradicts Levin's study. Having five siblings in one family, all younger than age 6 years, jumping on a bed or sofa in a tiny apartment commonly produces a limb fracture in the youngest one. Your detective work becomes more complex. Hennrikus and Shaw, in Fresno, have directly refuted Levin's study.

Lack of Tenderness. Parents are gentle as they handle an injured child. "Battering" parents sometimes handle the child like a sack of potatoes and are oblivious of his cries. Once in an interview, I (M.R.) asked the parents, "Is he a good boy?" The father replied, "No, he is very bad." I then inquired, "What do you do when he is bad?" Father then grabbed the boy's arm—his thumb fitting exactly to a large bruise on the boy's arm—and shook his fist at him.

History of Previous Obvious Injuries. Some children are already known to the social service because of family problems. Others have been seen in emergency departments before. This information is difficult to obtain but sometimes emerges later.

Management

A high index of suspicion is warranted. Statistics suggests up to 10% of all injuries in children younger than the age of 2 years are due to inflicted injury. The doctor should approach all fractures in this age group as potential examples of abuse until he has been convinced otherwise. In much of the western world, doctors are required by law to inform the social services whenever there is a suspicion of child abuse. This law protects not only the child (and siblings) from further injury but the doctor from legal proceedings.

Whether or not the injury itself demands admission, the child should be admitted for protection and to provide time for investigation. The family can be advised that the child must be examined and tested to determine the cause of the fracture. Often, formal casting can be delayed (use traction or a splint) while awaiting full social services evaluation.

The doctor may find himself or herself in a strange position that of acquiring evidence against the parents as well as trying to provide them with counsel. The social science worker has much to offer in these circumstances but needs support from you. They will be able to alleviate the strains in the family by using community resources, educating the family in child rearing, and perhaps putting them in contact with Parents Anonymous, an organization of reformed child abusers. In the future parenting courses in schools may help to prevent child abuse in future generations.

If a child has been seriously injured, the parents may be charged with child abuse and the child temporarily placed in a foster home. In the end, a common judicial view is often taken that the child is better off with his or her own parents, even in an indifferent home, than in long-term foster care. Different states (United States) have differing philosophies in interpreting the rights of the biological parents to raise their child versus the states right to be sure that children are raised humanely. The size of the adult prison population in North America suggests that no state has a "clearly just right" philosophy on the matter.

The Battering Child

A 6-week-old child was brought to the emergency department with symmetrical spiral fractures of the humerus (Fig. 19-15). The parents thought the arms had been caught in the sides of the crib—an immediately suspicious explanation. Instead, the babysitter's children were the culprits—whether in play or in malice was never determined. Adelson has recently described cases where infants were killed by other children. Some of these killings were due to sibling rivalry.

Munchausen by Proxy Syndrome

Munchausen syndrome is named after Baron von Munchausen, a repeated teller of exaggerated tales. In the adult medical world, such patients are characterized by habitual presentation for hospital treatment of an apparent acute illness, the patient giving a dramatic and usually medically "correct" history, all of which in the end is untrue.

In the Munchausen by proxy syndrome, a parent creates such a disease in the child, mandating unneeded admissions, extensive workups, and unneeded operations. Orthopedics must be careful of this syndrome. The line between an overly demanding (but normal) parent and a Munchausen by proxy parent is sometimes narrow. A 2004 *New Yorker* magazine article brilliantly elucidates this puzzling condition.

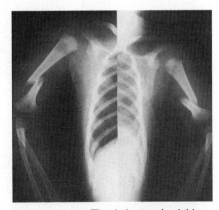

Figure 19-15. The babysitter's children, age 7, 5, and 2 years, had produced these symmetrical fractures.

The Skeletal Survey—When Is It Overdone?

This child had a simple ankle fracture but the inexperienced ER doctor wasn't clear on the history and called the social service team. A total of 18 films were taken with little else learned. Although generally indicated, the skeletal survey produces a great deal of irradiation. Some wonder if there is still a role for a "babygram" in the low index of suspicion case.

Overdiagnosis and Family Stress

As the child abuse syndrome has become better recognized, some families end up being falsely accused. For example, if an infant has one fracture (say humerus or femur) and the finding of "periostitis of the newborn" (a known phenomenon), the investigative team can be misled. Also, subtle forms of osteogenesis imperfecta may cloud the issue.

Sometimes the orthopedist needs to help educate the social worker regarding the potential for fracture associated with rough play. Hennrikus and Shaw have nicely illustrated this in their important 2003 publication. A team approach is required to best serve the family.

PATHOLOGIC FRACTURES

By definition, a pathologic fracture is one through weak bone of abnormal composition. There are multiple causes as noted.

Local Bone Lesions

Simple Bone Cyst. Most pathologic fractures in the upper humerus are caused by bone cysts. (Unicameral bone cyst (UBC)—simple bone cyst—the terms are used interchangeably.) Minimal displacement is the rule. Diagnosis can be confidently made on the radiologic appearance alone (Fig. 19-16). Although the term simple bone cyst is commonly used, it may lead you and the parents to underestimate the chemistry of the lesion. As one wit once said, "Don't call it a simple bone cyst until you have treated ten cases. They are very often not simple (to manage)."

The presence of the cyst does not interfere with healing, and the fracture is treated as if the cyst is not present. However, if nothing is done, refracture is likely.

Neer found that 80% of children had one to three refractures after the initial injury and that 10% had some deformity as a result. For this reason, he advocated treating all cysts.

Bone cysts occasionally produce fractures in weight-bearing bones such as the neck of the femur. Deformity is likely. Bone cysts may breach the growth plate. Growth disturbance and even collapse of the femoral head may follow. The same (growth arrest) can occur in the proximal humerus.

Treatment—Steroid Injection. The treatment of cysts has been transformed by the discovery that injection with methylprednisolone will produce healing (Fig. 19-17). Scaglietti, Marchetti, and Bartolozzi consider it important to use two

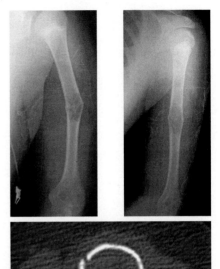

Figure 19-16. Midshaft unicameral bone cyst in a child. He had recurrent fractures despite steroid injection treatment. The CT scan shows the cortical break after his most recent fracture.

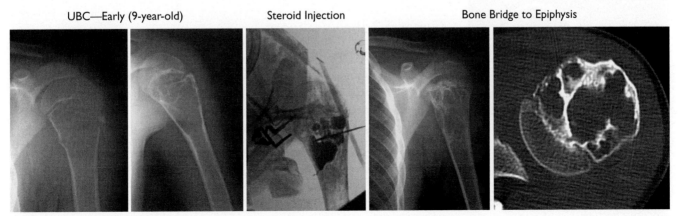

UBC—Early (9-year-old)	Steroid Injection	Bone Bridge to Epiphysis

Figure 19-17. Nine-year-old boy with a simple bone cyst (UBC). He has been treated with steroid injection three times. He has developed a physeal bridge and his humerus is now 2 cm short.

cannulated needles to enter the cyst under radiographic control in order to avoid hemorrhage. The exit of clear, yellow fluid confirms the diagnosis, so that biopsy is usually unnecessary.

Forty to 200 mg of methylprednisolone acetate (Depo-Medrol) is introduced, depending on the size of the cyst. We usually do this under anesthesia. If the cyst is showing no signs of healing at 3 months, the injection is repeated and may be repeated again. In 72 cases Scaglietti followed for more than 18 months, the results ranged from complete healing in 36% to a clearly positive result in 96%. Surgery for bone cysts is now much less common but is occasionally required.

Current methods to replace steroid injection with bone marrow injection and vigorous methods of breaking down the wall of the lesion with strong, curved needles (Weintraub) appear to be successful but are more complicated to perform than steroid injection. We have tried the new methods and found them unnecessarily complicated. We have reverted to steroid injection, which is very effective, providing you are very persistent (a somewhat un-American trait—at least for surgeons serving in an "injection only" role).

Curettement plus bone grafting may be required in the few cysts, which are large and recalcitrant. This is most commonly considered in large proximal femoral cysts, which risk intertrochanteric fracture (although even these lesions can heal with persistent steroid injections). Any curettement must be delayed until the cyst has grown away from the physis (otherwise physeal closure, which sometimes occurs even without curettement, will be attributed to your industrious scraping).

Nonossifying Fibroma. The distal tibia, followed by the distal femur, are the most common sites of the fracture through cortical nonossifying fibromas. Centrally placed lesions do not weaken bone. The risk for fracture is greater then one might think, especially in the distal femur and distal tibia (Fig. 19-18).

Most of these fractures are spiral and little displaced. Healing is accompanied by partial obliteration of the fibroma. Because the diagnosis is obvious, biopsy is not required. Refracture is unusual. A small series of large fibromas has been reported. Some of these were grafted initially because of their size and risk for fracture or because of the doubts about the diagnosis. CT scans are often performed in large lesions to clarify size and risk for fracture (cortical break, cortical thinning).

Miscellaneous. Almost every type of bone lesion has been associated with a pathologic fracture (Fig. 19-19). Fibrous dysplasia of the proximal femur is a typical example. Also, congenital pseudarthrosis of the tibia (often in a patient with neurofibromatosis) may present with pain and a pathologic fracture.

General Bone Weakness

Neuromuscular Disorders. In children, a major cause of pathologic fractures is osteoporosis resulting from neuromuscular disorders. Fractures are especially common in these patients after operation and cast immobilization (because of joint stiffness and disuse atrophy).

Cerebral Palsy. Fractures in children with cerebral palsy (CP) are uncommon, unless they are on anti-seizure medicines, which affect vitamin D metabolism. Children with CP who have had reconstructive surgery, and then are immobilized in a cast commonly develop fractures. Routine care is generally effective. However, in bed-fast patients, particularly those with contractures and convulsions, fracture is common. Very simple methods of treatment are needed for

At Injury

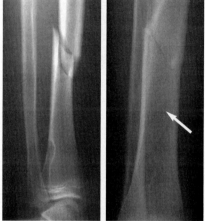

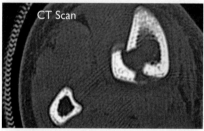

CT Scan

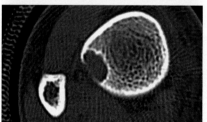

Figure 19-18. Ten-year-old male with a pathologic fracture of the tibia. The fracture line spirals from the distal nonossifying fibroma up to the main fracture. It is sometimes difficult to determine what size of cyst will weaken the bone enough to produce a fracture.

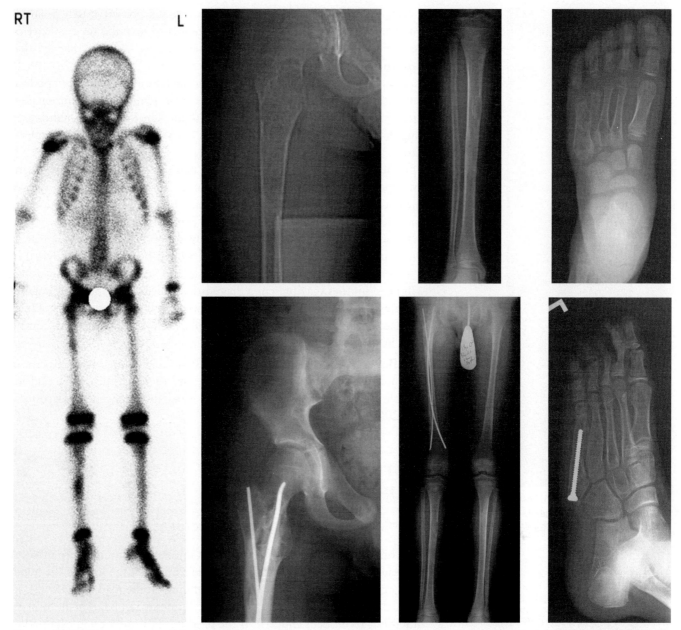

Figure 19-19. This eight-year-old boy presented with right hip pain and was found to have a subtle fracture line in a large bone lesion in the intertrochanteric area. Diagnosis was polyostotic fibrous dysplasia. The femur lesion was excised and bone grafted and fixed with flexible nails. The left foot was treated due to a recurrent fracture. His other lesions are being monitored.

these patients, because pressure sores are difficult to avoid. Referral to the metabolic bone disease unit may help in patients who get into a vicious fracture cycle (cast off-refracture-cast off-refracture).

Muscular Dystrophy. The policy of keeping children with Duchenne dystrophy on their feet as long as possible, by means of surgical releases and bracing, led to more lower limb fractures in this group. Fractures occur at all sites and require typical cast immobilization. The aggressive approach to encourage walking as long as possible has been tuned down in some centers (Children's Hospital—San Diego), resulting in fewer fractures.

Spina Bifida and Paraplegia. Diagnosis is often delayed when a fracture occurs in an anesthetic part of the lower limb. The surgeon is confronted with a swollen, hot, red limb in a child with a slight fever—symptoms that simulate

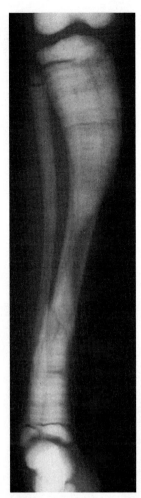

Figure 19-20. Fracture in osteopetrosis in a girl of 8 years. This family of affected children sustains frequent fractures.

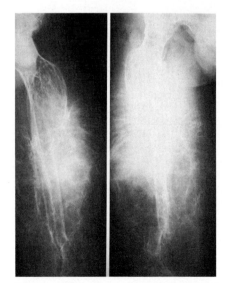

Figure 19-21. An extreme example of hyperplastic callus in osteogenesis imperfecta. This phenomenon has only been noted in association with dislocation of the radial head.

acute osteomyelitis especially in physeal fractures that present exactly as an infection. We have coined the term Charcot physis to describe the sequence of progressive pain—free physeal injury—partial healing—further damage that can close the physis.

Fracture is very common after orthopedic operations and cast immobilization; supracondylar and trochanteric fractures of the femur are so common after hip surgery that I warn the parents to expect them. The incidence is reduced by insisting that the child stand for a few hours every day while in the postoperative cast.

Rapid healing is the rule for fractures in neuromuscular conditions. Commonly, hyperplastic callus is seen. There is no single explanation for the massive volume of callus; repeated movement, unspecified neural influence on bone formation, and hyperphosphatemia are possible reasons.

Treatment should be simple and carefully supervised. An early return to brace-wearing for the tibia, or a well-padded weight-bearing cast, is advised in order to prevent further disuse osteoporosis and a succession of fractures. Growth plate injuries may present a diagnostic challenge. We noted premature growth arrest occurred in five of the nine patients with neurogenic physeal fracture (Charcot physis) and advised immobilization and non-weight-bearing until full healing has occurred.

General Bone Disease. Fractures in osteopetrosis and osteogenesis imperfecta are common. Displacement is usually slight, and there is much to be said for simple splinting. Air splints have also been tried for osteogenesis imperfecta (Fig. 19-20, 19-21).

FRACTURES IN SPECIAL GROUPS OF PATIENTS

Head Injuries with Long Bone Fractures

When a child is hit by a car, Waddell's triad of injuries is commonly produced. A child's femur is at the level of the bumper; the trunk is at the level of the hood; the child may receive a blow to the head on landing on the road (Fig. 19-22).

Fractures of the femur and the shaft of the humerus can be difficult to manage in restless, recumbent children. If the head injury is minor and expected to clear in a day or two, the fracture should be immobilized by simple splinting until routine methods may be employed. Fat embolism may be blamed for prolonged unconsciousness if this is not done.

When decerebration is likely to be prolonged beyond a few days, internal traction is advised (Fig. 19-23).

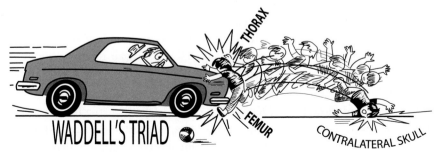

Figure 19-22. Waddell's Triad of injuries in children.

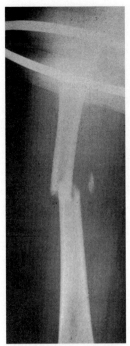
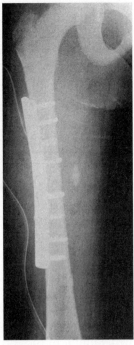
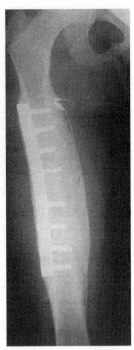

Figure 19-23. This fracture was uncontrollable owing to a severe head injury. Plating avoids the risk of producing avascular necrosis of the femoral head from damage of the epiphyseal arteries. Antibiotic cover is wise because poor nutrition and multiple tubes increase the risk of infection.

Fractures in the Newborn

The literature is full of birth injuries of every type. We still see a fair number (clavicle, humerus) in especially large babies (Fig. 19-24). Long bone fractures are easily recognized, but separations of unossified epiphysis present a challenge to diagnosis.

There may be difficulty distinguishing between a birth fracture and child abuse. Callus appears within 7 to 10 days around a birth fracture. Truesdall, in 1917, analyzed 33,000 deliveries for skeletal injury and found 85 injured children. There were no greenstick fractures, and only 10% were epiphyseal separations. The humerus and clavicle were most commonly fractured, and a Velpeau bandage controlled these well. Fractures of the midshaft of the femur accounted for 12%, and traction was required to prevent gross overriding and anterior angulation.

Hemophilia

A well-controlled hemophiliac today is free of crippling deformities and can lead quite an adventurous life. Fractures present no special problem if cryoprecipitate is administered. Fractures heal at the normal rate.

The child should be either admitted or monitored by a well-run hematology service, which can monitor the factor levels, and carefully watched for a few days.

A greater risk than fractures, which provoke immediate attention, is a slow bleed into a closed compartment, which results in Volkmann's contracture. This obviously demands urgent decompression.

Renal Dystrophy and Rickets

Children waiting for a kidney transplant may develop profound osteodystrophy. A slow slip of the upper femoral epiphysis should be pinned as soon as it is noted. Dialysis is no bar to anesthesia (Fig. 19-25).

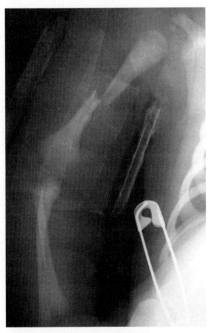

Figure 19-24. This type of humeral fracture is common in the newborn. Large babies seem to be at greater risk.

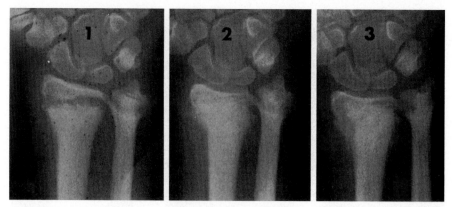

Figure 19-25. (1) Vitamin D-resistant rickets. This child was receiving insufficient vitamin D. (2) A slight fall produced a pathologic epiphyseal separation. The dosage of vitamin D was increased. (3) At 2 months, the separation has healed.

STRESS FRACTURES

The most common sites of stress fracture in children are the upper third of the tibia, the lower half of the fibula, followed by metatarsal, rib, pelvis, femur and humerus. They are particularly common in the spring, when children become active after a winter of inactivity. The radiographic appearance may be confused with a neoplasm or an infection, but the distinction is usually clear. If the diagnosis is in doubt, serial radiographs should be obtained over a short period of time (Fig. 19-26). A bone scan will demonstrate a stress fracture earlier than a radiograph and occasionally a CT scan or MRI is needed to differentiate a subtle, healing stress fracture from a Ewing's sarcoma.

Stress fractures through the distal femoral growth plate have been described in athletes. Abstinence from a sport may be sufficient treatment, but a cast is helpful if a child is overly active, if pain is marked, or if the fracture looks as if it may become complete. All stress fractures of the femoral neck should be immobilized in a spica or fixed with threaded pins.

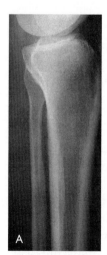
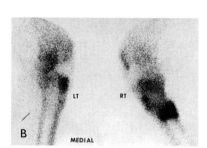
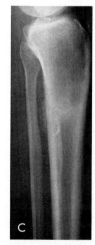

Figure 19-26. This runner had recently increased his mileage to 30 miles per week. One day, the right upper tibia became tender and the patient began to limp. A) The x-ray film at this time was normal. B) Bone scan showed a hot transverse bar—the typical first sign of a stress fracture. Later, periosteal new bone forms and the hot area becomes more diffuse and less characteristic. C) After 3 weeks, the diagnosis can be made radiographically. Two years later, the patient developed the same symptoms in the other leg. The radiograph was normal at Elsewhere General Hospital and the patient was told there was nothing the matter. When his request for a scan was turned down he went elsewhere. (Courtesy of David Gilday, MD.)

Suggested Readings

Vascular and Compartment Syndromes

Hargens AR, Mubara SJ: Current concepts in pathophysiology, evaluation, and diagnosis of compartment syndrome. Hand Clin 1998 Aug:14(3):371–83

Holden CEA. The pathology and prevention of Volkmann's ischemic contracture. J Bone Joint Surg 61B:296,1979

Isaacson J, Louis DS, Costenbader JM: Arterial injury associated with closed femoral-shaft fracture. Report of 5 cases. J Bone Joint Surg 57A:1147, 1975

Karlstrom G, Lonnerholm T, Olerud S: Cavus deformity of the foot after fracture of the tibial shaft. J Bone Joint Surg 57A:893, 1975

Matsen FA, Mayo KA, Krugmire RB et al: A model compartmental syndrome in man with particular reference to the quantification of nerve function. J Bone Joint Surg 59A:684, 1977

Mubarak SJ, Carroll NC: Volkmann's contracture in children: Aetiology and prevention. J Bone Joint Surg 61B:285, 1979

Mubarak SJ, Owen CA, Hargens AR et al: Acute compartment syndromes. Diagnosis and treatment with the aid of the wick catheter. J Bone Joint Surg 60A:1091, 1978

Nonaccidental Trauma

Adelson L: The battering child. JAMA 222: 159, 1972

Caffey J. Multiple fractures in long bones of infants suffering from chronic subdural hematoma. Am J. Roentgonol. 56:163–173, 1946

Hennrikus WL, Shaw BA. Injuries where children repeatedly fall from a bed or couch. Clin Orthop 407:148–151, 2003

Kempe CH, Silverman FN, Steele BF, Droegemueller W, Silver HK. The battered-child syndrome. JAMA 1962 Jul 7;181:17–24.

King J, Dietendorf D, Apthorp J et. al. Analysis of 429 fractures in 189 battered children. J Pediatr Orthop. 8:585–589, 1988.

Levin S: Infant fall-out. South African Med J 46:586, 1972

Loder R, Bookout C. Fracture patterns in battered children. J Pediatr Orthop. 5:428–433, 1991.

Van Stolk M: The Battered Child in Canada. Toronto, McClelland & Stewart, 1972

Pathologic Fractures

Devas MB: Stress fractures in children. J Bone Joint Surg 45B:528, 1963

Drennan DB, Fahey JS, Maylahn DJ: Fractures through large nonossifying fibromas. J Bone Joint Surg 54A:1794, 1972

Engh CA, Robinson RA, Milgram J: Stress fracture in children. J Trauma 10:532, 1970

Fry K, Hoffer MM, Brink J: Femoral shaft fractures in brain-injured children. J Trauma 16:317, 1976

Godshall RW, Hansen CA, Rising DC: Stress fractures through the distal femoral epiphysis in athletes. Am J Sports Med 9:114, 1981

Neer CS, Francis KC, Marcove RC et al: Treatment of unicameral bone cyst. J Bone Joint Surg 48A:731, 1966

Petersen EA, Haase J: Unstable fractures in children with acute, severe brain injury. Acta Orthop Scand 45:321, 1974

Scaglietti O, Marchetti PG, Bartolozzi P: The effects of methylprednisolone acetate in the treatment of bone cysts. J Bone Joint Surg 61B:200, 1979

Sillence DO. Osteogenesis imperfecta; an expanding panorama of variance. Clin Orthop 159:11–25, 1981.

Traub J, O'Connor W, Musso P. Congenital pseudarthrosis of the tibia: A retrospective review. J Pediatr Orthop 19:735–740, 1999.

Wenger DR, Jeffcoat BT, Herring JA: The guarded prognosis of physeal injury in paraplegic children. J Bone Joint Surg 62A:241, 1980

20

Accident Prevention, Risk, and the Evolving Epidemiology of Fractures

Dennis Wenger

ACCIDENT PREVENTION

In the last edition of this text, considerable attention was given to accident prevention strategies. Mercer Rang became a leader in promoting the concept of safer playgrounds, better sports equipment, and auto safety issues (both for passengers and pedestrians).

Tremendous progress has been made. Automobiles are much safer (better design [structural "cage"], airbags [front, side], better brakes [ABS] and better seat belts—plus laws that mandate their use). The routine (and usually legally

> "The great end of life is not knowledge but action"
> —THOMAS HENRY HUXLEY

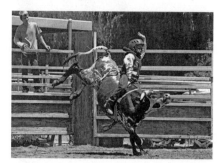

Figure 20-1. Helmet wear is fortunately becoming the standard for many sports. Efforts to prevent head injury have been a huge success. (Photo courtesy of R. Knudson.)

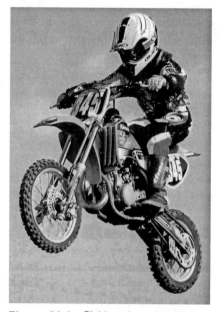

Figure 20-2. Children love the thrill of riding motorized vehicles. (Photo courtesy of R. Knudson.)

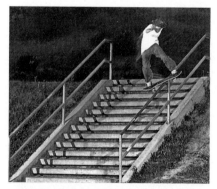

Figure 20-3. Skateboarding is a spectacular American-born sport that not only improves one's sense of balance but also increases the chance of fracture. (Photo courtesy of T. Hooker.)

mandated) requirement for helmet use in bicycling and other sports (Fig. 20-1) has been of immense value in reducing head injuries. In many neighborhoods, the playgrounds are safer, due to better design and soft surfaces (replacing compacted dirt).

Furthermore, in developed countries, the establishment of effective trauma systems including, in many cases, pediatric trauma centers has helped reduce the morbidity and mortality associated with severe musculoskeletal injury. Also, the rapid growth of pediatric orthopedics as a subspecialty of orthopedic surgery has been of great value in reducing fracture morbidity because of research produced by the major pediatric orthopedic centers that have an interest in trauma. The concentration of experience in treating severe fractures has greatly improved the quality of fracture care in North America. The methods learned by fellows who have trained in these centers are now available to injured children, not only in large but also in medium-sized cities.

Despite this great progress, not all the news is good regarding risks to children and the incidence of fractures.

ACCIDENT OR CULTURAL CONSEQUENCE?

The term accident is defined in the Oxford American Dictionary as follows:

1. An unexpected or undesirable event, especially one causing injury or damage
2. Chance, fortune (we met by accident)

We continue to marvel at how our culture uses the term in reference to children's fractures (Fig. 20-2). Parents will bring in a 6-year-old boy who was driving his own mini-racing motorcycle in the desert with a large number of family members. The child has multiple fractures (one open) with the parents distraught over the "accident." In many cases, the term "accident" has become a euphemism for failure to act in a responsible manner. When small children and powerful machines are involved, this failure borders on neglect.

Vitale and colleagues at Columbia suggest that the incidence of fractures is increasing in our culture (rather than decreasing) due to cultural patterns that will be discussed later in this chapter (Galano et al.—see Suggested Readings).

As sports become safer (helmets, pads, etc.), children (and adults) are more likely to perform with greater speed or at greater risk to achieve the same satisfaction (Fig. 20-3). The concept of "risk homeostasis" will be discussed later.

Brent and Weitzman, in the *Journal of Pediatrics* (2004), recently presented a comprehensive analysis of the environmental risks of childhood in North America. They noted that accidents are the leading cause of death in children younger than age 15 years and that many are preventable with safety education. Leaders in pediatric orthopedics have made a concerted effort to work on developing methods that might prevent fracture. Yet the incidence of fractures appears to be increasing rather than decreasing in our culture.

Brent and Weitzman group environmental risks to children with the major ones as noted below. Many of these subgroups can lead to musculoskeletal injury.

- Trauma from falls
- Vehicular accidents
- Burns
- Choking, strangulation
- Drowning
- Bicycling
- Pedestrian injuries
- Guns

- Sports injuries
- Power tools/farm tools
- Obesity
- Alcohol, smoking, drug use

In this chapter, we will focus on the categories with risk for musculoskeletal injury in children; that is falls, vehicular accidents, sports injuries, and power tools. A growing, but less easily categorized group, not clearly demarcated in the review by Brent and Weitzman, includes wheeled vehicles that are not formally vehicular (skateboards, rollerblades, "wheelie" shoes, etc.) that can be used in very dynamic (even aggressive) ways. Also, the use of gasoline-powered mini-bikes and scooters by even the very young is in a "growth pattern."

"In California, a parent who fails to properly restrain a child is fined $350 (per child)"

Falls

Infants can suffer head injuries when falling down stairs, off of beds, or against sharp, pointed furniture. Toddlers and children aged 5 to 19 years often fall from windows, stairs, trees, garage roofs, and ladders. Trampoline injuries produce many fractures (as well as head and neck injuries). More than 60,000 children had emergency room visits for trampoline injuries in 2002. When multiple children jump at once, injury is more likely and younger children are at greater risk for fracture.

Histories for falls can be so odd as to confound those trying to separate ordinary trauma from nonaccidental trauma. A parent of one of our patients said that she dropped her child (wet from a bath) into a toilet with a resulting limb fracture. She proved to be a sound, loving mother and her rapid retrieval skills kept the child off the drowning list!

Vehicular Accidents

Passenger injuries are extremely common in children younger than age 10; these children should never ride in the front seat of a car. Education and regulations regarding properly installed car and booster seats have improved this circumstance.

Safety—Children in Cars

Motor vehicle crashes are a leading cause of injuries and death for children.

When used correctly, child safety seats can reduce fatal injuries in cars by 71% for infants and 54% for children from age 1-4.

More than 95% of child safety seats are **NOT** used correctly.

IT IS THE LAW that children must ride in a safety seat or booster, properly used, until they are at least **6 YEARS OR WEIGH AT LEAST 60 POUNDS.**

Courtesy of Trauma Department—
Children's Hospital—San Diego,
reproduced with permission.

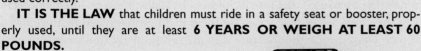

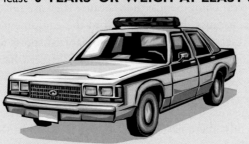

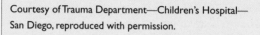

Safety Seat Guide

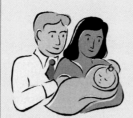

Children must ride in a rear-facing (facing toward the back of the car) safety seat until they are at least 1 year AND weigh 20 pounds.

Kids over 1 year and between 20-40 pounds may be in forward-facing safety seats.

Young children between 40 and 60-80 pounds (usually 4 to 8 years old) MUST ride in a booster.

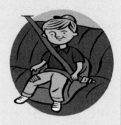

Children who are over 4 feet 8 inches AND at least 80 pounds can fit correctly in lap/shoulder belts.

Courtesy of Trauma Department—Children's Hospital—
San Diego, reproduced with permission.

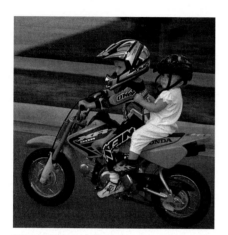

Figure 20-4. Younger and younger children are participating in motorized vehicle activities. (Photo courtesy of S. Nelson.)

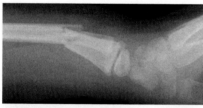

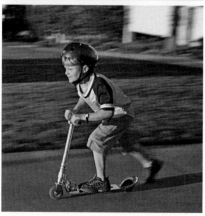

Figure 20-5. The razor scooter has proven to be a great source of new fractures. The nature of the fall provides a "Smith pattern" injury of the distal radius. The tiny wheels, and large sidewalk cracks are not a good mix. (See Kiely et al.—Suggested Readings.)

New government-mandated latch systems, which allow a nationally standardized method for attaching child seats to the automobile frame, will make auto travel safer. Legislation-mandated child car seat use also helps. In California, a parent who fails to properly restrain a child is fined $350 (per child).

Also, children younger than age 10 are at great risk for death from pedestrian accidents including being run over by the family car in their own driveway (lack of vision from the height of the new, taller SUVs have added to the problem). For teenagers, impulsive behavior, speeding, and inattentive driving as well as drunken driving make auto accidents a leading cause of death in this age group. The Europeans may have a better pattern (drink early and with family, drive late—age 18 years).

We see many young patients whose parents have aspirations for their children to become professionals in motorcycle racing and/or daredevil motorcycle jumping activities. If you are good enough you can "get a sponsor" (equipment, etc.) at a very young age (Fig. 20-4).

Sports Injuries, Bicycling

Children riding a bicycle, tricycle, scooter, or skateboard or using a razor scooter (Fig. 20-5) should use a well-fitted helmet to reduce the risk for head injury. Bicycling is a risk for children and ideally would be restricted to daylight use, in safe areas, with helmet use. Children who play football, baseball, soccer, hockey, and lacrosse are advised to always wear proper protective equipment and be properly supervised.

Such reports and recommendations represent the ideal and are a bit like recommending a balanced diet for all children. In reality, most children who skateboard, ride bicycles, or play sports do them in an unsupervised manner and do not wear equipment either because they are not properly educated or in many cases, because they cannot afford the equipment. It would appear that fracture risk is reasonable controlled in organized sports for children but is increasing in the uncontrolled environment of the "street wheel scene."

Playgrounds and Sport

Recently, there has been a substantial focus in the first world on the risks that poorly designed playgrounds provide to children, thus increasing their risk for

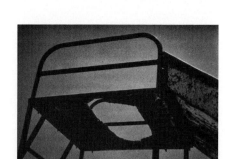

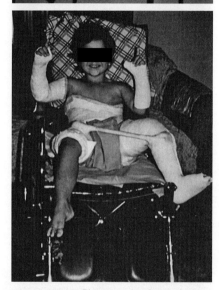

Facts About Bike Safety

Head injury is the leading cause of death in bicycle crashes.

Using a helmet can lower death rate by 75%.

Only about 15% to 20% of children wear helmets.

Courtesy of Trauma Department—Children's Hospital—San Diego, reproduced with permission.

fracture (Fig. 20-6). Poor landing surfaces such as hard-packed dirt or asphalt can be changed to surfaces such as rubber mats, wood shavings, or soft sand. Slowly, we are beginning to see playgrounds becoming safer. (Perhaps plaintiff attorneys can be given a bit of credit—once the issue of poor playground design and fracture risk became apparent, successful lawsuits against schools and parks ensued.) Now the playgrounds are safer. Unfortunately, the pendulum has swung too far and now some organizations are unwilling to provide playgrounds because of insurance cost (due to legal risk).

Negative Effects of "Very Safe Playgrounds"

A second, and less well-understood consequence of the move toward low-height, low-risk playgrounds is the denial of athletic freedom and risk that some believe develop balance and physical dexterity in childhood. The traditional view of child development included that playgrounds should include adventuresome swinging ropes, relatively high slides, and swings with long ropes or chains and a large arc. Complex climbing devices, such as monkey bars, were common (Fig. 20-7).

The idea behind such equipment included that the activity developed a child's dexterity, physical stamina, and ability to face risk. It was accepted that an unwary child might be injured but the risk-benefit ratio favored adventurous design. The Boy Scouts and Outward Bound have this focus for older children. In summary, modern super safe, "low rise" playground equipment may decrease the injury rate but at the same time prevent a child from achieving his or her full physical abilities by limiting play experiences that demand judgments regarding distance, height, timing, etc.

In our culture, the need for adventuresome play that involves risk has to a great degree moved from the playground to other venues such as small-wheeled scooters, rollerblades, skateboards, racing bicycles, motorized scooters, and small motorcycles, which have proven to be a prolific new cause for fractures.

Power Tools

Brent and Weitzman noted that nearly 10,000 children, age 15 and younger, are injured by lawn mowers each year (Fig. 20-8). Young children should not be nearby when a power mower is used and these experts suggest that children younger than 12 years should not be allowed to operate a walk-behind mower and children younger than 14 should not operate a riding mower. Physicians with agricultural roots in America, understanding the benefit of responsibility learned at an early age, might quarrel with this advice.

Figure 20-6. Playground safety is important. This boy was enjoying a day at the park when the weathered plywood at the top of a slide finally failed. He had fractures in three limbs.

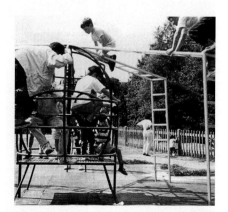

Figure 20-7. More complex, high off the ground playground equipment helps to develop balance and judgement (in a Darwinian way). In the modern era, such playgrounds are being reigned in because of the risk of injury. Lawyers have helped to guide this trend. Is it really a good trend for our children?

Other Risks—Aggressive Sport or Calcium Deficiency?

A recent study, utilizing the population base of Olmstead County, Minnesota and surrounding communities, suggested that the incidence of childhood forearm fracture was increasing: 263 per 100,000 population—1969; 372 per 100,000 population—1999 (30 years later).

Although uncertain of the cause, they suggested a changing pattern of physical activity or decreased bone acquisition due to poor calcium intake or perhaps both.

They also noted a greater rate of fracture increase in girls (52%) as compared to boys (32%) with the largest increases in pubertal age children. This female over male increase led to speculation regarding calcium intake. On the other hand, another report estimated that in 1971, only 31,000 girls participated in organized high school sports, whereas 3 million girls participated in 2003. Although increased numbers wouldn't necessarily increase the risk for forearm fractures, increased numbers also means that more girls are competing at high levels (premier leagues), which may increase the speed and ferocity of sport collision. Also, in our experience, girls also love the thrill of the new variety of motorized off-road vehicles.

In our center, we are experiencing an epidemic of repeat fractures in the same bones (Fig. 20-9). We attribute this to aggressive lifestyle rather than "soft bones."

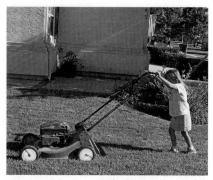

Figure 20-8. Young children should not use dangerous rotary lawn mowers. The risk for soft tissue injury and scalping type fractures is great, especially if the grass is wet. (Photo courtesy of C. Farnsworth.)

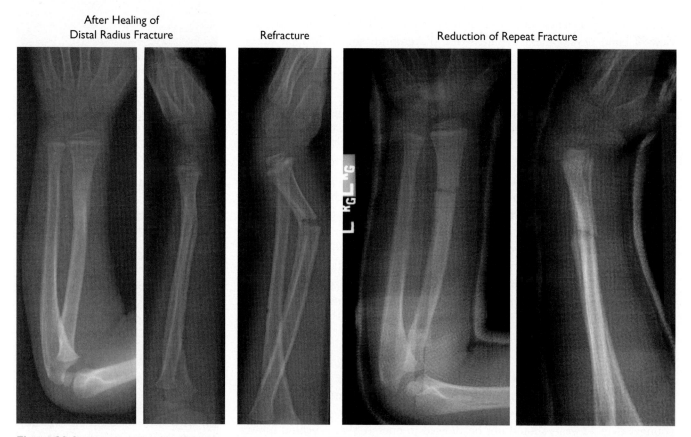

After Healing of
Distal Radius Fracture   Refracture   Reduction of Repeat Fracture

Figure 20-9. We now see about 50 recurrent fractures per year. This case is typical with the refracture occuring 6 months after the original injury—skateboarding was the cause of both.

CULTURAL PATTERNS AND FRACTURE RISK

Throughout history, children likely suffered injuries while working with their parents, hunting, and in adventuresome play. With the evolution of advanced economies, children have had more leisure time allowing play in formal playgrounds, vigorous sport, as well as exposure to both wheeled and then motorized wheeled vehicles. As already noted, we are now experiencing an increasing incidence of fractures in children.

Our profession's reaction to this changing childhood risk has been laudable with the American Academy of Orthopaedic Surgeons, the American Academy of Pediatrics, the Pediatric Orthopaedic Society of North America, the European Pediatric Orthopaedic Society, and parallel organizations devoting resources and research toward accident and injury prevention. The goal has been to decrease the incidence and severity of fractures by methods ranging from playground design, seat belt use, mandated car seat use, mandated helmet use, the wearing of proper protective devices for sports, and age and location risks for all-terrain vehicle (ATV) use.

Unfortunately, the exponential growth of use of automobiles in large cities in the world have made progress in accident prevention difficult. The number of vehicles on the streets each day in Cairo, Shanghai, Jakarta, and São Paulo has skyrocketed over the last 20 years and the design and construction of safe, well-designed streets and highways has not kept pace. The result is a radical increase in musculoskeletal injuries, both for drivers and pedestrians. Thus industrialization, the growth of cities, and the use of gasoline-powered vehicles of all types (automobiles to "pocket" scooters) have made life more risky for a child.

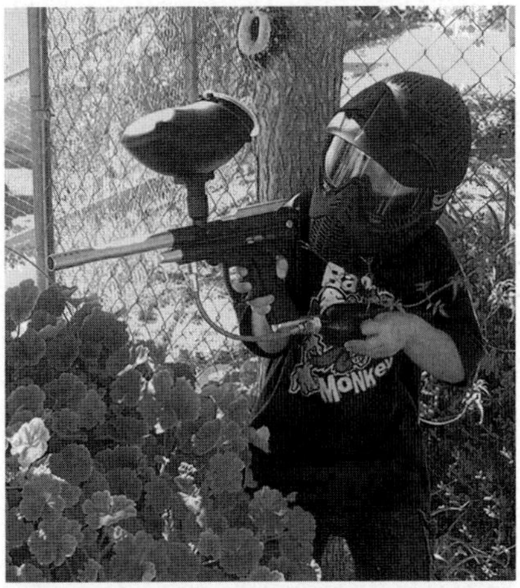

Figure 20-10. Children and adolescents love to sense risk and danger. The growth of the "paint ball gun industry" clarifies the issue. (Photo courtesy of A. Jacobson.)

HUMAN NEED FOR RISK—WAR VERSUS SPORT?

Perhaps, an underappreciated reason for an increase in childhood fractures is the innate pleasure that comes from risk-taking activities (Fig. 20-10). In the historical era, a large percentage of young males in a culture marched off to war with often much of the army decimated in a few days (Peloponnesian Wars, American Civil War—Grant's army lost 7,000 men in 20 minutes at Cold Harbor; World War I trench warfare—thousands of men killed within a few days' time).

It would appear that the adolescent brain (particularly male) has an innate need to experience risk and that the traditional risks (tribal warfare, hunting wild game with a spear) have been replaced with modern counterparts. The increased risk for fractures in male children will be discussed later.

Risk Homeostasis—Helmets and Pads Yet More Fractures

Advanced cultures have tried to make sports safer with helmet wear for bicycling, well-padded surfaces on ideally designed playgrounds, and strict rules regarding protective gear for organized sport, yet the fracture incidence is increasing. It would appear that risk seekers have found a need for new outlets. Thus the rapid growth of "extreme" sports throughout the world, particularly in North America.

Recommendations by the American Academy of Pediatrics

No use of ATVs by children or adolescents younger than 16.

Use of ATVs should require automobile driver's license and, preferably, special certification in ATV use.

No use of ATVs on public streets or highways.

No passengers on ATVs.

No operating of ATVs under the influence of alcohol.

No use of ATVs between sundown and sunrise.

Courtesy of Trauma Department—Children's Hospital—San Diego, reproduced with permission.

*"As helmets, protective
splints, and rules evolve, the
participants simply crank to
a higher level of performance,
speed, and risk"*

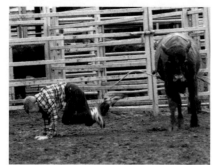

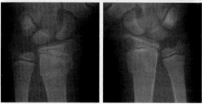

Figure 20-11. Children of every age enjoy a variety of sports. The forearm serves its programmed shock absorbing, collapse role, much like the hood of a Volvo in a head-on collision. Better an arm fracture than a skull or neck fracture. This youthful bull rider suffered bilateral distal radius fractures with a balanced, symmetric fall, avoiding more serious injury. (Photo courtesy of R. Knudson.)

This began with rollerblading, skateboarding, and aggressive bicycle and motorcycle riding. Large numbers of the population enjoy participating in these sports with a focus on speed and risk. A concept known as the "Extreme Games" focuses on high-risk sports and is televised internationally each year. Even the complexity level of gymnastic activities, diving activities, etc., as seen during the recently televised Olympic games, has escalated to a startling degree.

Each year, we see hundreds of children who have suffered fractures while attempting to mimic the extreme sporting activities that they have seen on television. These include skateboarding stunts and motorized vehicle activities. Even in the well-structured sports (BMX bicycle racing), the development of new helmets, pads, etc., have been superceded by the demands of the extreme stunts that the children attempt. Supercross, a popular dirt bike (motorized bike) competition, is now held in stadiums throughout North America. A professional circuit has evolved and parents are told that training should start early if their child is to be competitive—thus the 5-8 year olds that we see (often with serious fractures) who have been emulating their professional supercross idols.

Risk Homeostasis

This increase in fracture incidence, despite the best intended advice of organizations regarding safety rules, helmet wear, protective equipment wear, and rules for organized sports, may represent a variation of what the Dutch (now Canadian) psychologist Gerald Wild has coined "risk homeostasis." As vehicles are made safer (air bags, ABS brakes, etc.), drivers drive more rapidly and have more accidents. A study of taxi drivers, who were rotated between "safety performance vehicles" (air bags, ABS, better suspension) and standard vehicles, found a higher accident rate in the "safety" vehicles. The drivers simply drove faster and took more risks!

The same phenomenon is likely in play regarding both official and particularly unofficial childhood "sport" (Fig. 20-11). As helmets, protective splints, and rules evolve, the participants simply crank to a higher level of performance, speed, and risk. The helmets remain up to the task, but the limbs serve as "crumple zones" (to protect the central, vital organs). Thus human reflexes and protective limb extension (with a fall) serve much like the hood and engine mounts of a safe Volvo vehicle (front collapses—central "cage" remains intact). These patterns in no way question the value of protective helmets, protective splints, and sport rules. Their routine application has greatly improved the injury environment in organized sports. Mandated helmet wear for bicycling children, preventing brain injury, is perhaps the most profound example. However, the limb fracture epidemic continues.

ANALYSIS OF PEDIATRIC ORTHOPEDIC MUSCULOSKELETAL INJURIES

Vitale and colleagues at Columbia University, through the International Center for Health Outcomes and Innovation Research, provide additional data on children's musculoskeletal injuries. A recent paper from their center clarifies pediatric trauma as the leading cause of death and disability in children, accounting for 11 million hospitalizations, 100,000 permanent disabilities, and 15,000 childhood deaths each year in the United States. The direct cost of pediatric trauma is over $8 billion per year, which is only a fraction of the true total cost because indirect costs to families and society are impossible to estimate.

They note that the incidence of pediatric trauma in the United States is among the world's highest, likely because of the dangers associated with our

Off-Road Vehicle Injuries—Pediatric Trauma Patients

Average hospital length of stay = 3.8 days

Hospital length of stay range = 0–21 days

Average hospital charge for hospitalized ATV trauma patients = $27,000

Hospital charge range = $5,500 to $299,289

Courtesy of Trauma Department—Children's Hospital—San Diego, reproduced with permission.

highly mechanized society as well as the gravity of urban violence. Although the overall death rate of children in the United States has decreased over the past two decades, much of this was due to a decline in deaths from natural causes whereas traumatic causes have increased in children.

Vital and colleagues use the 1997 Kids Inpatient Data Base (KID) to examine orthopedic trauma as it occurred in a national pediatric inpatient population. They noted that a femur fracture was the most common reason for hospitalizing a child with a musculoskeletal injury, followed by tibial-fibular fracture and humerus fracture (including distal elbow fractures). Closed supracondylar fractures accounted for 59% of all humerus fractures. Next in frequency for admission were fractures of the radius and ulna followed by vertebral fractures, pelvic fractures, and hand fractures (hand fractures are very common but few require hospital admission).

Gender Issues

In support of the general sense that males are likely to participate in more risky activities, Vitale et al. found that 78% of hand and finger fractures, 72% of forearm fractures, 71% of tibia and fibular fractures, 71% of femoral fractures, 58% of humeral fractures and 56% of vertebral fractures occurred in males. The only type of fracture to have a higher incidence in females were pelvic fractures, but this was by only a miniscule amount (50.1% female—49.9% male).

This clear gender disparity, with males were more likely to sustain orthopedic injuries, was proposed to be due to participation in high-injury contact sports such as football and hockey (Fig. 20-12). Also, extreme motorized sports, bicycling sports, skateboarding sports, etc., are pursued more aggressively by males.

Interestingly, when one gets to the college athletic level, with a specific focus on anterior cruciate ligament injuries, the female to male ratio reverses with an anterior cruciate ligament injury ratio 2:1 for college soccer and 8:1 for college basketball. These are related to male to female anatomic differences in the human knee (shape of the intercondylar notch) as well as hormonal issues and training techniques that make female college athletes at great risk for knee ligament injuries.

MANDATED SPORT FOR EVERY CHILD— RISKS AND BENEFITS

The idea that all children should participate in vigorous physical education and pursue sports during their growing years has been historically powerful in advanced cultures, suffering a fall-off in the 1960s and 1970s but has been recently revived. In the United States Title IX legislation, mandating sport opportunity equality, greatly increasing female participation.

Percent of Fractures in Males (vs. Females)

Hand and finger—78%

Forearm—72%

Tibia, fibula—71%

Femur—71%

Galano, Vitale et al.

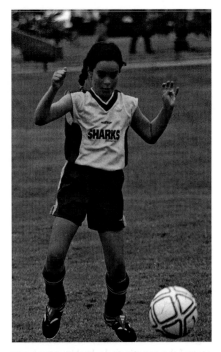

Figure 20-12. Sport for females has been a great 20th (and 21st) century advance. The increase risk for ligament injury (knee) was a bit of a cultural surprise. (Photo courtesy of L. Manhiem.)

Coda

OTHER TEXTS

Ours is a basic text that covers common problems. To see the future, we have stood on the shoulders of giants. These "giants" are the comprehensive children's fracture texts from around the world that have helped us to understand the nuances of fracture care. We present a short list.

1. Benson MKD, Fixsen JA, Macnicol MF (eds) Children's Orthopaedics and Fractures. London: Churchill Livingston, 1994.
2. Blount WL Fractures in Children. Baltimore: Williams and Wilkins, 1955.
3. Dimeglio A, Herisson C, Simon P: Les Traumatismes de l'enfant et leurs sequelles. Paris: Masson, 1993.
4. Green NE, Swiontkowski MF (eds): Skeletal Trauma in Children, 3rd ed. Philadelphia: Saunders, 2003.
5. Letts RM (ed): Management of Pediatric Fractures. New York; Churchill Livingstone, 1994.
6. MacEwen HF, Kasser JR, Heinrich SD (eds): Pediatric Fractures: A Practical Approach to Assessment and Treatment. Philadelphia: Williams and Wilkins, 1993.
7. Hefti F: Kinderorthopadie in der Praxis. Springer; Berlin, 1998.
8. Metaizeau JP. Osteosynthese Chez L'enfant. Montperlier: Sauramps Ed, 1988.
9. Morrissy RM and Weinstein S (eds): Pediatric Orthopaedics, 5th ed. Philadelphia: Lippincott, 2001.
10. Ogden JA: Skeletal Injury in the Child. Philadelphia: Lea and Febiger, 3rd ed. 2000
11. Rang M: The Growth Plate and its Disorders. Baltimore: Williams and Wilkins, 1969.
12. Rang M: Children's Fractures, 2nd ed. Philadelphia: Lippincott, 1983.
13. Rockwood CA Jr, Wilkins KA, Beaty KH (eds): Fractures in Children, 5th ed. Philadelphia: Lippincott-Raven, 2001.
14. Sharrard WJW: Paediatric Orthopaedics and Fractures. Oxford: Blackwell, 1971.
15. Tachdjian M: Pediatric Orthopaedics (J. Herring, editor, 3rd ed). Philadelphia: Saunders, 2002.
16. Von Laer L: Pediatric Fractures and Dislocations. New York: Georg Thieme Verlag, 2004.
17. Weber BG, Brunner C, Freuler F: Die Frakturenbehandlung bei Kindern und Jugendlichen. Berlin: Springer-Verlag, 1978.

We thank these authors for their immense contributions. We also apologize for not listing other texts that are also available. We would simply state that "if you can't find it in this list, it likely doesn't exist."

MR

MP

DW

305

Index